Optimal Treatment Strategies in End-stage Renal Failure

Edited by

CLAUDE JACOBS

*Professor of Nephrology (Emeritus), Service de Néphrologie,
UFR Pitié-Salpêtriere, Paris, France*

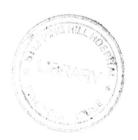

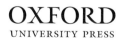

OXFORD

UNIVERSITY PRESS

OXFORD

UNIVERSITY PRESS

Great Clarendon Street, Oxford OX2 6DP

Oxford University Press is a department of the University of Oxford.
It furthers the University's objective of excellence in research, scholarship,
and education by publishing worldwide in

Oxford   New York

Auckland   Bangkok   Buenos Aires   Cape Town   Chennai
Dar es Salaam   Delhi   Hong Kong   Istanbul   Karachi   Kolkata
Kuala Lumpur   Madrid   Melbourne   Mexico City   Mumbai   Nairobi
São Paulo   Shanghai   Taipei   Tokyo   Toronto

and an associated company in Berlin

Oxford is a registered trade mark of Oxford University Press
in the UK and in certain other countries

Published in the United States
by Oxford University Press Inc., New York

British Library Cataloguing in Publication Data
Data available

Library of Congress Cataloging in Publication Data
(Data available)

ISBN 0 19 262971 9
10 9 8 7 6 5 4 3 2 1

Typeset by Cepha Imaging Pvt. Ltd.

Printed in Great Britain
on acid-free paper by
T.J. International Ltd, Padstow

PREFACE

The twentieth century is quite rightly deemed as the most barbaric in human history. More than 50 million people have perished in two World Wars of unprecedented savagery, to whom countless more have to be added who have been killed or disabled in conflicts of lesser magnitude or media coverage. Hundreds of million people worldwide still cannot get the daily caloric supply required for achieving little more than just surviving for a short lifespan, and the abyss between the economically developed, wealthy countries, and the so-called 'developing' countries has never been wider.

In absolute contrast with this dismal state of affairs, more advances for prolonging life and alleviating human suffering have been made available to the economically privileged populations of the Western world during the past 100 years, than in any other period in history. Public health measures, vaccinations, and antibiotics have eradicated many formerly lethal infectious diseases. From corticosteroids to recombinant human erythropoietin, as well as from Röentgen X-rays to magnetic resonance imaging, the combined efforts of the scientific, medical, and industrial communities have indeed revolutionized the profile of human life. The greatest challenge ahead in the Western developed countries lies in finding acceptable solutions for addressing the social and economical problems raised by the rapidly growing number of centenarians.

Among all these tremendous changes in the domain of healthcare, the replacement of renal function by extra- or intra-corporeal depurative methods and kidney transplantation have coined a particularly remarkable landmark in medical history. The development of the artificial kidney and of peritoneal dialysis have demonstrated, for the first time, that vital functions performed by a human organ could be replaced in case of total and irreversible failure for an unlimited period of time by human-built devices or by adapting a component of the body for achieving a task completely different from its normal function. The kidney has also been the initiator in the field of organ transplantation, and the clinical experience gained in kidney transplantation has acted as a springboard for the further development of liver, pancreas, and heart transplantation. Forty years ago, when the undersigned was a young nephrologist in training, he had to learn how to ensure patients with terminal uremia a peaceful, painless death within a few weeks' time. At present, he enjoys meeting some of his patients who are alive and well several decades after having started some form of renal replacement therapy, while more than a million patients world-wide are currently benefiting from these life-saving procedures. This contrast well illustrates the acceleration of history in the domain of healthcare. The challenge for the medical community in the years to come will be to exert the necessary economic and political pressures for extending the availability of renal replacement therapies to all those people world-wide who still are dying from not having access to them.

Preface

The contributors to this volume have all participated very actively in the fascinating adventure of the development of renal replacement therapies, which actually has been one of the core issues of their professional life. The editor is most grateful to them for having devoted much of their time and effort in order to enable the readers to benefit from their long-term experience in their respective area of expertise.

Data reported in several chapters of this book are based on (or taken from) the annual reports of the United States Renal Data System. The interpretation and reporting of these data are the responsibility of the authors and in no way should be seen as an official policy or interpretation of the US Government.

March 2002
C. Jacobs MD, FRCP

CONTENTS

Dedication

To my wife, Janine

my children, Valérie and Frédéric
and my mentors in Nephrology

Marcel Legrain and Belding H. Scribner

CONTRIBUTORS

Rashad Barsoum The Cairo Kidney Center, Bab-El-Louk, Cairo, Egypt

Michel Broyer Hôpital des Enfants Malades, Paris, France

Giovanni C. Cancarini Ospedale Spedali Civili, Brescia, Italy

Pierre Cochat Hôpital Edouard Herriot, Lyon, France

Alex M. Davison St James's University Hospital, Leeds, United Kingdom

Ulrich Frei Virchow Klinikum, Berlin, Germany

Eric Goffin Cliniques Universitaires Saint-Luc, Brussels, Belgium

Claude Jacobs Hôpital de La Pitié, Paris, France

Carl Kjellstrand Loyola University, Chicago, USA

Cecilia Kjellstrand Annex Teen Clinic, Minneapolis, USA

Kar Neng Lai Queen Mary Hospital, Hong-Kong

Rosario Maiorca Ospedale Spedali Civili, Brescia, Italy

Krishnan Mani Apollo Hospitals, Chennai, India

Françoise Mignon Hôpital Bichat-Claude Bernard, Paris, France

Zaki Morad Hospital Kuala Lampur, Kuala Lampur, Malaysia

Thierry Petitclerc Hôpital de La Pitié, Paris, France

Yves Pirson Cliniques Universitaires Saint-Luc, Brussels, Belgium

Boleslaw Rutkowski Medical University, Gdansk, Poland

1

Extra-corporeal renal replacement therapies

Thierry Petitclerc and Claude Jacobs

Introduction

The survival for an unlimited period of time of patients suffering from end-stage renal failure (ESRF), by the means of blood-purification systems, is a true and important landmark in medical history insofar as it represents the first successful long-term replacement of a human vital organ by a human-built machine. Barely four decades separate us from the pioneering endeavour undertaken by B.H. Scribner and associates, in their first attempt to apply intermittent hemodialysis to a single patient with non-reversible terminal renal insufficiency, from the contemporary scene where hundreds of thousands of patients worldwide benefit from the prolongation of their lives thanks to the ongoing advances made all over this timespan in the conceptual, pathophysiological, and techical aspects of this completely novel area of clinical medicine.

This chapter aims at briefly describing the main components and modes of utilization of extra-corporeal the blood-purification systems most widely used for the treatment of terminally uremic patients at the beginning of the third century. In spite of their formidable success in terms of preservation of life, their technical complexities, together with their basically unphysiological characteristics, account for a very imperfect replacement of the native kidney and explain why their application remains quite a sophisticated and demanding medical exercise that requires a good technical training along with a broad knowledge in large areas of internal medicine.

Components of extra-corporeal systems for replacement of renal function

Vascular accesses

Permanent access

Chronic extra-corporeal dialysis was not feasible until the introduction of the external arteriovenous shunt by the team of Scribner (1) and afterwards the endogenous fistula by Brescia *et al.* (2). This fistula consists of a subcutaneous anastomosis of the radial artery to the cephalic vein at the level of forearm. After several weeks, the venous limb of the fistula dilates, permitting repeated punctures with dialysis needles.

Creation of an arteriovenous fistula may be not possible in patients with a poor arterial system (patients with diabetes or severe atherosclerosis), or with very small or deep veins in markedly obese or older patients, or in patients whose veins have thrombosed and recanalized as a result of multiple punctures. In these cases, arteriovenous connection can be performed via a graft made from an autogenous saphenous vein, an allogenous vein, or from synthetic material (mainly polytetrafluoroethylene: PTFE). The most common initial site of graft placement is the non-dominant forearm from the radial artery at the wrist to the basilic vein.

Provided the availability of a cephalic vein of adequate size, a native arteriovenous fistula should be preferred to an arteriovenous graft as a first procedure because of its longer lifespan (approximately 70% vs. 30% at 3 years), and lower incidence of thrombosis and infection (3). Native arteriovenous fistulas are the most common initial accesses in Europe (about 2/3), but not in the USA (about 1/3).

Temporary access

Central venous catheters are widely used as temporary access methods in patients in whom blood access has failed or was not created sufficiently in advance to be functioning when renal replacement therapy is required. The internal jugular vein should be preferred to the subclavian vein because of the incidence of post-catheter partial or total occlusion of the subclavian vein, which can interfere with the future creation of an arteriovenous fistula or graft in the ipsilateral arm or which may cause edema of the arm. Tunnelized double-lumen or twin catheters inserted in the jugular vein can be used for several months or even years as permanent access in aged or severely ill patients.

Specially designed devices have been recently proposed. For example, the Hemasite[R] consists of a biocarbon implant mounted on a bovine graft or a PTFE vascular prosthesis with a self-sealing valve avoiding the need of needle punctures. The Dialock[R] is a subcutaneously implantable chamber connected to permanent silicone twin catheters (4–5). The Lifesite[R] is a membraneless titanium device with a mechanical valve and an internal pinch clamp (6). The place of these devices in the vascular access armamentorium remains to be determined.

Surveillance and monitoring of vascular access

A successful dialysis treatment rests heavily on a properly functioning vascular access. Unfortunately, the first sign of an upcoming dysfunction is all too often thrombosis and flow cessation. In order to screen the patients at high risk of thrombosis, monitoring of vascular access is important. This monitoring includes physical examination, record of venous pressure, duplex ultrasonography, and measurements of access recirculation and flow rate.

The physical examination (inspection, palpation, auscultation, and possibly manual occlusion of the fistula during dialysis) should not be underestimated, since it can be useful to detect early potentially failing fistulas. Recording changes in the venous pressure, systematically measured at each dialysis session by the dialysis monitor, should contribute to detecting potential outlet stenoses. However, venous pressures may not rise because of access recirculation relieving the pressure increment, which would otherwise occur due to flow resistance caused by access outlet stenosis (7).

Recirculation is defined as the fraction of cleared extra-corporeal blood flow that returns to the inlet of the extra-corporeal blood-lines without systemic equilibration. The level (in term of percentage) of recirculation depends:

(1) upon the configuration of the vascular access and placement of the access needles; and
(2) on a cardio-pulmonary component the arteriovenous access blood flow bypassing systemic tissue components. Identification of specific access problems requires the separation of these two components by various dilution techniques.

The magnitude of vacular access recirculation is often overestimated with the use of conventional urea-based methods (8). Some devices have been recently proposed for an instantaneous and more accurate measurement of recirculation. Usually, a bolus of saline is injected into the venous return line and changes in ultrasound velocity (9), conductivity measured magnetically (10), or hemoglobin dilution measured optically, are all non-invasively monitored on both the arterial and venous sides. The use of a thermal bolus induced by a change in dialysate temperature precludes the injection of a saline bolus into the blood and enables full automatization of the procedures.

Duplex ultrasonography provides for both a two-dimensional image and a pulsed-wave Doppler analysis of flow velocity. This technique can detect stenosis and predict thrombosis (11), but is expensive and highly operator-dependent.

New techniques have recently been proposed for the non-invasive measurement of access flow from the recirculation induced by the reversal of blood-lines. All the methods designed for recirculation measurement can be used when blood-lines are in reversed position. Ultrasound dilution (12), conductivity dilution (13), and hemoglobin dilution (14) allow non-invasive measurements of access flow by injection of a saline bolus with similar results. A transient change in ultrafiltration rate (0–30 ml/min) (15), in temperature dialysate (16) or in conductivity dialysate (17, 18) has been recently proposed for avoiding the injection of a saline bolus. The infusion of a small bolus of hypertonic glucose solution allows the level of recirculation to be quantified at the bedside (19).

Filters

Dialyzers

Two types of dialyzers are currently used: parallel flat-plate dialyzers and hollow-fiber dialyzers (Table 1.1).

Parallel flate-plate dialyzers are composed of sandwiched sheets of membrane in a parallel plate configuration. As blood and dialysate flow, resistances are low; no backfiltration occurs with this type of dialyzer. A shortcoming of parallel flat-plate dialyzers is their high weight and a relatively high volume of their blood compartment (70–120 ml), even if a reduction in size has been achieved by the use of thinner membrane support plates.

Table 1.1 Some types of currently available hemodialyzers

Name	Identification	Manufacturer	Membrane	Type of membrane	Type of dialyzer	Geometry	Sterilization
Crystal	2800 to 4000	Hospal	PAN (AN69XS)	Synthetic	High–flux	Parallel plate	Gamma
Nephral	200 to 500	Hospal	PAN (AN69XT)	Synthetic	High–flux	Hollow fiber	Gamma
Filtryzer	BK–1.3F to BK–2.1F	Toray	PMMA	Synthetic	High–flux	Hollow fiber	Gamma
Filtryzer	B3–0.5A to B3–2.1A	Toray	PMMA	Synthetic	Low–flux	Hollow fiber	Gamma
Hemoflow	F 40S to F 80S	Fresenius	Polysulfone	Synthetic	High–flux	Hollow fiber	Steam
Hemoflow	F4HPS to F8HPS	Fresenius	Polysulfone	Synthetic	Low–flux	Hollow fiber	Steam
Polyflux S	PF 11S to PF 21S	Gambro	Polyamide S	Synthetic	High–flux	Hollow fiber	Steam
Polyflux L	PF 6L to PF 8L	Gambro	Polyamide S	Synthetic	Low–flux	Hollow fiber	Steam
Tricea	90G to 210G	Baxter	Triacetate	Cellulosic	High–flux	Hollow fiber	Gamma
Dicea	90G to 210G	Baxter	Diacetate	Cellulosic	Low–flux	Hollow fiber	Gamma
LunDia Pro	500G to 800G	Gambro	Gambrane	Synthetic	Low–flux	Parallel plate	Gamma
GFS Plus	12 to 20	Gambro	Hemophan	Cellulosic	Low–flux	Hollow fiber	Steam

Hollow-fiber dialyzers are the most popular dialyzers today. They comprise bundles of 10 000–15 000 capillary tubes through which blood circulates. Blood velocity and pressure drops should be optimized for ensuring an even distribution of the blood in the fiber bundle. Hollow-fiber dialyzers have a low priming volume (40–80 ml).

Hemofilters use highly permeable membranes. They are predominantly of a hollow-fiber type.

Dialysis membranes

Like the glomerular basement membrane, the dialysis membrane should be non-permeable to albumin and all the solutes with a molecular weight higher than albumin. The cut-off of the membrane is defined as the highest molecular weight of a solute that can pass through the membrane and depends on the maximal diameter of the pores. Dialysis membranes can be classified according to their chemical nature, their permeability characteristics, or their 'biocompatibility' (Table 1.1).

Chemically, the membrane is either of natural origin (cellulosic membranes), non-substituted such as Cuprophan or substituted such as Hemophan or cellulose-acetate and thus hydrophilic, or synthetic and thus either hydrophobic (such as poly-sulfone, polyamide, polyacrylonitrile, polymethylmetacrylate), or hydrophilic (such as polycarbonate-polyether, ethylvinyl-alcohol). In addition, some membranes (such as polyacrylonitrile AN69) are negatively charged.

The permeabilities of dialysis/filtration membranes are two-fold. The diffusive permeability is characterized by the mass transfer coefficient K_0A, which rapidly decreases according to the solute molecular weight. High-efficiency dialyzers are fitted with a thin membrane and a large surface area and have a high K_0A for urea. The convective permeability is characterized by the hydraulic permeability and the solute sieving coefficient. High-flux dialyzers have a high hydraulic permeability and a high sieving coefficient for solutes with molecular weights in the range of 1500 to 5000 Da (middle molecules).

Biocompatibility is defined as the ability of a material (e.g. a dialysis membrane), a device (e.g. a dialyzer), or a system (such as a dialysis circuit including dialysis membrane, dialyzer, and dialysis fluid) to perform without a clinically significant host response. Regarding the dialysis membranes, complement activation, with the generation of anaphylatoxins C3a and C5a and subsequent dialysis-induced leukopenia, is commonly considered as an index of bio-incompatibility.

Synthetic hydrophobic membranes are generally considered more biocompatible. In addition, these membranes are usually more porous, with a higher hydraulic permeability. However, there are currently no universally convincing clinical data from prospective and randomized studies to support the systematic use of these much more expensive membranes in terms of long-term morbidity or mortality. Despite several hundreds of papers published on this subject, an unequivocal beneficial effect of the use of highly permeable/biocompatible membranes on chronic hemodialysis–patient survival remains an ongoing very debated issue on both sides of the Atlantic Ocean (20–22). About the only clearly demonstrated advantage of the use of biocompatible membranes is the reduction of occurrence of carpal tunnel syndromes in patients treated with these types of membranes for more than 6–8 years (23).

Different procedures are used for the sterilization of dialyzers: chemical (with ethylene oxide, ETO), physical (gamma radiation), or heat (steam). ETO-sterilization does not affect the dialyzers' performances, but may be responsible for acute hypersensitivity reactions. Gamma sterilization is increasingly employed, but aromatic polyurethane compounds may release methylene dianiline—a potentially carcinogenic substance—following irradiation. Steam sterilization allows the absence of chemical residues, but is not possible for all types of membrane because degradation may occur.

Dialyzer re-use

Hemodialyzer re-use refers to the processing of a used dialyzer cartridge with or without connecting lines, for repeated hemodialysis sessions performed for the same patient. The advantages of re-use include a reduction in the treatment cost or the possibility to use more expensive, high-flux dialyzers within a non-expanded budget. Re-use results also in an improvement in biocompatibility, especially for the non-substituted cellulosic membranes, and a reduction in the occurrence of the first-use syndrome, especially for ETO-sterilized membranes.

The disadvantages of re-use are the possible exposure to disinfectants if the rinsing/priming procedures of the dialyzers are insufficient, the risk of hemolysis, and of development of anti-N antibodies if formalin is used. Occurrence of pyrogenic reactions, or even septicemias secondary to bacterial contaminations, are potential risks, which are not reported as occuring with an increased frequency in centres practising re-use of dialyzers compared with those which do not.

A risk of underdialysis (see below) may be related to an undetected decrease in dialyzer efficiency. However, the decrease in urea clearance is usually very slight, 1–2% for ten re-uses (24). A careful testing of the effective permeability of more than 80% of the fiber bundles of reprocessed capillary dialyzers is a standard procedure to be carried out prior to each re-use of a given dialyzer.

A possible increase in mortality remains a highly debated issue. Actually, recent large-scale surveys have shown that after careful adjustments for patient and dialysis procedure characteristics no differences emerge in mortality risks between Dialysis Units which re-use dialyzers and that which do not practice re-use (25).

Anticoagulation

Standard procedure consists of general heparinization, but regional anticoagulation or absence of anticoagulation may be required in patients at high risk of bleeding or who are actively bleeding.

General heparinization

Unfractioned heparin is the anticoagulant most widely used to prevent clotting in the extra-corporeal blood circuit during hemodialysis. The standard procedure consists of administring an initial bolus (usually 50IU/kg of dry body weight) of unfractioned heparin into the arterial line immediately after its connection to the patient.

This initial bolus is followed by a half-dose injected mid-dialysis or by a continuous infusion (500–1000 IU/h) facilitated by the use of an heparin pump that is integrated in to the modern dialysis monitors. Undesired effects of heparin include hyper-lipidemia, thrombocytopenia, osteoporosis, and allergy.

The use of low molecular weight heparin (LWMH) is slightly more expensive, but has several advantages:

(1) longer half-life allows anticoagulation with a single dose at the start of dialysis;
(2) less derangement of serum triglycerides; less risk of bleeding and consequently fewer blood-transfusions or less erythropoetin requirements;
(3) the possibility of using a standard dose for all adult patients;
(4) less incidence of thrombocytopenia.

Regional anticoagulation

Regional anticoagulation can be obtained by a constant infusion of heparin into the arterial line neutralized by a constant infusion of protamine into the venous line before return of the blood to the patient. The difficulty is to determine the adequate respective doses of heparin and protamine to achieve extra-corporeal, but not systemic, anticoagulation.

With the use of sodium citrate, blood is anticoagulated by chelating ionized calcium with citrate and using a calcium-free dialysate. Calcium chloride is infused into the venous line. Disadvantages of this method include the need for additional equipment and the potential risk of calcemia disorders and metabolic alkalosis (26).

Hemodialysis without anticoagulation

Heparin-free hemodialysis can be successfully performed by rinsing the extra-corporeal blood circuit every 30 min with about 100 ml saline, together with an adequate increase of the ultrafiltration rate. The advantages of this method are its safety and simplicity. Disadvantages include the need of a close monitoring of the venous and arterial pressure alarms, a careful monitoring for early signs of clotting, the requirement of high blood flow (>250 ml/min) and low weight loss, the impossibility to transfuse via the hemodialysis circuit.

Dialysis fluids

Water treatment

Tap water is unsuitable for the preparation of dialysis fluids because its mineral and organic solutes contents are both variable and excessive. Table 1.2 indicates the highest concentrations of contaminants allowed in water used for dialysate preparation.

Bacterial contamination of the dialysate and the potential transfer of endotoxin from dialysate into the blood result in the repeated stimulation of several biological and immunological systems by long-term endotoxin challenge and have been recognized as factors predisposing to clinical complications, such as the β_2m-amyloidosis,

Table 1.2   Maximum contaminant levels allowed in water used for dialysate preparation according to European Pharmacopeia (1993)

Total bacterial count (CFU/ml)	<100
Endotoxins (IU/ml)	<0.25
Sodium (mg/l)	<50
Potassium (mg/l)	<2
Calcium (mg/l)	<2
Magnesium (mg/l)	<2
Chloride (mg/l)	<50
Total CO_2 (mg/l)	<5
Chlorine (mg/l)	<0.1
Sulfate (mg/l)	<50
Nitrate (mg/l)	<2
Fluoride (mg/l)	<0.2
Ammonia (mg/l)	<0.2
Aluminum (mg/l)	<0.01
Heavy metals (mg/l)	<0.1
Total solids (mg/l)	<10

atherosclerosis, and malnutrition (27). Concerning the microbiological quality of water, the standards of European Pharmacopoeia (Table 1.2) seem not sufficiently rigid, particularly for high-flux hemodialysis or online convective procedures. The present aim of water treatment is to obtain ultrapure water defined by upper levels of bacteria and endotoxins at 0.1 micro-organism/ml and 0.05 IU endotoxin/ml, respectively, in order to enhance the biocompatibility of dialysis treatment and to offer the possibility of treating patients with convective procedures using online re-infusion of the dialysis fluid into the bloodstream (28, 29).

Water treatment is usually performed in two steps: pre-treatment and purification.

Pre-treatment   This consists of:

1. Pre-filtration using cartridge filters designed to clean raw supply water by eliminating the large-size particules (5–500 μm) and consequently prevent fouling of the downstream equipment.
2. It is followed by filtration on an activated-carbon filter for eliminating the dissolved organic contaminants, chlorine and chloramine. Periodically, when its adsorptive capacity is exceeded, the activated charcoal has to be replaced. Overall efficacy of

the charcoal filter is dependent upon cartridge geometry, incoming water flow, and content of chlorine and chloramine, but the most critical factor is the water contact time with the charcoal bed.

3. Microfiltration using membrane filters for eliminating the low-size particles (0.45–5 μm).
4. Water softening is then required for preventing hard-water syndrome by reducing the divalent ion charge in exchanging two Na^+ ions for Ca^{++} and Mg^{++} using a cationic resin. It protects membranes of equipment downstream—and particularly membrane of reverse osmosis units—from build-up and scaling. Undetected saturation of the softener may result in massive release of calcium and aluminum, a potentially life-threatening event.

Purification   The second step of water treatment consists of a reverse osmosis procedure, through a semi-permeable membrane, to repel ions according to their valence, and screening out organic particles. The obtention of ultrapure water requires two reverse osmosis units placed in series and a microfiltration through a 0.1 μm pore-size filter.

Electrolytes

Dialysis fluids contain only the four quantitatively most important cations (sodium, potassium, calcium, and magnesium) and the two quantitatively most important anions (chloride and bicarbonate) present in plasma with a composition close to that of extracellular fluid, but with variations specified in order to correct the abnormalities developed during the interdialytic period. A typical dialysate composition is shown in Table 1.3. This formula can be slightly modified for individual patients

Table 1.3   An example of standard dialysate composition

	Concentrate after dilution (mmol/l)		Final dialysate (mmol/l)
	Acid concentrate	Bicarbonate concentrate	
Cations			
Sodium	107	33	140
Potassium	2	–	2
Calcium	1.75	–	1.75
Magnesium	0.5	–	0.5
Anions			
Bicarbonate	–	33	29
Chloride	113.5	–	113.5
Acetate	–	–	4
Other solutes			
Acetic acid	4	–	–
Carbon dioxide	–	–	4
Glucose	5	–	5

(see Prescription and quantification of dialysis: the concept of dialysis adequacy). The dialysis fluids are obtained by diluting concentrates of electrolytes with purified water.

Because the bicarbonate precipitates as carbonate in the presence of divalent cations (calcium or magnesium), the suggestion has been made to substitute bicarbonate with an organic anion (acetate or lactate), which is metabolized in liver and muscle, in order to regenerate bicarbonate. However, acetate has an important vasodilator effect, which induces hemodynamic unstability. Hence, some patients tolerate acetate dialysis poorly, particularly those patients with cardiac failure, malnourishment, or liver failure, and also patients treated by high-efficiency dialysis, which provokes a too rapid transfer of acetate into the bloodstream to be adequately metabolized by the liver. The use of a bicarbonate buffer, more physiological but requiring the use of two concentrates, is now standard with the presently available dialysis monitors. The presence of a small amount of acid (in the bicarbonate-free concentrate) is required for obtaining (during the mixing) the carbon dioxide (about 2–7 mmol/l) that permits, as in plasma, the simultaneous presence of calcium and bicarbonate. When acetic acid is used, it entails the presence of 2–7 mmol/l of acetate in the final dialysate. The use of chlorhydric acid avoids this drawback, but the very low pH of concentrate containing chlorhydric acid makes these concentrates not easy for routine use.

The presence of glucose at a physiologic plasma concentration (5–7 mmol/l) in the dialysate avoids the waste of about 300 mmol of glucose per session, and is furthermore mandatory for diabetic patients. The use of dialysate, enriched with glucose, is recommended for old or malnourished patients. It tends to become increasingly systematic, in order to prevent denutrition—a major complication in ESRD-patients.

The use of concentrates in sterile bags or in powder cartridges allows a high bacteriological quality. However the use of concentrate in powder form is possible only if the cartridge contains one single constituent (e.g. sodium bicarbonate).

Dialysis machines and monitors

The functions of dialysis machines consist in the delivery of quantitatively and qualitatively appropriate dialysis fluid to the dialyzer (see previous section), and in the monitoring of the circulation of dialysate and extra-corporeal blood flow. In the case a fall of blood-flow rate, or of variations in arterial or venous pressures detected by dedicated sensors, or in case of blood leak into the dialyzer detected by dialysate photometry, the blood pump will be stopped with blood-lines clamped and alarms will flash and sound. Dialysate composition is usually monitored by conductimetry, dialysate temperature by specific sensors, and dialysate flow by flowmeter. Whenever one of these parameters wanders out of the preset limits, the dialysate will be derived in by-pass and alarms will flash and sound.

The dialysate delivery system must be disinfected after each dialysis by chemical agents or heat. Chlorine or peracetic acid are now often preferred to formalin. The presence of residual disinfectant in the dialysate should be carefully checked by an appropriate test before the start of the dialysis session.

Modes of utilization of extra-corporeal blood-purification systems

In all extra-corporeal blood-purification systems, like in the native kidneys, waste products are removed through a semi-permeable membrane. However, in contrast with native kidneys, the solute transfer through the semi-permeable membrane is not necessarily a convective transfer due to ultrafiltration. In conventional hemodialysis the transfer is mainly diffusive but in other techniques (hemofiltration, hemodiafiltration), the convective transfer plays a predominant role.

Conventional hemodialysis

In conventional hemodialysis, the circulation of the dialysate/dialysis fluid allows the diffusion of solutes between the blood and the dialysate compartment of the dialyzer. Waste products (urea, creatinine, uric acid, etc.) are absent from the dialysate delivered by the dialysis machine in order to maximize the transmembrane concentration gradient and thus their removal.

The removal of water is obtained by filtration (called ultrafiltration when the filtration occurs across a semi-permeable membrane). This water transfer by ultrafiltration is responsible for the convective transfer of solutes from plasma to dialysate. In conventional hemodialysis, the convective transfer of a given solute is negligible for small molecular weight solutes (such as urea), compared to the diffusive transfer, being proportional to its transmembrane concentration gradient. On the other hand, it can be of importance for small molecular weight solutes with a high plasma concentration and a low transmembrane concentration gradient (such as sodium).

Convective transfer is practically exclusive for middle molecular weight solutes such as β2-microglobulin, because diffusion is negligible when molecular weight is high. With a membrane having a high sieving coefficient for middle molecular weight solutes (high-flux dialyzers), this convective transfer can even occur for zero or low net ultrafiltration, if backfiltration (i.e. dialysis fluid entering into the bloodstream from the dialysate compartement), occuring in the distal end of the dialyzer, partially compensates for the fluid lost by the ultrafiltration taking place in the proximal part of the dialyzer.

Convective techniques

Hemofiltration

In hemofiltration, the transport of water and solutes is purely convective. In contrast with the diffusive transfer, convective transfer is practically independent of molecular weight within the limits of the membrane pore size. Consequently a high-flux membrane is required. The total ultrafiltration is much higher than the desired weight loss and the perfusion of a sterile and pyrogen-free substitution fluid is mandatory for preventing dehydration. Fluid substitution can be performed before (pre-dilution) or after (post-dilution) the hemofilter.

Pre-dilution hemofiltration is less efficient than post-dilution hemofiltration and requires approximately twice as much substitution fluid, increasing excessively the cost, as long as the availability of substitution solutions is dependent on industrially manufactured bags. On the other hand, pre-dilution hemofiltration allows an increase in the volume of substitution fluid, and thus dialysis efficiency, without the risk of clotting due to high hematocrit inside the hemofilter, as observed in the post-dilution mode. Because it is now technically possible to prepare online and without additional cost, a sterile and pyrogenic-free substitution fluid, pre-dilution hemofiltration could be more widely used in future years (30).

Hemodiafiltration

Hemodiafiltration is a hemodialysis procedure carried out with highly permeable membranes, in which fluid removal exceeds the desired weight loss: fluid balance is maintained by the infusion of a sterile and pyrogen-free substitution solution. Hemodiafiltration provides the possibility for delivering renal replacement therapy with the largest solute removal over a wide molecular weight spectrum. With online preparation of substitution fluid, hemodiafiltration can be performed at a cost similar to that of high-flux hemodialysis (31).

Other procedures

In the above described diffusive and convective procedures, the composition of dialysis and substitution fluids is similar to that of physiologic extracellular fluid. Newer dialysis procedures, often called biofiltration, use dialysis and substitution fluids with a non-physiologic composition.

In acetate-free biofiltration, the dialysis fluid is base-free (without acetate nor bicarbonate). The bicarbonate repletion of the patient is obtained by infusion in a post-dilution mode of sodium bicarbonate (32, 33). Acetate-free biofiltration offers some technical advantages: total absence of acetate, no precipitation of calcium carbonate and thus no limitation in bicarbonate supply, and easier cleansing of the dialysis monitor. Compared with conventional bicarbonate dialysis, acetate-free biofiltration is associated with improvements in protein intake, control of acid–base balance, dialysis efficiency, and in hemodynamic tolerance (34).

In duocart-biofiltration, the dialysate contains only sodium chloride and bicarbonate obtained from two powder cartridges. The ionic complement (potassium, calcium and magnesium chlorides) and glucose are perfused in a post-dilution mode (35). Compared with acetate-free biofiltration, duocart biofiltration offers several additional advantages: components presented in powder form, absence of glucose in the dialysate, lower cost of the reinfusion (1.5 l of cheap solutes instead 6–8 l of more expensive sodium bicarbonate).

Prescription and quantification of dialysis: the concept of dialysis adequacy

Adequacy of dialysis can be defined as a determination made by clinical assessment of the patient's clinical status and well-being. This frequently debated parameter is based on the currently accepted criteria shown in Table 1.4.

Control of depuration: the dialysis efficiency

Frank Gotch has coined the concept of dialysis dose by comparing dialysis treatment with a pharmacological treatment. With urea being taken as a surrogate for uremic toxins accumulated during the interdialytic period, the dialysis dose is defined as the product (Kt) of the whole body urea clearance (K) by the effective duration of the dialysis session (t). It represents the volume of body fluid depurated from urea. The optimization of the dialysis dose needs to answer the two following questions:

1. What is the dialysis dose to be prescribed for a given patient? (Medical problem.)
2. Is the prescribed dialysis dose actually delivered to the patient? (Technical problem.)

Like a pharmacologic drug, the dialysis dose has to be normalized to the patient's personal criteria and thus take into account a distribution volume. Because the distribution volume of urea, taken as a surrogate for waste products, is the total body water (V), the dialysis dose is usually normalized to V and the dimensionless index (Kt/V), directly related to the equations of urea kinetics, is called normalized dialysis dose.

Table 1.4 Usually accepted criteria for adequate dialysis

Interdialytic weight load $< 5\%$ of body weight
Kt/V >1.2 or urea reduction ratio $>65\%$
nPCR >1 g/kg/day
Pre-dialytic parameters:
BP $<150/90$ mmHg
Potassium <6.5 mmol/l
Calcium: 2.2–2.5 mmol/l
Bicarbonate >20 mmol/l
Phosphate <1.8 mmol/l
Albumin >37 g/l
Hemoglobin: 11–12 g/dl

Since the National Cooperative Dialysis Study, and some more recent studies, have demonstrated a relationship between the normalized dialysis dose (Kt/V) and patient morbidity and mortality, Kt/V is considered as a reference index for determining the adequate dialysis dose (Kt) to be prescribed to the patient and for verifying its effective delivery (36, 37). For a Kt/V value ranging between 0.6 and 1.6, mortality and normalized dialysis dose are significantly and inversely correlated (38). Recent guidelines set the minimal value of dialysis dose at Kt/V 1.2–1.3 with no further reduction in mortality rates being observed for Kt/V>1.3 or a urea reduction rate (URR) >70% (39, 40).

Two types of methods are used for assessing the efficacy of dialysis. The indirect methods provide a global estimation from the observation of the change in the blood urea concentrations during the session by using urea kinetic modeling. The measurement of URR is the easiest method for estimating the dialysis efficacy: a minimal value of 65% is usually recommended. However the immediate post-dialysis urea or blood urea nitrogen (BUN) is often an unreliable parameter, since it is influenced by vascular access and cardiopulmonary recirculation, and by the dilution of the blood sample with the restitution fluid administered intravenously at the end of the dialysis session. In addition, post-dialysis BUN is relatively unstable because of an hemodialysis-induced disequilibrium between the body fluid compartments of the patient, and should actually be substituted by an estimate of an equilibrated post-dialysis BUN. This can be accomplished by directly measuring the BUN at least 30min after end of dialysis (which creates inconvenience for the patient and staff), or by predicting the equilibrated post-dialysis BUN according to a specific mathematical model of urea rebound (41). Whether the online recording of the changes in urea concentration, in the spent dialysate during the dialysis session, and the analysis of this urea profile by a multicompartmental model can indeed provide a reliable estimation of the normalized dialysis dose remains debatable (42).

Direct methods are based on the independent measurement of the three parameters K, t, and V. The calculation of K, from the predialysis BUN and the value of the total urea nitrogen removed during the session, is usually considered as the gold standard. Because the ionic dialysance, calculated from measurements of dialysate conductivity, is a reflect of the instantaneous effective urea clearance, its repeated measurement during dialysis has been shown as a reliable, automatic, and inexpensive method for calculating the delivered dialysis dose at each session (43).

Control of fluid balance: assessment of dry weight

In hemodialysis and derived techniques, fluid removal from the patient is obtained by ultrafiltration due to a transmembrane gradient of hydraulic pressure. In modern dialyis machines, the hydraulic pressure is automatically adjusted by a feedback system called ultrafiltration controller. The physician only prescribes the desired weight loss, the ultrafiltration controller then automatically determines the adequate value of the transmembrane pressure required, depending on the hydraulic permeability of the dialyzer. The desired ultrafiltration is routinely reached with an accuracy better than 50 ml.

However two problems are still debated:

1. What is the true dry weight for a given patient?
2. How can this value be reached without inducing untoward symptoms of clinical intolerance?

Dry weight is clinically defined as the lowest weight a patient can tolerate at the end of a dialysis session without the development of symptoms and, particularly, arterial hypotension. Consequently the dry weight in hemodialysis should theoretically be lower than the physiologic dry weight resulting from normal renal function and body volume regulation, allowing a better tolerance to the interdialytic fluid overload. However, the routine evaluation of dry weight from clinical examination is very imprecise and it is thus very difficult to determine, with a low margin of error, whether a patient is over or underhydrated (44). Different techniques have recently emerged for better assessing post-dialysis dry weight:

(1) measurement of concentrations of biochemical markers, such as atrial natriuretic peptide (ANP) or cyclic guanidine monophosphate (cGMP);
(2) measurement of vena cava diameter by ultrasound (45);
(3) bioimpedance analysis (46).

Unfortunately no method has yet emerged as a gold standard.

Because the fluid removal is performed only from the patient's blood compartment, ultrafiltration, by inducing a drastic decrease in blood volume, is the major determinant of hypovolemia-induced symptoms and particularly symptomatic hypotension. Recent technological advances allow a routine, non-invasive monitoring of blood volume changes by measuring hematocrit (using optical or impedancemetric methods) or total protein concentration (by ultrasonic method). With these monitoring devices, it should be possible to predict hypotensive episodes and, by using a feedback between the measured blood volume reduction and the prescribed ultrafiltration rate and/or dialysate sodium concentration, to prevent hypovolemia-induced symptoms (47). However, the reduction in blood volume during hemodialysis is subject to considerable intra- and inter-individual variations, and consequently blood volume monitoring seems, at least at present, of limited interest in the prevention of dialysis-related hypotension (48).

Control of sodium balance

As in plasma, sodium is the major determinant of dialysate osmolality. The sodium transfer during the dialysis session is principally convective, due to the prescribed ultrafiltration, but its diffusive component is of greatest interest, because the physician can control it by prescribing the dialysate sodium concentration. However, the determination of the optimal dialysate sodium concentration is still debated. Too low a sodium dialysate is responsible for intradialytic discomfort (including symptomatic hypotension, cramps, nausea). Too high a sodium concentration is responsible for interdialytic morbidity and mortality secondary to chronic sodium overload.

Thus the role of dialysate sodium concentration should not be seen in terms of acting on intradialytic tolerance alone. Prescribing adequate sodium dialysate concentration requires that the entirety of short- and long-term side-effects of dialysis treatment be taken into account. The usual dialysate sodium concentration is in the 138–145 mmol/l range.

The optimal value of dialysate sodium concentration is that which allows the physiological value of the exchangeable sodium pool to be restored at the end of dialysis. This value depends on predialytic natremia. Specially designed software, based on biofeedback techniques using online sensors and kinetic modeling, have been recently developed for the fully automatic determination of the optimal dialysate sodium concentration (49, 50).

The use of a decreasing profile of dialysate sodium during the dialysis session can be useful for improving intradialytic tolerance. A decreasing profile induces a diffusive sodium influx during the early period of the session, in order to prevent the rapid fall in osmolality due to the loss of urea and other small molecular weight solutes across the dialyzer. During the remaining period, a low dialysate sodium concentration allows the avoidance of chronic sodium overload. The association of a decreasing ultrafiltration profile can be useful for preserving plasma volume during the phase of lower sodium supply (51).

Control of potassium balance

During the dialysis session, the interdialytic potassium load should be removed by using a low potassium dialysate. A 2 mmol/l potassium dialysate is a standard value generally permitting the removal of the potassium overload. However, a possibly abrupt decrease of kalemia during the early period of the session can trigger the occurrence of cardiac arrythmia in some patients, particularly in elderly or critically ill patients, or patients receiving digitalis and prone to cardiac arrythmia. For these patients, a dialysate concentration of potassium up to 3 mM, combined with the prescription of Kayexalate[R], can be useful. A recently proposal is to profile the dialysate potassium concentration during the dialysis session: a relatively high level during the early period, when serum potassium level is high avoids a too dramatic fall in kalemia and thus prevents cardiac arrythmia. A lower dialysate potassium concentration during the remaining period allows the subsequent removal of the remaining potassium overload (52).

Control of acid–base balance

End-stage renal failure induces metabolic acidosis and thus a fall in plasma bicarbonate during the interdialytic period. Consequently a buffer-reload is necessary during the dialysis session. Bicarbonate-buffer is more physiological and is thus currently preferred over other alkalating agents (see Electrolytes).

The bicarbonate supply should allow a predialytic plasma bicarbonate level not lower than 20 mmol/l, but with a post-dialytic plasma level not higher than 30 mmol/l, because of the risk of metabolic alkalosis and of its induced symptoms (nausea, hypertension, headaches). Usually, sufficient bicarbonate concentrate is supplied to provide a final concentration in the dialysate in the range of 28–36 mmol/l, taking into account the amount of bicarbonate consumed by the acid required for generating carbon dioxide (see Electrolytes).

Control of calcium phosphate metabolism

In order to avoid a negative calcium balance during hemodialysis, dialysate calcium concentration is usually in the range 1.5–1.75 mmol/l. Dialysate with a 1.5 mmol/l calcium content is more physiological but it usually renders an important interdialytic supplementation necessary (53). Lower levels (1.25 mmol/l) are used in patients who tend towards predialysis hypercalcemia.

Phosphate is normally absent from the dialysate because ESRF patients typically have hyperphosphatemia. An adequately treated patient should have a predialytic serum phosphorus level lower than 1.8 mmol/l. Hyperphosphatemia can be induced by too high an interdialytic dietary intake, an insufficient delivered dialysis dose, or uncontrolled hyperparathyroidism. On the other hand, malnourished patients or those being intensively dialysed (such as patients on long nocturnal dialysis) may become hypophosphatemic and need a phosphate-enriched dialysate obtained by addition of phosphorus to the bicarbonate concentrate (54).

Complications related to extra corporeal dialysis equipments

Acute complications and/or accidents

Dialysate-induced complications

Dialysate temperature is normally regulated at about 37 °C by a thermostat. Malfunctions of the thermostat, or of another component of the monitoring system, can result in abnormaly high or low dialysate temperatures with consequent change in body temperature. Too low a temperature increases secretion of catecholamines and can induce shivering. Too high a temperature can induce massive hemolysis. However, in the conscious patient, a sensation of warm or cold will occur before a dangerous change in body temperature.

Dysfunction of the water-treatment system can be responsible for several, sometimes severe and even life-threatening, accidents. Failure in softening results in an increase of dialysate calcium concentration up to 3.6 mmol/l, inducing a hard-water syndrome: nausea, vomiting, hypertension, progressive lethargy. Defection in charcoal filters can result in contamination of water by chloramine, inducing methemoglobinemia and hemolysis. Faulty reverse osmosis units can cause contamination of water by aluminum responsible for bone disease, microcytic anemia, and chronic encephalopathy with dementia. Contamination of the water used for preparing the dialysate by metals present in the pipes of the distribution system (lead, copper, aluminium) can provoke various and sometimes severe clinical reactions, which may affect several or all the patients treated in a given dialysis facility. Expert installation and maintenance of the water-treatment system is crucial for the safety of extra-corporeal dialysis treatments.

Dialyzer-induced complications

Anaphylactoïd reactions within the first 5 min of dialysis can be the result of residual amounts of ethylene oxyde (ETO) used during sterilization by the manufacturer. Such acute reactions are identified as first-use syndrome, since reprocessed cellulosic membranes generally do not induce this type of reaction. In order to avoid the occurrence of this syndrome, the use of ETO-sterilization is progressively substituted by gamma-ray or steam sterilization.

More recently, acute allergic reactions have been reported with the use of the AN69 polyacrylonitrile membrane in patients treated with angiotensin-converting enzyme inhibitors (ACEI). This reaction is related to an early and vigorous production of bradykinin induced by the contact of the blood with the negatively charged AN69 membrane. In such patients, bradykinin accumulates in the blood because ACEIs block the action of the enzyme responsible for its degradation (55, 56).

Chronic complications related to dialysis components

Some chronic complications are related to the long-term consequences of the bio-incompatibiltiy of the components of the blood-purification systems. Complement activation with generation of the anaphylatoxins C3a and C5a, activation of the contact phase with bradykinin release, contamination of dialysate by bacteria and lipopolysac-charide (LPS) endotoxins, or use of acetate dialysate resulting in IL-1 production by monocytes, induce a chronic inflammatory state. Such a disorder may favor dialysis-related amyloïdosis, increased susceptibility to infections, increased muscle protein catabolism, malnutrition, atherosclerosis, and finally increased mortality (57–59). The use of biocompatible dialysis membranes (with minimal activation of complement and bradykinin generation) and of sterile, non-pyrogenic dialysate containing a minimal concentration of acetate are currently the means considered as probably the most efficient for preventing or minimizing these long-term complications.

Complications of vascular access

Vascular access failures remain a major cause of morbidity (and cost) in hemodialyzed patients.

Clotting

Clotting is the most frequent cause of access failure. It is rarely related to a coagula-tion disorder: repeated clotting of the vascular access needs extensive coagulation testing including determination of protein C, total and free protein S, search for circulating anticoagulant and for anticardiolipid antibodies. Antivitamin K therapy or antiplatelet agents may be indicated in these cases.

Clotting is most often related to an insufficient flow rate in the vascular access due to a stenosis induced by intimal hyperplasia. The mechanism of smooth muscle-cell hyperplasia that causes these intimal abnormalities is an area of active research (60).

Prevention of thrombosis is based on the early detection of stenosis in order to intervene before the access fails and to prolong the useful life of the access. The radiographic angiogram of the access shows whether or not a stenosis is present, but this technique is too invasive and too expensive for routine screening.

Reduction of access flow limits the blood flow to the dialyzer and can induce access recirculation if the access inflow rate (Q_A) becomes lower than the blood flow (Q_B) in the extra-corporeal circuit. An accurate measurement of access recirculation would thus seem a better technique than recording venous pressure for detecting the risk of thrombosis.

However, the predictive value of access recirculation measurement with regard to future access thrombosis is poor because recirculation does not occur unless access blood flow is lower than Q_B and thus markedly impaired, especially in patients treated by low-flux techniques (61). A recent prospective study has failed to find any correlation between the incidence of thrombosis and the percentage of recirculation (62). In addition, a location of the stenosis between the two needles could induce low blood flow without recirculation. Thus, absence of access recirculation does not necessarily mean the absence of access problems (63).

Measurement of access blood flow seems to provide the most performant means to monitor vascular access (64). The detection of a flow rate below 600 ml/min or of a decrease in blood flow higher than 15%, evidenced from serial measurements, is associated with an increased risk of thrombosis, even if recirculation access does not occur at this level (65, 66). When a reduction in access flow is evidenced, the systematic prescription of a radiographic angiogram associated with early angioplastic or surgical treatment would decrease the risk of clotting and/or losing vascular access in these patients.

Bacterial infections

Bacterial infections occuring in hemodialysis patients are located at, or starting from, the vascular access in more than half of the cases. They are usually due to staphylococci (*Staphylococcus aureus* or *S. epidermidis*). Diagnosis is based upon the finding of local signs of inflammation, but septicemia may occur even in the absence of overt local signs. Prompt, vigorous therapy with antibiotics is mandatory. Infection of a temporary access (IV catheter or other device) requires its removal most of the time. In a patient with an infected vascular graft, the access may have to be occluded or removed.

Other complications

Excessive flow rate in the vascular access may lead to limb distal ischemia, edema or high-output cardiac failure, and requires surgical revision. Distal ischemia is favored by atherosclerosis, especially in diabetics. Aneurysms and pseudo-aneurysms should be surgically repaired if a marked thinning of the overlying skin develops.

The underdialysis syndrome

The underdialysis syndrome is the consequence of an insufficient efficacy of the dialysis system and is responsible for increased mortality. It may be due to an inadequate blood flow in the dialyzer, too small a membrane surface area, access recirculation, or insufficient duration of the sessions.

Underdialysis results in accumulation of uremic toxins, both in the low and in the middle molecular weight ranges. This accumulation provokes anorexia, one of the symptoms of uremia only partially corrected by dialysis. This appetite loss, especially for protein-containing food, results in decreased protein intake and muscle mass inducing spurious low predialysis urea and creatinine levels, that may erroneously incite to decrease the prescribed dialysis dose, thus aggravating malnutrition with the creation of a highly hazardous vicious circle.

Anorexia, due to underdialysis or to another cause (depression, disequilibrium syndrome, gastro-intestinal disorders, social problems, etc.), is often combined with increased catabolism (due to metabolic acidosis, infection, etc.). The resulting malnutrition is a major cause of morbidity and mortality.

The underdialysis syndrome is suspected on clinical signs of malnutrition and on the irrespect of usually accepted criteria for adequate dialysis (Table 1.4): serum albumin $<35\,g/l$, $Kt/V<1$, normalized protein catabolic rate (nPCR) $<0.8\,g/kg/day$. Patients who display rather low plasma levels of urea, creatinine, and phosphate should be carefully discussed, because malnutrition may mask underdialysis.

The prevention of the underdialysis syndrome is based on dialysis sessions with a high urea clearance ensuring an optimal efficacy for removal of low molecular weight uremic toxins and of sufficient duration ($<12\,h/week$) for allowing optimal clearance of uremic toxins in the middle molecular weight range. Careful attention should be given to overweight patients (defined as having a body mass index >27.5), in whom the dialysis dose considered as correct for non-obese patients may turn out as insufficient with a creeping development of an underdialysis syndrome (67).

Indications and contra-indications to extra-corporeal renal replacement therapy

Initiation of extra-corporeal renal replacement therapy

The patient's clinical status at the start of dialysis is a major factor of morbidity and mortality during the future course of renal replacement therapy (RRT). An example of a desirable clinical and biochemical profile of patients at the time of initiation of dialysis is summarized in Table 1.5. In addition, taking into account the highly detrimental effect of malnutrition in these patients, dialysis should be started when the spontaneous dietary protein intake falls below $0.8\,g/day/kg$ of body weight (68). The

Table 1.5 Desirable clinical and biochemical profile of patients with chronic renal failure at the time of initiation of dialysis

Glomerular filtration rate (estimated as (Clcr+Clurea)/2): 8–10 ml/min/1.73 m²

Absence of fluid overload

Blood pressure < 140/90 mmHg

Serum albumin > 35 g/l

Dietary protein intake > 0.8 g/kg/day

Serum potassium < 5 mmol/l

Serum bicarbonate > 22 mmol/l

Serum calcium: 2.3–2.5 mmol/l

Serum phosphate < 1.6 mmol/l

Serum PTH: 90–150 pg/l

respect of this profile should entail the construction of the vascular access early enough to avoid the placement of a temporary access in an emergency situation which all too often generates various complications, prolonged hospital stays and soaring costs.

The concept of incremental dialysis is based on the principle that a weekly global Kt/V for urea higher than 2 should be maintained in patients with advanced chronic renal failure by adding to the renal residual function an adequately titrated dose of dialysis. This dose has to be increased over time—according to the progressive fall of the residual renal function—by increasing the duration of sessions and their weekly frequency (69). However, logistical problems in many overcrowded centers do not allow individual tailoring of the dialysis schedules, which explains the currently limited application of this concept.

From a practical point of view, timely initiation of renal replacement therapy (RRT) should be decided according to the overall clinical tolerance of each individual patient to his or her advanced stage of CRF, with a special regard for blood pressure and nutritional status (70).

Technical contra-indications to extra-corporeal renal replacement therapy

There are almost no absolute contra-indications to extra-corporeal dialysis therapy. Dementia or advanced malignancy can militate against the initiation or more often the pursuit of chronic dialysis. These situations raise social and ethical issues which will be dealt with in Chapter 10. From a purely technical point of view, there are only few contra-indications to extra-corporeal RRT and their number is decreasing according to technologic advances.

Contra-indication to heparin administration is only a relative contra-indication to extra-corporeal RRT. Hemodialysis can be performed without anticoagulation or with local citrate anticoagulation and low molecular weight heparin can often be used in patients at hemorragic risk.

Hemodialysis is responsible for rapid correction of electrolyte imbalance and can be contra-indicated in patients with cardiac arrythmias who are poorly responsive or intolerant to antiarrythmic drugs. Rapid correction of fluid overload can be contra-indicated in patients with severe hemodynamic instability, especially in diabetic or amyloïd patients. In severely ill patients requiring intensive care (for example, following a recent myocardial infarction), a slow continuous veno-venous procedure is best indicated.

Hemodialysis needs a well-functioning vascular access and cannot be performed in patients without venous puncture access sites. However, the large number of prosthetic vascular devices now available makes a transfer of patients to an alternative dialysis technique (peritoneal dialysis), because of extinction of all accesses to the bloodstream, a very rare event.

The unphysiology of extra-corporeal renal replacement therapy

Native kidneys have three functions: depuration of waste-products, regulation of water and electrolyte balance, endocrine secretion. With regard to these three functions, all the modes of extra-corporeal RRT are unphysiological.

The depurative action of extra-corporeal RRT is very efficient for low molecular weight solutes. Intradialytic clearances of urea and creatinine are higher than that provided by native kidneys. However, the efficacy of conventional hemodialysis dramatically falls as the molecular weight of waste products increases, because of the diffusive nature of the transfer across the dialysis membrane. The convective techniques, whose depuration process is similar to that of the glomerular basement membrane, are to some extent more physiological, thus explaining their good tolerance and highly satisfactory results on several biochemical criteria.

Extra-corporeal RRT is intermittent, not continuous like the native kidney or continuous peritioneal dialysis: too abrupt a fall of waste-product concentrations and/or of weight is responsible for various signs and symptoms of intolerance, mainly hemodynamic or neurological perturbations, which develop particularly in elderly or severely ill patients. Hence the recent interest in the revival of daily dialysis schedules performed five or six times a week, either on a short-high efficiency mode or, preferably in frail patients, on long-slow nightly schedules (71–72).

There is no regulatory function in extra-corporeal RRT for providing accurate control of electrolyte balance, in contrast with the native kidneys, which ensure a very sophisticated permanent fine-tuning of electrolyte and acid–base balance by the means of feedback loops monitored by hormonal secretions. Only a self-limitation, similar to that for urea and other wastes, allows a relative stabilization of electrolyte concentrations: the higher the electrolyte plasma concentration, the greater the electrolyte removal for a given dialysate composition. The recent development of biofeedback techniques, based on the use of online sensors, should provide the blood-purification system with some regulatory functions, especially concerning the regulation of blood volume changes and sodium balance.

Extra-corporeal blood-purification systems are deprived from any endocrine function. The pharmacological availability of some hormones normally synthesized by native kidneys (active vitamin D, erythropoetin) provide a partial compensation for this absence. Finally, the unphysiology of RRT is also a consequence of the bio-incompatibility of several components of the dialysis/filtration systems, which stimulate chronic inflammatory reactions and long-term complications.

Logistical aspects of extra-corporeal renal replacement therapy

The saga of maintenance hemodialysis for sustaining life in patients with end-stage renal disease (ESRD) began in March 1960 when a single patient started on such a treatment in a clinical research unit of the Department of Medicine at the University of Washington, USA (73). The feasibility of this revolutionary therapy spread very quickly, but also simultaneously with its major stumbling block, namely its tremendous cost. Within only a few months it became obvious for the promoters of maintenance hemodialysis that, all the more in the absence of an unlimited medical insurance coverage, long-term hemodialysis treatment could not be delivered in a hospital-based setting to every uremic patient who needed it. Finding an alternative, less expensive way for providing long-term dialysis was felt as an absolute prerequisite for any future development in the area. Thus, the first out-of-hospital free-standing dialysis unit was established as soon as 1962, along with a home hemodialysis program pioneered mainly in the USA by the Seattle group (Scribner, Blagg, and Eschbach) and in the united Kingdom by Shaldon and colleagues (74, 75). In 1966, Scribner warned the author of this chapter that 'maintenance hemodialysis will have to be performed in the home or will have no future'. The subsequent decades have proven this prediction unfounded.

Where do we stand 40 years later? We shall consider in this section the facts and figures that have developed and currently stand in the economically developed countries of the Western World. The specific aspects pertaining to the provision of RRT in the emergent/developing countries are reviewed in Chapter 11.

Many different factors have played a key role in the evolving spectrum of the provision of dialysis methods in the developed countries. Among them have to be cited the impact of medical options (which are largely influenced by the type of medical education delivered to nephrologists in training), the more or less strong determination of medical and administrative partners for diversifying the modes of delivery of RRT, ongoing technical advances, important changes over time in the demography and epidemiology of ESRD patients, and, quite universally, economic constraints, which in many countries were and are actually the quantitative and quite often qualitative limiting factors for meeting appropriately the needs of the population of patients with ESRD. A global view of the distribution of the main modes of renal replacement

Table 1.6 Global profile of renal replacement therapies applied to patients with ESRD in six Western European countries in 1998 (Germany, Netherlands, United Kingdom, Spain, Italy, France)

	n	%
Hemodialysis	129 472	59.5
Peritoneal dialysis	19 324	8.9
Transplantation	68 673	31.6
Total	217 469	100

Adapted from Locatelli *et al.* (2000). Nephrol. Dial. Transplant, **15**, 1133–39.

therapy as it stood at the end of the last decade in six West European countries is displayed in Table 1.6.

Back in the 1960s, there were only two options for long-term hemodialysis therapy: either in-center hemodialysis (located in academic or community hospitals, or free-standing units) or home hemodialysis. In more recent years, the panel of options has much enlarged, comprising in-center, satellite, self/limited care hemodialysis units, and home hemodialysis, which have been challenged since the mid-1980s by home-practised peritoneal dialysis techniques (see Chapter 2). The advantages of home hemodialysis over all other hemodialysis methods have been clearly demonstrated in many studies, yielding the best results in terms of patient-survival, professional and social rehabilitation, and (at least in some studies) quality of life (72, 76, 77) through maintenance of a greater independance compared to the numerous constraints in life-style suffered by in-center patients due to sometimes long and troublesome travels required twice or thrice weekly to and from overbusy dialysis centers, difficulties in getting acceptance for temporary hemodialysis treatments during vacations or professional trips, etc.

However, the enthusiasm for home hemodialysis had to be somewhat tempered, taking into account that this method can be practised optimally only by a subgroup of carefully selected, highly motivated, psychologically stable, and well-trained patients, without severe co-morbidities, and favored by a well-supporting familial environment. Experience has universally shown that many of these mandatory features change over time as the patients get older and/or sicker, and many familial partners successively feel tired, later exhausted, and finally burn-out.

Between December 1988 and December 1997, in the USA, the percentage of patients treated with home hemodialysis among the whole population of patients submitted to all methods of dialysis combined, has fallen from 2.18% (2194 out of 100 480 patients) down to 0.78% (1729 out of 221 596 patients) (78). Whereas home hemodialysis accounted for more than 15% of the ESRD population in the European countries contributing to the EDTA Registry in 1975, this percentage decreased steadily over the years, reaching barely 3% in 1994 (79). The causes for this disfavor of home hemodialysis are multi-fold. The (fortunate) development of renal transplantation takes away a large part of the elective recruitment of home dialysis patients, i.e. the young and fittest subgroup. Since the mid-1980s, the development of home-practised peritoneal dialysis methods, which have gained much in efficacy and safety, have cannibalized a substantial fraction of potential home hemodialysis candidates. More fundamentally, four decades of experience have clearly shown that only a relatively small proportion of patients do really and truly volunteer for home hemodialysis on grounds of medical or socio-professional advantages, whereas this mode of RRT has been more or less overtly imposed upon a much larger group of ESRD patients due to economic constraints that prevent the expansion of the number of dialysis centers. Indeed, the sharp decline of home hemodialysis in the USA began almost immediately after the implementation of the coverage of ESRD treatments by Medicare in 1973, which led to a huge increase in 'for profit' and 'non-profit dialysis' facilities. In the United Kingdom, where healthcare resources are still among the lowest in the Western World, home hemodialysis has always largely predominated over center hemodialysis, but has been strongly challenged by home peritoneal dialysis in recent year. Thus, the majority of the United Kingdom patients with ESRD remain treated with methods alternative to hemodialysis in contrast with other large European Countries, such as Germany (Table 1.7).

The recent revival of daily hemodialysis, first pionneered in Italy (80) in the late 1970s and technically updated in Canada (54, 81), currently stimulates a reniewed interest in home hemodialysis. This is in line with the concept of ideal dialysis, which should deliver high doses through frequent sessions (72); this goal being achieved thanks to advances in technology, which render frequent hemodialysis less cumbersome and safer than 20 years ago. Although the debate between the promoters of nightly-long versus daily-short dialysis schedules remains unsettled, the results reported thus far, in rather small series of patients with either modality of daily dialysis, show unequivocal improvements versus conventional, thrice-weekly hemodialysis regarding vascular stability during dialysis sessions, better control of blood pressure, greater removal of phosphate and β2-microglobulin, reduction of erythropoietin requirements, liberization of diet with greater protein intake, improvement in quality of life, and vocational rehabilitation (81–83). A larger and longer experience with daily hemodialysis is clearly required for a more comprehensive, long-term

Table 1.7 Distribution of renal replacement therapies in six Western European countries in 1998

	Highest rate of all patients treated	Lowest rate
Transplantation	54% UK	20% Italy
Hemodialysis	71% Germany	28% UK
Peritoneal dialysis	18% UK	5% Germany and Spain

Adapted from Locatelli *et al.* (2000). Nephrol. Dial. Transplant., **15**, 1133–39.

evaluation of the medical advantages of the method. A wider implementation of daily dialysis will depend to a large extent on the patients' and families' acceptance, (which may not be much more enthusiastic than for any other home-practised dialysis method), as well as on not yet well-defined financial feasibility. Re-use of disposable supplies, first of all dialyzers, is an absolute economical prerequisite, but is still considered illegal in several countries. Home daily hemodialysis will remain cheaper than thrice-weekly in-center dialysis due to savings in labour costs, transportation, etc., but peritoneal dialysis, even automated peritoneal dialysis will for certain remain a challenging financial competitor.

Reimbursement/funding of dialysis, that is its cost to the healthcare budget, varies considerably between the countries of the Western World, ranging between 0.7% and 1.8% of the total annual healthcare expenditure for less than 0.05% of the nations' global population (84). Hence, selecting out-of-center dialysis modalities is a universal priority pursued for as many as possible of the patients having to be treated with RRT. A recent comprehensive international review based on data collected in European Countries, Canada, and USA well confirms the results of numerous studies published previously by individual groups or regional, national surveys: costs of dialysis treatment are highest when delivered in public hospitals, followed by private centers, they are lower in limited-care hemodialysis centers, and lowest for home hemodialysis and peritoneal dialysis—the latter two methods being at a similar level (85). The cost of automated peritoneal dialysis is close to that of limited-care hemodialysis. Of note, the precise definition of limited-care hemodialysis varies according to different countries, their common denominator being, however, not to be located physically or financially in a major academic or community hospital. Aside from these financial aspects, the clinical results and outcomes achieved by highly experienced groups of patients treated with out-of-center hemodialysis are among the best reported in the literature for patients submitted to maintenance dialysis, even in those qualified as 'at risk' who are not accepted for transplantation because of old-age and/or medical contra-indication (85).

The very wide variations that exist in clinical practice relating to renal replacement therapy are little supported by evidence-based information. Rather, the split between hemodialysis (and related techniques) and peritoneal dialysis is dictated in several countries by available hemodialysis facilities. The distribution between home, satellite, and in-center hemodialysis is determined by the demography of the patient group, and social factors such as the type of housing and distance from main center. The duration of hemodialysis sessions is often a mix of patient preference and physician bias, together with an element of resource availability. The guiding inspiration for clinicians involved in the provision of end-stage renal failure support has been, and is, to provide benefit for the maximum number of patients, and it is this that has dictated the varying evolution of the service between centers and countries.

References

1. Quinton, W.E., Dillard, D.H., and Scribner, B.H. (1960). Cannulation of blood vessels for prolonged hemodialysis. *Transactions of the American Society of Artificial Internal Organs*, **6,** 104–7.

2. Brescia, M.J., Cimino, J.E., Appel, K., and Hurwich, B.J. (1966). Chronic hemodialysis using venipuncture and a surgically created arteriovenous fistula. *New England Journal of Medicine*, **275**, 1089.

3. Stehman-Breen, C.O., Sherrard, D.J., Gillen, D., and Caps, M. (2000). Determinants of type and timing of initial permanent hemodialysis vascular access. *Kidney International*, **57**, 639–45.

4. Levin, N.W., Yang, P.M., Hatch, D.A., Dubrow, A.J., Caraiani, N.S., Ing, T.S. *et al.* (1998). Initial results of a new access device for hemodialysis. *Kidney International*, **54**, 1739–45.

5. Canaud, B., My, H., Morena, M., Lamy-Lacavalerie, B., Leray-Moragues, H., Bosc, J.Y. *et al.* (1999). Dialock: a new vascular access device for extra-corporeal renal replacement therapy. Preliminary clinical results. *Nephrology Dialysis Transplantation*, **14**, 692–8.

6. Buerger, T., Gebauer, T., Meyer, F., and Halloul, Z. (2000). Implantation of a new device for hemodialysis. *Nephrology Dialysis Transplantation*, **15**, 722–4.

7. Depner, T.A. (1994). Techniques for prospective detection of venous stenosis. *Advances in Renal Replacement Therapy*, **1**, 119–30.

8. Hester, R.L., Curry, E., and Bower, J. (1992). The determination of hemodialysis blood recirculation using blood urea nitrogen measurements. *American Journal of Kidney Disease*, **20**, 598–602.

9. Depner, T.A., Krivitski, N.M., and Mac Gibbon, D. (1995). Hemodialysis access recirculation measured by ultrasound dilution. *ASAIO Journal*, **41**, M749–753.

10. Lindsay, R.M., Burbank, J., Brugger, J., Bradfield, E., Kram, R., Malek, P. *et al.* (1996). A device and a method for rapid and accurate measurement of access recirculation during hemodialysis. *Kidney International*, **49**, 1152–60.

11. Strauch, B.S., O'Connell, R.S., Geoly, K.L., Grundlehner, M., Yakub, N., and Tietjen, D.P. (1992). Forecasting thrombosis of vascular access with Doppler color flow imaging. *American Journal of Kidney Diseases*, **19**, 554–7.

12. Krivitski, N.M. (1995). Theory and validation of access flow measurement by dilution technique during hemodialysis. *Kidney International*, **48**, 244–50.

13. Lindsay, R.M., Blake, P.G., Malek, P., Posen, G., Martin, B., and Bradfield, E. (1997). Hemodialysis access blood flow rates can be measured by a differential conductivity technique and are predictive of access clotting. *American Journal of Kidney Diseases*, **30**, 475–82.

14. Lindsay, R.M., Rothera, C., and Blake, P.G. (1998). A comparison of methods for the measurement of hemodialysis access recirculation: an update. *ASAIO Journal*, **44**, 191–3.

15. Yarar, D., Cheung, A.K., Sakiewicz, P., Lindsay, R.M., Paganini, E.P., Steuer, R.R. *et al.* (1999). Ultrafiltration method for measuring vascular access flow rates during hemodialysis. *Kidney International*, **56**, 1129–35.

16. Schneditz, D., Wang, E., and Levin, N.W. (1999). Validation of hemodialysis recirculation and access blood flow measured by thermodilution. *Nephrology Dialysis Transplantation*, **14**, 376–83.

17. Gotch, F.A., Buyaki, R., Panlilio, F., and Folden, T. (1999). Measurement of blood access flow rate during hemodialysis from conductivity dialysance. *ASAIO Journal*, **45**, 139–46.

18. Mercadal, L., Hamani, A., Béné, B., and Petitclerc, T. (1999). Determination of access blood flow from ionic dialysance: theory and validation. *Kidney International*, **56**, 1560–5.

19. Magnasco, A., Alloatti, S., Bonfant, G., Copello, F., and Solari, P. (2000). Glucose-infusion test: a new screening test for vascular access recirculation. *Kidney International*, **57**, 2123–28.

20. Locatelli, F., Bloembergen, W., Hakim, R.H., Stannard, D.C., Held, Ph.J., Wolfe, R.A. *et al.* (1999). Relationship of dialysis membrane and cause specific mortality. *American Journal of Kidney Diseases*, **33**, 1–10.

21. Leypoldt, J.K., Cheung, A.K., Carroll, C.E., Stannard, D.C., Pereira, B.J.G., Agodoa, L.Y. *et al.* (1999). Effect of dialysis membranes and middle molecule removal on chronic hemodialysis patient survival. *American Journal of Kidney Diseases*, **33**, 349–55.

22. Locatelli, F., Valderrabano, F., Hoenich, N., Bommer, J., Leunissen, K., and Cambi, V. (2000). Progress in dialysis technology: membrane selection and patient outcome. *Nephrology Dialysis Transplantation*, **15**, 1133–39.

23. Kuchle, C., Fricke, H., and Schiffl, H. (1996). High-flux hemodialysis postpones clinical manifestations of dialysis-related amyloidosis. *American Journal of Nephrology*, **16**, 484–88.

24. Cheung, A.K., Agodoa, L.Y., Daugirdas, J.T., Depner, T.A., Gotch, F.A., Greene, T. *et al.* and the Hemodialysis (HEMO) Study Group. (1999). Effects of hemodialyzer re-use on clearances of urea and β2-microglobulin. *Journal of the American Society of Nephrology*, **10**, 117–27.

25. Ebben, J.P., Dalleska, F., Ma, J.Z., Everson, S.E., Constantini, E.G., and Collins, A.J. (2000). Impact of disease severity and hematocrit level on re-use associated mortality. *American Journal of Kidney Diseases*, **35**, 244–49.

26. Janssen, M.J., Deegens, J.K., Kapinga, J.H., Beukhof, J.R., Huijgens, P.C., Van Loewen, A.C. *et al.* (1996). Citrate compared to low molecular weight heparin anticoagulation in chronic hemodialysis patients. *Kidney International*, **49**, 806–13.

27. Lonnemann, G. (2000). Chronic inflammation in hemodialysis. The role of contaminated dialysate. *Blood Purification*, **18**, 214–23.

28. Ledebo, I. and Nystrand, R. (1999). Defining the microbiological quality of dialysis fluid. *Artificial Organs*, **23**, 37–43.

29. Canaud, B., Bosc, J.Y., Leray-Moragues, H., Stec, F., Argiles, A., Leblanc, M. *et al.* (2000). On line hemodiafiltration-safety and efficacy in long-term clinical practice. *Nephrology Dialysis Transplantation*, **15**, 511–16.

30. Ledebo, I. (1999). Hemofiltration redux. *Blood Purification*, **17**, 178–81.

31. Ledebo, I. (1999). Online hemodiafiltration: technique and therapy. *Advances in Renal Replacement Therapy*, **6**, 195–208.

32. Van Stone, J.C. and Mitchell, A. (1980). Hemodialysis with base-free dialysate. *Proceedings of the Clinical Dialysis and Transplantation Forum*, **10**, 268–71.

33. Man, N.K., Ciancioni, C., Perrone, B., Chauveau, P., and Jehenne, G. (1989). Renal biofiltration. *Transactions of the American Society of Artificial Internal Organs*, **35**, 8–13.

34. Movilli, E., Camerini, C., Zein, H., D'Avolio, G., Sandrini, M., Strada, A. *et al.* (1996). A prospective comparison of bicarbonate dialysis, hemodiafiltration and acetate-free biofiltration in the elderly. *American Journal of Kidney Diseases*, **27**, 541–7.

35. Mercadal, L., Petitclerc, T., Béné, B., Jaudon, M.C., and Jacobs, C. (1999). Duocart biofiltration: a new method of dialysis. *ASAIO Journal*, **45**, 151–6.

36. Gotch, F.A. and Sargent, J.A. (1985). A mechanistic analysis of the National Dialysis Cooperative Study (NCDS). *Kidney International*, **28**, 526–34.

37. Held, P.J., Port, F.K., Wolfe, R.A., Stannard, D.C., Carroll, C.E., Daugirdas, J.T. *et al.* (1996). The dose of hemodialysis and patient mortality. *Kidney International*, **50**, 550–6.

38. Clark, W.R., Rocco, M.V., and Collins, A.J. (1997). Quantification of hemodialysis: analysis of methods and the relevance to patient outcome. *Blood Purification*, **15**, 92–111.

39. Wolfe, R.A., Ashby, V.B., Daugirdas, J.T., Agodoa, L.Y.C., Jones, C.A., and Port, F.K. (2000). Body size, dose of hemodialysis, and mortality. *American Journal of Kidney Diseases*, **35**, 80–8.

40. Owen, W.F. (2001). Hemodialysis adequacy. *American Journal of Kidney Diseases*, **37**, 181–8.

41. Smye, S.W., Tattersall, J.E., and Will, E.J. (1999). Modeling the post-dialysis rebound: the reconciliation of current formulas. *ASAIO Journal*, **45**, 562–7.

42. Depner, T.A., Greene, T., Gotch, F.A., Daugirdas, J.T., Keshaviah, P.R., Star, R.A., and the Hemodialysis Study Group. (1999). Imprecision of the hemodialysis dose when measured directly from urea removal. *Kidney International*, **55**, 635–47.

43. Di Filippo, S., Andrulli, S., Manzoni, C., Corti, M., and Locatelli, F. (1998). Online assessment of delivered dialysis dose. *Kidney International*, **54**, 263–7.

44. Jaeger, J.Q. and Mehta, R.L. (1999). Assessment of dry weight in hemodialysis: an overview. *Journal of the American Society of Nephrology*, **10**, 392–403.

45. Katzarski, K.S., Nisell, J., Randmaa, I., Danielsson, A., Freyschuss, U., and Bergström, J. (1997). A critical evaluation of ultrasound measurement of inferior vena cava diameter for assessing dry weight in normotensive and hypertensive hemodialysis patients. *American Journal of Kidney Diseases*, **30**, 459–65.

46. Fisch, B.J. and Spiegel, D.M. (1996). Assessment of excess fluid distribution in chronic hemodialysis patients using bioimpedance spectroscopy. *Kidney International*, **49**, 1105–9.

47. Santoro, A., Mancini, E., Paolini, F., Cavicchioli, G., Bosetto, A., and Zucchelli, P. (1998). Blood volume regulation during hemodialysis. *American Journal of Kidney Diseases*, **32**, 739–48.

48. Krepel, H.P., Nette, R.W., Akçahüseyin, E., Weimar, W., and Zietse R. (2000). Variability of relative blood volume during hemodialysis. *Nephrology Dialysis Transplantation*, **15**, 673–9.

49. Locatelli, F., Andrulli, S., Di Filippo, S., Redaelli, B., Mangano, S., Navino, C. *et al.* (1998). Effect of online conductivity plasma ultrafiltrate kinetic modeling on cardiovascular stability of hemodialysis patients. *Kidney International*, **53**, 1052–60.

50. Petitclerc, T. (1999). Recent developments in conductivity monitoring of hemodialysis session. *Nephrology Dialysis Transplantation*, **14**, 2607–13.

51. Coli, L., Bonomini, M., La Manna, G., Dalmastri, V., Ursino, M., Ivanovich, P. *et al.* (1998). Clinical use of profiled hemodialysis. *Artificial Organs*, **22**, 724–30.

52. Redaelli, B., Locatelli, F., Limido, D., Andrulli, S., Signorini, M.G., Sforzini, S. *et al.* (1996). Effect of a new model of hemodialysis potassium removal on the control of ventricular arrythmias. *Kidney International*, **50**, 609–17.

53. Nappi, S.E., Saha, H.H.T., Virtanen, V.K., Mustonen, J.K., and Pasternack, A.I. (1999). Hemodialysis with high-calcium dialysate impairs cardiac relaxation. *Kidney International*, **55**, 1091–6.

54. Pierratos, A., Ouwendyk, M., Francoeur, R., Vas, S., Laj, D.S., Ecclestone, A.M. *et al.* (1998). Nocturnal hemodialysis: three-year experience. *Journal of the American Society of Nephrology*, **9**, 859–68.

55. Verresen, L., Fink, E., Lemke, H.D., and Vanrenterghem, Y. (1994). Bradykinin is a mediator of anaphylactoïd reactions during hemodialysis with AN69 membranes. (1994). *Kidney International*, **45**, 1497–503.

56. Renaux, J.L., Thomas, M., Crost, T., Loughraieb, N., and Vantard, G. (1999). Activation of the kallikrein-kinin system in hemodialysis: role of membrane electronegativity, blood dilution and pH. *Kidney International*, **55**, 1097–103.

57. Pérez-Garcia, R. and Rodriguez-Benitez, P. (2000). Why and how to monitor bacterial contamination of dialysate? *Nephrology Dialysis Transplantation*, **15**, 760–4.
58. Bergström, J., Lindholm, B., Lacson, E.J.R., Owen, J.R., Lowrie, E.G., Glassock, R.J. *et al.* (2000). What are the causes and consequences of the chronic inflammatory state in chronic dialysis patients? *Seminars in Dialysis*, **13**, 163–75.
59. Brunet, Ph. and Berland, Y. (2000). Water quality and complications of hemodialysis. *Nephrology Dialysis Transplantation*, **15**, 578–80.
60. Sukhatme, V.P. (1996). Vascular access stenosis: prospects for prevention and therapy. *Kidney International*, **49**, 1161–74.
61. Besarab, A. and Sherman, R.A. (1997). The relationship of recirculation to access blood flow. *American Journal of Kidney Diseases*, **29**, 223–9.
62. May, R.E., Himmelfarb, J., Yenicesu, M., Knights, S., Alp Ikizler, T., Schulman, G. *et al.* (1997). Predictive measure of vascular access thrombosis: a prospective study. *Kidney International*, **52**, 1656–62.
63. Schneditz, D. (1998). Recirculation, a seemingly simple concept. *Nephrology Dialysis Transplantation*, **13**, 2191–3.
64. Lindsay, R.M., and Leypoldt, J.K. (1999). Monitoring vascular access flow. *Advances in Renal Replacement Therapy*, **6**, 273–7.
65. Bosman, P.J., Boereboom, T.J., Eikelboom, B.C., Koomans, H.A., and Blankestijn, P.J. (1998). Graft flow as a predictor of thrombosis in hemodialysis grafts. *Kidney International*, **54**, 1726–30.
66. Roxana Neyra, N., Alp Ikizler, T., May, R.E., Himmelfarb, J., Schulman, G., Shyr, Y. *et al.* (1998). Change in access blood flow over time predicts vascular access thrombosis. *Kidney International*, **54**, 1714–9.
67. Salahudeen, A.K., Fleischmann, E.H., and Bower, J.D. (1999). Impact of lower delivered Kt/V on the survival of overweight patients on hemodialysis. *Kidney International*, **56**, 2254–59.
68. Hakim, R.M., and Lazarus, J.M. (1995). Initiation of dialysis. *Journal of the American Society of Nephrology*, **6**, 1319–28.
69. Keshaviah, P.R., Emerson, P.F., and Nolph, K.D. (1999). Timely initiation of dialysis. A urea kinetic approach. *American Journal of Kidney Diseases*, **33**, 344–8.
70. Jacobs, C. (2000). At which stage of renal failure should dialysis be started? *Nephrology Dialysis Transplantation*, **15**, 305–7.
71. Woods, J.D., Port, F.K., Orzol, S., Buoncristiani, U., Young, E., Wolfe, R.A. *et al.* (1999). Clinical and biochemical correlates of starting daily hemodialysis. *Kidney International*, **55**, 2467–76.
72. Raj, D.S.C., Charra, B., Pierratos, A., and Work, J. (1999). In search of ideal hemodialysis: is prolonged frequent dialysis he answer? *American Journal of Kidney Diseases*, **34**, 597–610.
73. Scribner, B.H. (1990). A personalized history of chronic hemodialysis. *American Journal of Kidney Diseases*, **16**, 511–19.
74. Murray, J.S., Tu, W.H., Albers, J.B., Burnell, J.M., and Scribner, B.H. (1962). A community hemodialysis center for the treatment of chronic uremia. *Transactions of the American Society for Artificial Internal Organs*, **8**, 315–20.
75. Shaldon, S. and Oakley, J.J. (1966). Experience with regular hemodialysis in the home. *British Journal of Urology*, **38**, 616–20.
76. Shaldon, S. and Crockett, R.E. (1975). The past, present and future of home dialysis. *Kidney International*, **7**, S418–S21.

77. Mailloux, L.U., Kapikian, N., Napolitano, B., Massey, R.T., Bellucci, A.G., Wilkes, B.M. *et al.* (1996). Home hemodialysis: patient outcome during a 24 year period of time from 1970 through 1993. *Advances in Renal Replacement Therapy*, **3**, 112–9.

78. U.S. Renal Data System. USRDS Annual Data report (1999). *Treatment Modalities for ESRD Patients.* National Institutes of Health, National Institute of Diabetes and Digestive and Kidney Diseases. Bethesda, Maryland, USA.

79. Feraud, P. and Wauters, J.P. (1999). The decline of home hemodialysis: how and why? *Nephron*, **81**, 249–55.

80. Buoncristiani, U. (1998). Fifteen years of clinical experience with daily hemodialysis. *Nephrology Dialysis Transplantation*, **13**, (Suppl. 6), 148–51.

81. Pierratos, A. (1999). Nocturnal home hemodialysis: an update on a 5 year experience. *Nephrology Dialysis Transplantation*, **14**, 2835–40.

82. Kooistra, M.P., Vos, J., Koomans, M.A., and Vos, P.F. (1998). Daily home hemodialysis in the Netherlands: effects on metabolic control, hemodialysis and quality of life. *Nephrology Dialysis Transplantation*, **13**, 2853–60.

83. Traeger, J., Sibai-Galland, R., Delawari, E., and Arkouche, W. (1998). Daily versus standard hemodialysis: one year experience. *Artificial Organs*, **22**, 558–63.

84. De Vecchi, A.F., Dratwa, M., and Wiedemann, M.E. (1999). Health care systems and end-stage renal disease therapies. An international review: costs and reimbursement / funding of ESRD therapies. *Nephrology Dialysis Transplantation*, **14**, (Suppl. 6), 31–41.

85. Arkouche, W., Traeger, J., Delawari, E., Sibai-Galland, R., Abdullah, E., Galland, R., *et al.* (1999). Twenty-five years of experience with out-center hemodialysis. *Kidney International*, **56**, 2269–75.

2

Peritoneal dialysis methods

Giovanni C. Cancarini and Rosario Maiorca

Until the introduction of hemodialysis, peritoneal dialysis (PD) was the only method used for the treament of end-stage renal disease (ESRD). Performed intermittently (IPD), in an inadequate and unstandardized way, it gave, however, unsatisfactory results, so that the introduction of hemodialysis (HD) led to its decline.

In 1976, Popovich and Moncrief described a simplified theoretical model to evaluate the mass-transfer in PD, and the results of a preliminary clinical study, predicting that the intraperitoneal infusion of 2l of dialysate, changed five times a day, would be able to maintain the blood levels of metabolites, such as urea and creatinine, as stable and acceptable (1). The introduction of continuous ambulatory peritoneal dialysis (CAPD) was a turning point in the history of peritoneal dialysis (PD) and nowadays, CAPD, and its automated form, APD, are reliable alternative treatments to HD, at least for the first years of treatment.

In this chapter, the present state of PD treatment and some clinical indications are outlined. For PD use in special conditions, the reader is referred to the relevant chapters of this volume.

Peritoneal dialysis solutions

Table 2.1 reports the standard formulation of peritoneal dialysis fluids. There are only minor changes among the different brands and they concern above all the dextrose concentration.

Electrolytes

Sodium concentration ranges from 132 to 140 mmol/l. In CAPD, the long lasting dwells allow greater sodium removal by both convection and diffusion, but this raises the risk of hypotension, which is higher with the lowest sodium concentration. For this reason the sodium concentration has been increased in CAPD solution to 140 mmol/l, which is still lower than the sodium concentration in plasma water.

Potassium is not normally contained in the dialysis solution. In this way 38–48 mmol of potassium are removed per day.

Table 2.1 Standard peritoneal dialysis solutions, range of concentrations of solute, pH, and osmolality

Sodium	(mmol/l)	132–140
Potassium	(mmol/l)	0–2.4
Calcium	(mmol/l)	1.00–1.75
Magnesium	(mmol/l)	0.25–0.75
Chloride	(mmol/l)	101–107
Lactate	(mmol/l)	35–40
pH	(pH units)	5.0–5.5
Dextrose	(g/dl)	1.36, 2.27, 3.86[*]
		1.5, 2.5, 4.25[+]
Osmolality	(mOsm/kg)	340–507

[*]Anhydrous dextrose; [+]monohydrated dextrose.

The usual concentration of calcium in PD fluids was commonly 1.75 mmol/l. The wide use of oral calcium salts as phosphate binders increases the risk of hypercalcemia and has led to solutions with a calcium concentration of 1.25 mmol/l.

PD fluids have a magnesium concentration ranging from 0.25 to 0.75 mmol/l, the former being indicated in patients given magnesium containing phosphate binders.

Osmotic agents

An osmotic agent is added to all peritoneal dialysis solutions to avoid its rapid absorption, and to favor water and solute ultrafiltration in the peritoneal cavity. So far, dextrose has been the molecule used routinely, since it is a normal component of the blood and is rapidly metabolized, once reabsorbed. Three different concentrations are commercially available: 1.5, 2.5, and 4.25 g/dl (or 1.36, 2.27, and 3.86 g/dl in some countries).

Dextrose is rapidly absorbed thanks to its low molecular weight (180 Da). Glucose absorption reduces the osmotic gradient between peritoneal cavity and blood, and in long dwells some backfiltration occurs (Fig. 2.1).

Ultrafiltration capacity is, thus, time-limited and even a 4.25 g/dl solution of dextrose is often unable to remove fluid after a 10–12 h dwell. The high dextrose concentration of dialysis fluid, has some disadvantages. First, it glycosilates structural proteins and enzymes, with duplication of the peritoneal capillary basal membrane, similar to that seen in diabetic microangiopathy (2). Second, the pH of the solution must be lowered to 5.0–5.5 to avoid generation of dextrose degradation products during heat sterilization; the low pH has negative effects on viability and function of mesothelial cells, neutrophils, and monocytes.

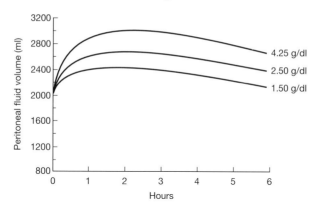

Fig. 2.1 Changes in intraperitoneal fluid volume during a standard dwell time with 1.5, 2.5, and 4.5 g/dl dextrose.

These negative effects have led to the search for different low molecular weight osmotic agents in substitution for dextrose. So far, only glycerol and amino acid-based solutions have come into clinical use. Glycerol has a molecular weight about one-half that of dextrose, thus it is rapidly absorbed. It has been used mainly in diabetics (3), since it avoids the detrimental glucose load.

Amino acids can be used as osmotic agents, but they also act as nutritional supplements and are useful in patients with low protein intake. One commercially available bag provides about 15 g of amino acids, equivalent to one-fifth of the recommended daily nitrogen intake (4). If the caloric intake is sufficient, these amino acids are synthesized into proteins, otherwise they enter the glucidic metabolical pathways after removal of the amino group that generates urea. The amino acid metabolism generates hydrogen ions (5), so only one or two amino acid bags a day can be used to avoid acidosis.

Clinical studies using amino acid solutions have brought contrasting results, probably due to different amino acid composition, insufficient correction of acidosis, and different baseline nutritional status of the patients.

Other attempts have tested high molecular weight osmotic agents, among which only polyglucose has come into clinical use. Polyglucose is a mixture of glucose polymers containing from few to more than 250 glucose molecules joined by 1–4 and, rarely, 1–6 bonds. Their molecular weight ranges from 960 to 19000 Da. The polyglucose molecules that pass into the blood circulation are hydrolyzed to maltose by the circulating amylase (6). Maltase, the enzyme able to hydrolyze maltose, is not present in plasma, but it is contained in many tissues where it hydrolyzes maltose to glucose, thus avoiding its accumulation in plasma. Thanks to its high molecular weight, only a little amount of polyglucose is absorbed and the osmotic gradient between dialysate and plasma is preserved for more than 12 h (Fig. 2.2). Moreover, thanks to the low number of big molecules, the osmolality of the polyglucose solution is similar (282 mOsmoles) to that of plasma, which avoids the negative effects of hyperosmolality on peritoneal cells.

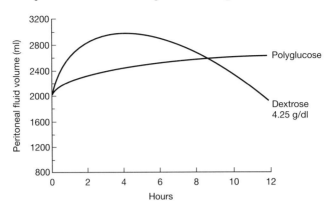

Fig. 2.2   Changes in peritoneal volume over time with Dextrose g/dl and polyglucose.

The caloric intake due to the polyglucose absorbed in each exchange is lower than that of dextrose 3.86 g/dl. Plasma levels of both polyglucose and maltose increased significantly, but do not cause an increase in plasma osmolality. Diabetics tolerate well the solution and their insulin requirement does not increase (6). In some patients maintained on polyglucose, the osmotic agent kept its effectiveness for 6 months and even after 30 months (7). Polyglucose was also used as compassionate therapy for ultrafiltration loss and enabled 60% of 36 patients with ultrafiltration loss, remaining on CAPD, to stay on the method for more than one year (7). Polyglucose, thanks to the higher ultrafiltration volume, removes 60% more β2-microglobulin than dextrose without increasing the albumin loss (8). The drawback of this solution is the risk of hyperosmolality when used for more than one exchange per day. Anedoctical cases of hypersensibility with skin reactions have been reported (9).

pH

The pH of peritoneal dialysis solutions is adjusted to 5.0–5.5, in order to avoid generation of dextrose degradation products during heat sterilization. This low pH impairs both viability and function of mesothelial cells, neutrophils, and monocytes, and its negative effects on peritoneal defense mechanisms are often synergistic with those of lactate (10).

Buffers

Acetate or lactate have been used as buffers for dialysis solutions. Both of them are vasodilators, impair myocardial contractility, and probably play a role in dislipidemia (11).

The first peritoneal dialysis solution contained acetate at a concentration of about 40 mmol/l. Due to its too important vasodilatory effect, stimulating action on the production of interleukin-1 favoring fibroblast proliferation, and its well-documented responsibility in the development of sclerosing peritonitis, leading to bowel obstruction and death, acetate is no longer used for peritoneal dialysis fluid.

Today, racemic lactate (i.e. equal amounts of D-lactate and L-lactate) is the standard buffer used in PD, at concentrations ranging from 35 to 40 mmol/l (12).

The best concentration of lactate, between 35 or 40 mmol/l, has not been established, due to the variations of other factors playing a role in the acid–base equilibrium, such as the organic acids introduced with the diet or deriving from tissue metabolism.

Lactate negatively affects mesothelial cells, as well as defense cells present in the peritoneal cavity, and its negative effect adds to those of the low pH and the high glucose concentration, in a synergistic way. To avoid this, pyruvate has been suggested as a possible substitute, which, *in vitro*, has been shown not to affect viability and function of mesothelial cells and peritoneal macrophages (13). Pyruvate has a very short half-life because, in the liver, it is rapidly transformed into bicarbonate without risk of lactic acidosis. However, commercial solutions with this buffer have not been available, so far.

Bicarbonate, as a buffer, should prevent the untoward effects of acetate and lactate on cell viability and function, on the cardiovascular system and on lipids. However, the precipitation of calcium carbonate, which occurs when bicarbonate and calcium are put into the same solution, has precluded its use, until recently.

Two methods have been suggested, and tested with positive results, to avoid calcium carbonate precipitation. Feriani *et al.* worked out a two-compartment bag, communicating through a breakable valve: one contains calcium chloride, magnesium chloride, acetic acid, and glucose; the other sodium chloride and sodium bicarbonate (14). A few minutes before filling the abdomen, the valve is broken by the patient, and the two solutions are allowed to mix. Acetic acid and sodium bicarbonate react developing CO_2, in the presence of which calcium and bicarbonate produce soluble, instead of insoluble, calcium bicarbonate. The pH of the final solution is close to the physiological range.

The second method has been suggested by Yatzidis and is based on the ability of glycylglycine to stabilize bicarbonate; a solution containing 30 mmol/l of bicarbonate and 10 mmol/l of glycylglycine, has a pH of 7.4 and is stable for more than 18 months (15).

Peritoneal permeability

Peritoneal dialyzing function can vary considerably among different patients due to differences in the surface area available for diffusion, in thickness, number of capillaries, and distance from capillaries to peritoneal cavity. Patients with low peritoneal permeability achieve with difficulty an adequate dose of dialysis (16), whereas those with high peritoneal permeability, which causes a rapid absorption of dextrose, do not get a sufficient ultrafiltration volume. The definition of the degree of permeability is of paramount importance in PD, because it allows one to choose the best PD treatment and to foresee the possibility of the patient to remain on PD, once residual renal function declines.

Many methods have been suggested, but the peritoneal equilibration test (PET) by Twardowski (17) has gained the greatest acceptance, thanks to its facility and simplicity. The test consists of a 4-h, 21 exchange with a 2.27 g/dl dextrose solution. Dialysate samples for creatinine and glucose are taken just after the inflow, and after 2 and 4 h. A blood sample for creatinine is taken during the second hour. At the end of the dwell, the patient fully drains and measures the effluent. The difference between the inflow and the outflow volume gives the net ultrafiltration volume, whereas the ratio between the dialysate and the plasma concentration of creatinine (creatinine D/P) allows an estimate of the permeability pattern. Dialysate concentration of creatinine must be corrected for the glucose concentration, since glucose partially reacts with the Jaffé reagent used to measure creatinine. Another index is the ratio between the concentrations of dextrose at 2 and 4 h, and at time zero. The two curves obtained have a different pattern, since creatinine increases in dialysate, with time, while dextrose decreases (Fig. 2.3). Twardowski has suggested dividing patients into four groups according to the D/P creatinine value at the fourth hour. The four groups are today indicated as high, high-average, low-average, and low permeability patterns.

Patients with a low permeability pattern might have to withdraw CAPD once residual renal function disappears but can derive benefit from the continuous modalities of APD (see below). Patients with a high permeability pattern might have poor ultrafiltration on CAPD and good results on APD, but they are at risk of malnutrition due to increased peritoneal protein losses (18).

Performing PET is not recommended in the first few weeks after the start of PD or after peritonitis, in order to avoid untoward effects on peritoneal function.

Measure of peritoneal dialysis dose

The dose of dialysis to be prescribed to a given patient should be adequate to his/her needs, similarly for every kind of therapy. Many attempts have been made to define

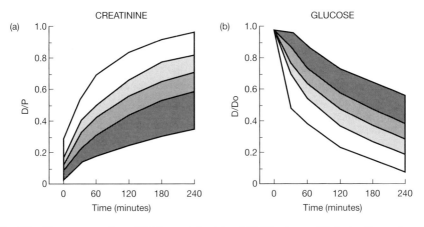

Fig. 2.3 Changes over time of D/P creatinine (a) and D/Do glucose (b) during the peritoneal equilibration test. Data from the Chair and Division of Nephrology, University of Brescia.

methods to measure the dose of PD and targets to reach to give an adequate dose (19–21). Two indices have progressively gained reliability among the many suggested: Kt/V and weekly creatinine clearance (wCcr). The first, derived from HD, measures the weekly clearance of urea; the second that of creatinine. Both of them are normalized to body size: total body water volume (i.e. the distribution volume of urea) is used for Kt/V, and body surface area (BSA) for wCcr. The contribution of residual renal function is added to them to measure the total blood purification. The validity of this sum is based on the not-demonstrated assumption that purification given by kidney and dialysis are equivalent.

Kt/V in PD

PD Kt/V is derived from the HD Kt/V, but, in PD, the urea clearance is directly measured and not calculated with mathematical formulae. The patient collects and measures both the daily total peritoneal drainage and urine output and takes samples from both of them. The multiplication of each volume by its urea concentration gives the amount of urea removed in one day through dialysate and urine; the sum of these gives the total amount of urea removed. Only one blood sample for blood urea nitrogen (BUN) is necessary since, in CAPD, serum urea has minimal changes during the day. Due to the slow rate of urea equilibration between blood and dialysis fluid, monocompartimental kinetics is assumed. The classical clearance formula measures the total dose of blood purification that is finally normalized to V, the total body water (Table 2.2). Many methods are available to estimate V; some of them use a fixed percentage of the body weight (58% for all or 60% for men and 55% for women), others use formulae based on sex, age, weight, and, in some cases, height (Table 2.2). The formula generally suggested is that of Watson (22). In these formulae the body weight considered is the actual body weight. However, this might be misleading in obese and wasted patients in whom the ideal or the desired body weight should be used.

Weekly creatinine clearance in PD

Creatinine clearance, the most customary for nephrologists, has been one of the first indices proposed in PD. Peritoneal creatinine clearance is calculated similarly to urea peritoneal clearance. The renal contribution to total blood purification is calculated as the mean between urea and creatinine clearance, to obviate the over-estimation of glomerular filtration rate due to tubular secretion of creatinine. This value is added to the peritoneal clearance to obtain the total creatinine clearance, which is then normalized to the body surface area (BSA) calculated according to the formula of Du Bois and Du Bois (23):

$$BSA \ (m^2) = 0.007184 \times weight \ (kg)^{0.425} \times height \ (cm)^{0.725} \tag{2.1}$$

The result is then multiplied by 10080, i.e. the minutes in a week, and divided by 1000 (to change from ml to l). So, wCcr is expressed as l/week/1.73 m^2 of BSA.

Table 2.2 Formulae to calculate Kt/V and to estimate V for the calculation of Kt/V

Weekly peritoneal Kt	=	(Durea/Purea)×DV×7
Weekly renal Kt	=	(Urea/Purea)×UV×7
Total weekly Kt/V	=	(peritoneal Kt+renal Kt)/V
Adults		
Watson formulae (98):		
Men		V = 2.447+0.3362 ×weight+0.1074×height−0.09516×age
Women		V = −2.097+0.2466×weight+0.1069×height
Hume formulae (99):		
Men		V = −14.012934+0.296785×weight+0.192786×height
Women		V = −35.270121+0.183809×weight+0.344547×height
Children		
Mellits-Cheek formulae (100)		
Boys		
If height ≤132.7 cm		V = −1.927+0.465×weight+0.045×height
If height >132.7 cm		V = −21.993+0.406×weight+0.209×height
Girls		
If height ≤110.8 cm		V = 0.076+0.507×weight+0.013×height
If height >110.8 cm		V = −10.313+0.252×weight+0.154×height

The urea concentrations are indicated as Durea for daily peritoneal effluent, Purea for plasma and urea for urine. DV is the daily volume of dialysate drainage; UV the daily urine output and 7 the number of days in one week. V is the water distribution volume of the total body. V is calculated in liters, weight is in kg, height in cm, and age in years.

Relationship between Kt/V and weekly creatinine clearance

The correct calculation of Kt/V and wCcr requires that the patient be edema-free and have no limb amputations. Some formulae allow adjustments for these cases (24).

The two indices are related to each other when an analysis of population is carried out, but each one is unable to predict the other in the same patient. This is due to the following reasons. Peritoneal clearance of creatinine is lower than that of urea because of its higher molecular weight (113 versus 60 Da). Moreover, the ratio between urea and creatinine peritoneal clearance is not always the same, since it increases as peritoneal permeability decreases (25). The renal contribution to the total blood purification is differently evaluated, urea clearance being lower than the mean of urea and creatinine clearance. Finally, whereas Kt/V is normalized to a volume proportional to the body weight, creatinine clearance is normalized to the BSA.

Continuous ambulatory peritoneal dialysis (CAPD)

CAPD, as proposed by Popovich and Moncrief, was founded on a model based on urea kinetics. These authors suggested that five 2-l exchanges a day for seven days a week were able to maintain stable BUN in a patient with a protein intake of 45 g/day. In the case of a residual renal function of 1.4 ml/min, the number of bags could be reduced to four a day. Recent studies on adequacy have underlined the importance of residual renal function and the need to increase the dialysis dose when renal function decreases.

Connection systems in CAPD

Many connection systems were proposed during the early years of CAPD. Nowadays, a great part of those in commerce derive from the Y-system and the twin-bag system, introduced in the late 1970s (26). Both of them reduce the risk of microorganism contamination by flushing the connection point with either fresh solution or the peritoneal effluent. This flushing is able to remove possible contamination at the time of connection. The connection deriving from the Y-system contains a little amount of disinfectant, sodium hypochlorite, in the lines during the dwell time to avoid bacterial growth following contamination at disconnection. The fear of causing peritoneal damage by using disinfectants within the connection has been proved to be justified only for chlorexidine, the use of which has been associated with sclerosing encapsulating peritonitis.

Other connection systems avoid the risk of contamination at disconnection by breaking the lines after having clamped them (27).

Thanks to these improvements, the incidence of peritonitis has dramatically dropped from one episode every few months in the early 1980s to one episode every 3 years in the more recent period.

Inflow volume

PD dialysis fluids are contained in bags whose volume ranges from 1 to 3 liters, to meet the peritoneal capacity of each patient.

In children, the volume of dialysis solution must be tailored to body size and varies from 10 ml/kg body weight in the first days, to 30–40 ml/kg body weight for standard PD. Also, in adult patients the volume is approximately prescribed according to body size and characteristics of the peritoneal cavity. A more accurate method measures the intraperitoneal pressure (28). Volumes that are too large may cause hernia, leakage, hemorrhoids, and can reduce the ultrafiltration volume.

Choice of solution

Initially, a PD solution containing 1.36–1.5 g/dl dextrose is sufficient, since the fluid balance is ensured by the residual renal function. Afterwards, when renal function decreases, a higher dextrose concentration is necessary, to avoid fluid retention. As the risk of damaging the peritoneal membrane grows along with the dextrose concentration, one should train the patient to reduce salt and fluid intake in order to use the lowest possible number of more concentrated solutions. Diuretics can be used to control fluid balance and reduce the use of hypertonic solutions.

The more frequent changes concern the calcium concentration, which needs to be reduced in patients taking calcium salts as phosphate binders.

In the case of inadequate protein intake, the substitution of a standard bag with an amino acid bag should be taken into consideration. Patients with a high permeability pattern absorb the dextrose rapidly, reduce the osmotic gradient, and can both reduce the ultrafiltration volume and cause a positive fluid balance. This is easier during the long nightly dwell. In this case the polyglucose solution is indicated (see p. 35).

The availability of the more biocompatible bicarbonate or bicarbonate/lactate solutions, so far limited to a few countries, should improve long-term survival of the peritoneum as a dialyzing membrane. The risk of lactic acidosis in patients with severe liver disease should be avoided. The only possible side-effect might be alkalosis, as observed in some patients using 39 mmol/l bicarbonate or 25 mmol/l bicarbonate plus 15 mmol/l lactate solutions.

Dialysis schedule at the beginning of CAPD

Once the peritoneal catheter has been introduced, CAPD can start after a break-in period of 2 weeks, a period necessary to allow healing of the surgical wound. During the first days of dialysis, it may be advisable to use low inflow volume (one-half or three-fourths of the adequate volume) to let the patient get accustomed to it. Three bags a day for 7 days, or four bags a day for 6 days a week, can be sufficient in the presence of some residual renal function. Residual renal function should be carefully monitored to find in time its reduction, if it is not compensated by increased dialysis administration, leading to inadequate blood purification. A check of Kt/V and wCcr every two to three months allows a timely adjustment of the dialysis dose, thus avoiding the risk of underdialysis.

Adequate dose of CAPD

Many clinical studies have shown that patient outcome depends on dialysis dose. The 'adequate' value should identify the dose beyond which there is no further improvement in clinical results.

The adequate value of weekly urea Kt/V has been suggested as 1.7–2.3 by theoretical models and clinical studies (29–30). Unfortunately, many of these studies were retrospective, with few patients and inappropriate statistical analysis. Two prospective studies have received the greatest consideration for the formulation of the DOQI guidelines (21): the CANUSA study (31) and that by Maiorca *et al.* (32).

The CANUSA study, based on a large population of patients, has strong statistical power. It suggests as adequate a Kt/V higher than 2.1, which, in the study, obtained an excellent survival. But this suggestion can be taken only as an indication: actually, the study design, and the lack of adjustment for the declining RRF, did not allow it to define the optimal Kt/V dose.

Maiorca *et al.* analyzed, in a prospective study, the outcome of a group of prevalent patients, on dialysis for different periods of time. Many patients had low or very low residual renal function. During the 3-year follow-up, the dialysis dose was modified to compensate for the loss of residual renal function, so that the total clearance had only few changes. That study demonstrated that a value of 1.96 of Kt/V was associated with the higher expectancy of life, and that further increases of dialysis gave no improvement in survival (32). This suggests that a Kt/V of 2.0 is currently considered as the optimal dose of dialysis.

In recent years, the weekly volume of dialysate has been progressively increased to 70l/week/1.73 m² BSA according to the results of CANUSA and Maiorca *et al.* (33). However, this target is not easily achievable in many patients, mainly in those with a large body size and no residual renal function. On the basis of the aforementioned studies, the DOQI guidelines, suggest that an adequate dose of blood purification in CAPD is obtained by a weekly urea Kt/V of 2.0 and 60l/week/1.73 m² BSA of wCcr (21, 34). In both cases the sum of renal and peritoneal contribution must be considered.

It is very important to underline that one should not restrict the concept of adequate dialysis to the amount of dialysis delivered. Correction of hypertension, calcium phosphate metabolism, calorie and protein intake, lipid profile, and frequent clinical assessment, all these are necessary to define adequate the dialysis.

Adjustment of the dialysis dose

The delivered dialysis dose can yield inadequate results if the prescribed dose is inadequate or the patient is not compliant with the prescription.

An inadequate dialysis dose can be improved by increasing the number or the volume of the exchanges or both. A number of bags higher than four has a negative impact on the quality of life, mainly in young and/or working people. More exchanges generally increase urea Kt/V, but have little effect on wCcr, more dependent on the dwell time, which decreases. Higher fluid volume per exchange increases the intraperitoneal pressure, raising the risk of hernia, leakage, hemorrhoids, and reduced ultrafiltration volume.

The attempt to increase the drain volume by using more hypertonic solutions has minor effect on the dialysis dose, but a negative effect on peritoneal membrane viability.

Automated peritoneal dialysis

Modalities of APD

APD indicates a family of PD modalities that uses a cycler to automatically exchange the dialysis solution. The cycler measures the appropriate volume of infusion, warms the solution up to a physiological temperature, inflows the solution into the abdominal cavity, controls the dwell time, drains the solution, and measures the drain volume. Measurements of inflow and outflow volume can be made by weighing the amount of fluid or by direct volume measurement.

APD is generally performed overnight to reduce its impact on the quality of life. However, many patients, mainly the anuric, need some additional daily exchanges, generally performed with the CAPD technique, to reach an adequate dialysis. Some cyclers allow a connection for one or two additional daily exchanges.

Table 2.3 summarizes the main APD modalities and Fig. 2.4 shows their schedules. All modalities can be done with the 'tidal' mode: the intraperitoneal volume is not completely drained (35, 36) and merges with the fresh solution. This method nullifies the 'dead time', i.e. the time during which the abdomen is empty, and there is no dialysis.

In the tidal mode, the first entry of the solution is prescribed according to the patient's abdominal capacity. Draining volume is 50–80% of that infused (tidal volume) plus the ultrafiltration volume obtained. The next fresh solution, amounts to the tidal volume.

Even if useful, the mode 'tidal' does not dramatically increase the urea and creatinine clearance, since the solute content of the residual peritoneal volume reduces the gradients of diffusion between plasma and solution. When used with the tidal mode, the NPD and CCPD are called NTPD and CTPD (37).

Solutions for APD

The solutions used for APD do not differ from those for CAPD but, in some cases, only solutions with 1.5 and 4.25 g/dl of dextrose are available in 5 l bags. Due to the sieving coefficient, a lower concentration of sodium (132 meq/l) is often used to reduce the risk of hypernatremia, as seen in the past on IPD. In fact, the ultrafiltration volume of the

Table 2.3   Main APD modalities currently used. All of them completely drain the fluid at the end of the dwell time. With all of them it is possible to use the 'tidal' system, which means partial draining (50–80%) of the peritoneal solution

	Abbreviation	When	Cycler	Supplementary bags during the day
Intermittent PD	IPD	Every other day/night	40 l	No
Nightly PD	NPD	Every night	6–12 nightly exchanges	No
Nightly PD + 1 daily exchange	NPD1	Every night	6–12 nightly exchanges	One 4- or 6-h daily dwell
Continuous cyclic PD	CCPD I	Every day	3–5 nightly exchanges	One 14-h daily dwell
Continuous cyclic PD type II	CCPD II	Every day	3-5 nightly exchanges	Two 6–8 h daily dwells

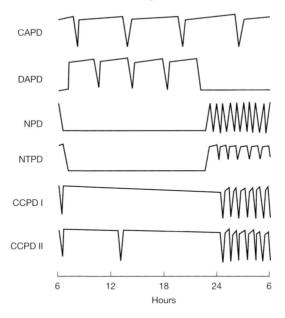

Fig. 2.4 Changes in intraperitoneal volume during different modalities of PD.

short dwells is hypotonic, due to the sieving coefficient, and a certain degree of hypernatremia could occur especially in patients using the highest dextrose concentration.

Adequate dose of APD

Kt/V and wCcr are used as indicators of the dialysis dose in APD. Their calculation is done as in CAPD. Errors in measuring the effluent volume, much higher than in CAPD, are one of the main causes of the wide variability of those indices. Continuous APD gives few changes in the serum concentrations of both urea and creatinine, while non-continuous APD, like IPD or NPD, gives greater changes. For this reason the average between pre- and post-dialysis serum concentrations of urea or creatinine must be included in the clearance formula. Otherwise, the calculation based on pre-dialysis values would decrease, and on postdialysis values increase Kt/V by 11% and wCcr by 5% (38). Also the body weight changes from pre- to post-dialysis. The post-dialysis weight, i.e. the 'dry weight', should be the weight used to normalize for the total body water or to calculate the BSA.

At present the targets of adequacy in APD are been derived from those accepted in CAPD. The ratio between urea D/P and creatinine D/P is different in CAPD and APD, due to their different molecular weight. In the short dwells, like those of APD, the clearance of urea, thanks to its lower molecular weight, is higher than that of creatinine. This, however, causes a faster dissipation of D/P gradient, so that, in the last hours of the long dwells, as on CAPD, urea diffuses less than creatinine

(Fig. 2.5). For this reason, in intermittent APD modalities, it is easier to achieve the urea Kt/V target than the desired wCcr. Achieving the targets is less difficult in continuous APD modalities. As a consequence, a 10% increase of adequacy targets (urea Kt/V = 2.2 l, wCcr = 66 l) has been suggested for intermittent APD, and a 5% increase for the continuous APD modalities (i.e. CCPD, CTPD) (39).

Another point that deserves some consideration is the inflow volume, even if its effect has been questioned. In the APD techniques, the patient supine position during treatment reduces the pressure on the abdominal wall and allows a higher inflow volume than in CAPD. An excessively high volume, however, might cause discomfort and reduce ultrafiltration. Moreover, even if wCcr should increase with the volume exchanged, if an excessively high volume requires more exchanges, the consequence is an increase in the 'dead time' and a decrease in the total creatinine clearance. This is especially true for patients with a low-average or low permeability pattern (40). Moreover, since the clearance of middle and large molecules is time-dependent, more than gradient-dependent, the clearance of these molecules is lower on discontinuous APD than on continuous APD or CAPD, and this requires to a more efficient schedule. The longer the nightly APD the more easily achievable the targets of adequacy, but a duration over 10h has a negative impact on the quality of life. Daily exchanges also have a negative impact, but they cannot be avoided if patients are anuric or have a large body size. For this population of patients, automated PD is the preferable method with large exchange volumes and as long as possible dwell times, but a combination of (daily) CAPD and (nocturnal) APD prescribed either empirically or with computer models may become necessary to achieve satisfactory results. If such regimens are not able to achieve the target clearances of fluid removal, transfer of the patients to hemodialysis should be considered. Addition of one or two weekly hemodialysis sessions to the PD schedule has also been suggested (41) but the ratio advantages/disadvantages of this choice remains to be defined.

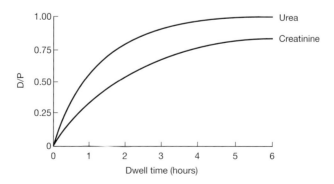

Fig. 2.5   Equilibration of urea and creatinine in dialysate with plasma concentration during a 6-h dwell.

An important help to APD comes from the recent availability of polyglucose solution, which allows sustained ultrafiltration for more than 12h, thus allowing long daily dwells. The patient can introduce this solution in the morning, at the end of an APD session, and can maintain it till the new APD session, at night.

Indications and contra-indications of PD

PD cannot be performed in patients with insufficient peritoneal patency or with reduced peritoneal surface area, i.e. patients with too large polycystic kidneys, severe peritoneal adhesions, former bowel resection, or prune-belly syndrome. Relative contraindications are recent major vascular surgery, hernias, peritoneal-pleural communication, urinary or intestinal diversion.

Some of the indications of PD derive from the need of ECV, electrolyte, and pH stability. Elderly patients are often burdened by myocardiosclerosis, atherosclerosis, and/or ischemic coronary disease. They have cardiac dysfunction, arrhythmia, and impaired sympathetic response to fluid removal. Hyperkinetic circulation, caused by the arteriovenous fistula, is usually not well-tolerated. PD may be preferred to HD in these patients. The oldest patients may be unable to dialyze themselves: in these cases a partner is necessary, and this availability or unavailability can influence the choice of treatment (see Chapter 5).

In patients with congestive heart failure refractory to diuretics, sometimes on a waiting list for heart transplantation, who can tolerate only minimal ECV changes, PD is the best way to maintain an acceptable equilibrium, thanks to its continuous fluid removal.

PD is indicated in uremic neonates in whom the vascular access is difficult to prepare and extra-corporeal treatment is problematic. PD is performed at home, without venipuncture, and with good cardiovascular and electrolyte stability. It requires less dietary restrictions, which are not well accepted by children (see Chapter 5).

The characteristic of PD, to be ambulatory and home-based, enables the patient to pursue his/her daily activities and this can be an important reason for its choice. The following choice is between CAPD and APD: it is based on the patient's clinical and social needs. The peritoneal permeability pattern is an important factor in the choice.

Indications and contra-indications of CAPD

The upright position increases the intra-abdominal pressure and the consequent risk of hernias, leakage, and hemorrhoids. Another limit for CAPD may come from the peritoneal permeability pattern. Patients with wide adhesions or high body size may not reach the targets of dialysis adequacy.

The peritoneal equilibration test defines the peritoneal transport pattern and helps foresee whether CAPD can be continued once the residual renal function disappears. The peritoneal equilibration test should be performed a few weeks (four or eight, according to different authors) after catheter implantation, when a steady state in peritoneal permeability has been reached.

Indications and contra-indications of APD

Patients with a peritoneal permeability pattern in the high and high average values are the best candidates for APD, since on CAPD they rapidly reduce the peritoneal osmolality gradient and are at risk of overhydration. On APD, the short dwells do not allow important reduction in peritoneal osmolality, while they allow sufficient blood purification. In children, APD, performed automatically during the night, helps the patient feel less ill and has a positive impact on parents' life.

Clinical assessment

Reaching the targets of an adequate dose of dialysis is not sufficient to assure a patient's good clinical status, many other factors have to be considered.

Hypertension occurs in many PD patients. It is often due to ECV expansion, decreased renal synthesis of anti-hypertensive prostaglandins and/or other vaso-dilating substances, and activation of the renin–angiotensin–aldosterone system. Treatment of hypertension requires a good ECV control and, often, anti-hypertensive drugs. Patients should moderate salt and fluid intake, and be trained to reach a correct balance of fluid by choosing the bags with the appropriate dextrose concentration. Anti-hypertensive drugs can have unfavorable side-effects in PD: beta blockers have been associated with peritoneal sclerosis; calcium antagonists can increase the peripheral edema; clonidine causes 'a dry mouth', which increases water intake; angiotensin-converting enzyme inhibitors may oppose the effect of recombinant human Erythropoietin and increase serum potassium.

The acid–base status is generally well-balanced in PD, and venous bicarbonate concentration ranges from 25 to 27 mmol/l, when 40 mmol/l lactate PD solutions are used. Supplements of sodium bicarbonate per os are often necessary when PD fluids with 35 mmol/l lactate are used. Nowadays, it is known that acidosis affects protein metabolism, by inhibiting their synthesis and stimulating catabolism, and impairs bone surface crystallization. So, two of the main problems of uremia, malnutrition, and osteodystrophy, can be negatively affected by inadequate acid–base balance (5).

Occurrence of hyperparathyroidism is prevented by a low phosphate diet and intake of phosphate binders, and by the use of vitamin D. Aluminum bone disease, anemia, and brain toxicity, due to aluminum accumulation, have progressively led to aluminum-containing phosphate binders being abandoned and, instead, calcium salts are used, i.e. carbonate or acetate and, more recently, Sevelamer hydrochloride—a non-aluminium, non-calcium containing phosphate binder, which, morover, has a favorable effect on the lipid profile of dialysis patients (42). Oral or intravenous Calcitriol, in appropriate doses, is another important means of preventing and curing hyperparathyroidism. Its main risk is the occurrence of hypercalcemia, which can be controlled by using dialysis solutions with low calcium content.

Anemia is less severe in PD than in hemodialysis patients, since blood losses in the extra-corporeal circulation and red cell trauma by pumps, do not occur. Four to eight thousand units of rhEPO per week generally achieve the desirable hematocrit target of 34–36%. Patients unable to reach these targets must be checked for inadequate dialysis (43), iron deficiency, infectious/inflammatory diseases, aluminum overload, or other anemia-causing diseases.

Complications of PD

Complications of PD are local or systemic. The local ones depend on physical or chemical effects of peritoneal solution on the peritoneal membrane and the abdominal wall, as well as on the risk of bacterial contamination. The systemic ones relate mainly to the metabolic effect of PD solutions.

Hernias

Many different kinds of hernias can occur in PD: umbilical, inguinal, diaphragmatic, and from surgical wounds. Predisposing factors are: old age, multiparity, reduced abdominal wall thickness. If present before the start of dialysis, a surgical correction of a hernia can be made simultaneously to the catheter insertion.

Hernias occurring during PD are frequently caused by the increase in intra-abdominal pressure caused by the PD solution, favored by coughing, vomiting, stipsis, contracture of the abdominal wall, polycystic kidney disease, and high inflow volume. Hernia prevalence is 9–24% in CAPD and 2–3% in APD. After the occurrence, the hernia can be repaired and PD restarted with a lower inflow volume.

Dialysate leak

This complication depends on the increased intra-abdominal pressure. It can manifest itself as an external leak through the tunnel, or as abdominal wall or genital edema. Sometimes it depends on inaccurate suture at the time of catheter in-dwelling. Replacement of peritoneal catheter and reduction of the inflow volume are generally effective.

Back pain

This complication depends on the weight of intra-abdominal fluid, which causes a change in the gravity center. As a consequence, lumbar lordosis increases, like in pregnancy, and causes back pain. This problem is more frequent in patients already affected by lumbar column diseases.

Chyloperitoneum

Appearance of lymph in the PD fluid causes an opalescent or milky-white drainage often mistaken for a sign of peritonitis: but, contrary to peritonitis, in chyloperitoneum there is no abdominal pain and effluent cultures are negative. Its occurrence is often intermittent. The differential cell count shows prevalence of lymphocytes. Opalescence often increases after meals and the color is due to chylomicrons.

Trauma at time of catheter insertion, pressure of catheter on the peritoneum, and peritoneal adhesions have been suggested as possible causes in PD. Other causes must not be forgotten: tuberculous peritonitis, peritoneal malignancy, lymphoma, and ovarian carcinoma.

Hemoperitoneum

One of the events that causes major alarm in PD patients is the appearance of blood in the effluent, and only very few milliliters of blood are sufficient to color it red. Hemoperitoneum in women of reproductive age is very often coincident with menstrual bleeding or ovulation. In the first case, peritoneal endometriosis or retrograde blood flow from the uterus have been supposed as a possible cause. In the second case, the folliculum rupture has been suggested. Other possible causes, not related to PD, are: trauma, malignancy or rupture of cysts of organs covered by the peritoneum, pancreatitis, rupture of the spleen, cholecystitis. Coagulation diseases, anticoagulant or anti-aggregant therapy can favor the appearance of bloody fluid.

The immediate risk in case of substantial bleeding is catheter obstruction by blood clots. Some authors suggest the use of heparin to avoid catheter obstruction. However, a safer approach might consist of rapid exchanges with dialysate lower than the body temperature, to induce vasoconstriction.

Pneumoperitoneum

Pneumoperitoneum occurs frequently in PD patients without symptoms or signs of bowel perforation; whereas, in the general population, when previous surgery is ruled out, 90% of cases are due to gastro-intestinal perforation. An upright chest X-ray differentiates true from false pneumoperitoneum. When post-operative pneumoperitoneum is ruled out, pneumoperitoneum occurs more often after catheter manipulation or with the use of cyclers.

Computed tomography is more sensitive than X-ray film in detecting sub-diaphragmatic free air; however, this technique is not done routinely and consequently the true prevalence of pneumoperitoneum might be underestimated. The amount of sub-diaphragmatic air might not allow one to differentiate between bowel perforation and other causes of pneumoperitoneum. The presence of air in the peritoneal cavity causes eosinophil appearance in peritoneal fluid, more often detected right after surgery. The air takes time to disappear, in fact 100 ml of intraperitoneal air takes about one week to resolve, and 800 ml take 23 days. Manual compression of the abdominal wall during drainage, while keeping the patient in the Trendelenbourg position, might favor air removal.

Peritoneal sclerosis

Some degree of peritoneal fibrosis is associated with long-term PD, and is attributed both to the unphysiology of the dialysis solution and to repeated episodes of peritonitis. Mesothelial cells undergo progressive microscopical changes and, eventually, cells detach from the basal membrane. Mesothelial basal membrane, but also the basal membrane of peritoneal capillaries, often duplicate. Since these changes are very similar to those of diabetic microangiopathy, a mechanism of non-enzymatic glycosilation, due to the high dextrose concentration in dialysate, could be involved (44). The thickness of the sclerotic tissue is about 20 mm.

Sclerosing peritonitis is, fortunately, a very infrequent complication of PD. Its macroscopic appearance has been defined as tanned and its thickness is some hundreds of millimeters. In the most severe cases, sclerosis conglutinates the intestinal loops and a new membrane encases the small bowel, which appears as a cocoon (sclerosing encapsulating peritonitis). Pathogenesis of sclerosing peritonitis is not fully defined, but a role has been ascribed to the unphysiology of dialysis fluids, acetate, multiple episodes of peritonitis, time on PD, beta blockers, chlorexidine, and plasticizers in the bags. Clinical manifestation consists in gastro-intestinal symptoms (nausea, vomiting, constipation), hemoperitoneum, changes in peritoneal permeability, and ultrafiltration. In the severest cases, bowel obstruction occurs and surgery becomes necessary. Operation can cause bowel perforation due to strong adhesions, and often bowel obstruction relapses after some time. Therapy with anti-inflammatory drugs, corticosteroid, and immunosuppressants has been reported to be effective in some cases. Prevention includes avoiding beta blockers, the introduction of disinfectants and drugs into the peritoneal cavity, and the shift to HD after multiple episodes of peritonitis or long lasting peritonitis (45).

Peritoneal calcification

Peritoneal calcifications are frequently reported in sclerosing peritonitis, but in some cases calcification seems to be independent of sclerosis. The typical radiological finding is the presence of eggshell-like calcification on a plain abdominal radiograph. Hyperparathyroidism and episodes of hemoperitoneum have been suggested as possible causes, the latter favoring iron deposits, which could act as nucleus of precipitation.

Hydrothorax

The presence of some diaphragm discontinuities can allow the passage of peritoneal fluid into the pleural cavity. When the hole is small, only little fluid flows and can be visualized with a chest X-ray. With larger defects, the pleural effusion can even reduce the respiratory capacity. Differential diagnosis with other causes of pleural effusion can be easily done by checking the glucose concentration in the thoracentesis fluid, which must be higher than in the plasma. D-Lactate, an isomer not present in the normal metabolism but present in dialysis fluid, is more specific. Alternative methods consist in putting methylene blue, or albumin labeled with radio-isotope, in the peritoneal fluid and searching it in the pleural effusion.

Thoracentesis, followed by a discontinuation of PD, make symptoms disappear. In the case of small diaphragm defects, the switch to HD for one month can help seal the hole. Subsequently, CAPD or APD with lower inflow volume can be tried. Major defects can be repaired in two ways: pleurodesis, by using oxytetracyclin, autologous blood, bacterial components, or fibrin glue; or by surgery. However, before undergoing these invasive therapies, the transfer to HD should be considered.

Exit-site and tunnel infection

The interruption of the body surface continuity, by the entrance site of the PD catheter, is at risk of bacterial contamination, favored also by the catheter movements especially during bag exchanges. The infection can be limited to the skin and the first few millimeters of the subcutaneous tunnel (exit-site infection), or can extend to part or all the tunnel (tunnel infection) and, from it, reach the peritoneal cavity and cause peritonitis.

Causative micro-organisms are generally gram-positive bacteria (especially *Staphylococcus epidermidis*), but also gram-negative bacteria can be involved. A pathogenetic role has been acknowledged in the nasal carriage of *Staphylococcus aureus*, since carriers are more often affected by gram-positive peritonitis.

Prevention of exit-site/tunnel infection starts during catheter in-dwelling and must continue during the break-in period and throughout the course of PD. Therapy consists in antibiotics as a first step, but in most severe cases 'shaving' of the external cuff of the catheter or catheter removal are indicated. Exit-site and tunnel infection have received much attention in the literature, for their risk of peritonitis and for their impact on the continuation of PD (21, 46).

Peritonitis

Peritonitis in PD is classified as infectious chemical and eosinophilic peritonitis.

Infectious peritonitis is the Achilles' heel of CAPD, mainly due to the risk of contamination during repeated bag exchanges. Besides this, there are many other possible routes of contamination, such as from the bowel wall in the presence of diverticula or bowel perforation, migration of bacteria from female genital organs, or secondary to an exit-site or catheter tunnel infection. Also the reduced resistance of peritoneal cavity to infection plays a role. This is due to the continuous lavage of peritoneal fluid, which removes opsonins, antibodies, complement, and defense cells, like neutrophils and macrophages. Moreover, the peritoneal solution has a negative effect on the function and viability of mesothelial cells, macrophages, and neutrophils.

All micro-organisms are able to cause peritonitis: virus, bacteria, yeast, protozoa, but bacteria, mainly gram-positive, are by far the most frequent. Diagnosis of infectious peritonitis requires the presence of two of the three following symptoms: abdominal pain with tenderness, cloudy fluid with a cell count higher than 100 leukocytes/mm^3 and prevalence of neutrophils, and a positive culture. To avoid false-negative results, it is advisable to grow some concentrated effluent in culture.

Therapy of infectious peritonitis consists of antibiotics given either intraperitoneally or through any other way of drug administration. The appropriate regimen is chosen according to the antibiogram results; to accelerate the treatment, however, an empiric therapy is generally used, while waiting for which is effective against gram-positive and gram-negative bacteria. This is an association between a first-generation cephalosporin plus ceftazidime, given intraperitoneally, without changing the CAPD schedule. Heparin is added to the dialysis fluid, to avoid fibrin clot, which can lead to obstruction of the catheter, reduced efficacy of antibiotics, and adhesion formation. Treatment of peritonitis should continue for at least 14–21 days, to avoid relapses. Peritonitis due to fungi and mycobacteria, typical and atypical, are more difficult to cure and discontinuation of PD is often necessary to avoid the negative effects of dialysis fluid on peritoneal defense mechanisms.

Detailed information about choice and dose of drugs goes beyond the limits of this chapter. Readers can refer to the periodical recommendation given by an *ad hoc* committee, the more recent published in 1996 (47).

An accurate choice of the connection system and a good training of the patient are of paramount importance in the prevention of peritonitis. Peritonitis can lead to peritoneal adhesions, diverticula perforation, discontinuation of PD and death, whose risk is 2–3% of peritonitis episodes. During the 1980s and the early 1990s peritonitis was the main cause of drop-out from CAPD. However, during the late 1990s, peritonitis as a cause for leaving PD was overcome by patient's choice (46) or inadequate dialysis (48, 49).

Chemical peritonitis

Contamination of dialysis fluid or accidental introduction of disinfectant used for connection can cause a chemical peritonitis, which generally resolves spontaneously in a short time.

Peritoneal pain can also occur in APD, due to the high dextrose and low pH of the dialysis fluid. The fluid exchange is too rapid to let pH equilibrate with plasma, and this continuous unphysiological exposure can cause serosal inflammation. The addition of a little amount of sodium bicarbonate to the bags relieves the pain.

Eosinophilic peritonitis

Cloudy fluid with a high percentage of eosinophils often occurs after catheter indwelling and in the first days of PD. It has been referred to allergy to catheter components or sterilizing agents, but can also occur after penetration of air into the peritoneal cavity. Eosinophilic peritonitis resolves nearly always spontaneously. In long-lasting cases, treatment with steroid has been suggested.

Loss of ultrafiltration

Difficulty in the control of fluid balance can occur in PD patients, over time. Once loss of residual renal function or excessive fluid intake have been excluded, attention must be drawn to peritoneal function. Loss of ultrafiltration has three different patterns (Table 2.4) and the peritoneal equilibration test (PET) helps to differentiate them (50).

Type I occurs in patients on PD for some years and has been related to the morphological changes of the peritoneum (loss of mesothelial cells, increased vascularization). One month of peritoneal resting, by shifting the patient to HD, can improve ultrafiltration and enable patients to continue on PD. Type I loss of ultrafiltration transiently occurs also during peritonitis.

Type II ultrafiltration loss is not frequent. In this type, not only fluid balance, but also adequacy of dialysis, can be impaired, and to maintain the patient on CAPD can become difficult. A shift to APD with two daily dwells, or to HD, should be considered. Sclerosing encapsulating peritonitis has been associated with both Type I and Type II loss of ultrafiltration.

Therapy of Type III depends on the problem diagnosed. Surgery, in case the cause is mechanical, can solve the problem. Excessive lymphatic absorption is diagnosed by evaluating the disappearance rate of some tracers (i.e. colloid, albumin) from the peritoneal fluid. Phosphatidylcholine or glycosaminoglycans have been suggested as possible therapy (51).

Malnutrition

In CAPD about 70% of dextrose contained in the dialysis solution is absorbed and enters the bloodstream. The continuous dextrose absorption reduces appetite, already

Table 2.4   Patterns of ultrafiltration loss in PD patients

Type I	Loss of ultrafiltration due to increased peritoneal permeability. Dextrose absorption is increased and, consequently, the dissipation of the osmotic gradient between dialysate and plasma more rapid. PET shows a high- or high-average permeability pattern.
Type II	Loss of ultrafiltration associated to reduction in peritoneal permeability. This depends on decreased peritoneal surface area (bowel resection and peritoneal adhesion). PET shows a low- or low-average permeability pattern.
Type III	Loss of ultrafiltration not associated with changes in peritoneal permeability. Causes are often mechanical (leakage, pleural effusion, increased residual intraperitoneal volume) or increased lymphatic absorption. PET does not show significant changes in permeability.

impaired by dysgeusia, abdominal distension, uremic gastro-enteropathy, or, possibly, masticatory defects. This loss of appetite does not affect the total carbohydrate intake, which is compensated by the peritoneal dextrose absorption, but lowers the protein intake; this in addition to the 1–4 g of amino acid and 5–12 g of proteins lost every day in the peritoneal effluent. Moreover, the losses, which are proportional to the degree of peritoneal permeability, can double during peritonitis.

The recommended protein intake is, in PD, 1.0–1.2 g/kg body weight, but many patients, especially the oldest, are unable to achieve these targets. Reduced protein intake and peritoneal loss of amino acids and proteins put the patient at risk of protein malnutrition, with decrease in lean body mass, sometimes undiagnosed because masked by an increase in body fat.

Malnutrition is an important risk factor for survival, thus its prevention and early diagnosis are of paramount importance (52). Methods to assess nutritional status consist of evaluation of serum concentration of some proteins or of nitrogen balance. Serum pre-albumin, albumin, transferrin, pseudo-cholinesterase, and IgG are checked; the earliest changes affect pre-albumin.

Normalized protein catabolic rate (NPCR) or, better, normalized protein nitrogen appearance (NPNA), measures the peritoneal and renal nitrogen excretion. The protein intake can be calculated by using various formulae, which give different results, since some of them measure, whereas other give a constant value of, the non-urea nitrogen losses. The formula suggested by Bergström, based on balance studies, is gaining consensus (53).

The main requirements for obtaining useful information in applying NPNA is that patients are metabolically stable, they are not affected by intercurrent diseases, and by including catabolic nitrogen in order to avoid over-estimating the protein intake. Normalization is done on actual body weight but, as for Kt/V, obese and wasted patients can generate problems, and they should be normalized to the ideal or desirable body weight.

NPNA is directly related to Kt/V (54), but it is not fully clarified whether this relationship has a physiological meaning (the higher KT/V the better NPNA) or merely depends on a mathematical coupling, since Kt/V and NPNA formulae are partially similar. However, favorable results on NPNA and, in some cases, on other nutritional indices like serum albumin, have been observed by increasing the dialysis dose; this effect takes some months to manifest (55). The relationship between Kt/V and NPNA from continuous becomes asymptotic when Kt/V rises above 2, suggesting that further increase in dialysis dose does not increase protein intake (56).

Anthropometric measures are subject to inter-observer variability, but can help an observer monitor the nutritional status over time. Subjective global assessment (SGA) is based on changes in body weight and appetite, and on changes in body fat and muscle. It has been validated for the assessment of nutritional status of CAPD patients (57), contrary to bio-impedance analysis, but not yet validated for PD patients.

Malnutrition occurs in about one-half of PD patients (58) and, as said above, is one of the main determinants of the outcome of uremic patients (31, 32, 59), and any effort to avoid it must be made. Adequate training of the patient, assessment of nutritional status, evaluation of dialysis dose (31, 32, 60), and acid–base balance (61, 62) are the main points to be considered. In the case of malnutrition, individualized diet counseling and amino-acid supplement should be given either per os or intraperitoneally, by using an amino acid-containing solution (4, 63).

Dyslipidemia

The continuous dextrose load in PD stimulates the secretion of insulin, which, in turn, increases serum triglycerides. After some months on CAPD, 60–80% of CAPD patients have hypertriglyceridemia, proportional to its serum concentration before CAPD and to the daily peritoneal absorption of glucose.

PD seems to be unable to correct 'uremic dyslipoproteinemia'. Very low-density lipoproteins (VLDL) are generally increased and apolipoprotein B has a major increase. Low-density lipoprotein cholesterol (LDL-C) and serum cholesterol are increased, whereas high-density lipoprotein cholesterol (HDL-C) and apolipoprotein A (apo A) are reduced. The following factors could play a role in causing such a hyperlipemia: glucose load, loss of apo A in the peritoneal effluent, impaired removal of triglycerides due to reduced activity of hepatic lipase and lipoprotein lipase. Moreover, CAPD patients have concentrations of serum lipoprotein (a) (Lp(a)) higher than HD patients, and this is a known risk factor for atherogenesis (64, 65).

The patient should be advised to maintain a diet containing unsaturated fatty acids and very few saturated fatty acids. Foods rich in, or supplemented with, omega 3-polyunsatured fatty acids can improve lipid abnormalities. Reduction of fluid intake helps to reduce the dextrose load of the hypertonic bags. Moreover, patients should stop drinking alcohol and should do regular exercise. Therapy with statins (inhibitors of the HMG CoA reductase) should be considered in cases refractory to.

References

1. Popovich, R.P., Moncrief, J.W., Decherd, J.P., Bomard, J.B., and Pyle, W.K. (1976). The definition of a novel/wearable equilibrium peritoneal dialysis technique. *Transactions of the American Society for Artificial Internal Organs*, **5** (Abstract), 64.
2. Dobbie, J.W. (1994). Ultrastructure and pathology of the peritoneum. In *Textbook of Peritoneal Dialysis* (ed. R. Gokal and K.D. Nolph), pp. 17–44. Kluwer, Dordrecht.
3. De Paepe, M., Matthys, E., Lameire, N. *et al.* (1983). Experience with glycerol as the osmotic agent in diabetic and non-diabetic patients.In *Prevention and Treatment of Diabetic Nephropathy* (ed. H. Keen and M. Legrain), pp. 299–313. MTP Press, Lancaster, UK.
4. Lindholm, B. and Bergström, J., (1994). Nutritional requirements of peritoneal dialysis patients. In *Textbook of Peritoneal Dialysis* (ed. R. Gokal, K.D. Nolph), pp. 443–72. Kluwer, Dordrecht.
5. Uribarri, J., Buquing, J., and OH, M.S. (1995). Acid–base balance in chronic peritoneal dialysis patients. *Kidney International*, **47**, 269–73.
6. Gokal, R., Mistry, C.D., Peers, E., and the MIDAS Study Group (1994). A United Kingdom multicenter study of Icodextrin in continuous ambulatory peritoneal dialysis. *Peritoneal Dialysis International*, **14**, (Suppl. 2), 522–7.

7. Stein, A., Peers, E., Hattersley, J., Harris, K., Feehally, J., Walls, J., and the MIDAS Study Group (1994). Clinical experience with Icodextrin in continuous ambulatory peritoneal dialysis patients. *Peritoneal Dialysis International*, **14**, (Suppl. 2), 551–4.

8. Mistry, C.D., O'Donohue, D.J., Nelson, S., Gokal, R., and Ballardie, F.W., (1990). Kinetic and clinical studies of b2-microglobulin in continuous ambulatory peritoneal dialysis, influence of renal and enhanced peritoneal clearances using glucose polymer. *Nephrology Dialysis Transplantation*, **5**, 513–19.

9. Fletcher, S., Stables, G.A., and Turney, J.H. (1998). Icodextrin allergy in a peritoneal dialysis patient. *Nephrology Dialysis Transplantation*, **13**, 2656–8.

10. Van Brownwswijk, H., Verburgh, H.A., Heezins, H.C., Van Der Meulen, J., Oe, P.L., and Verhoef, J. (1988). Dialysis fluids and local host resistance in patients on continuous ambulatory peritoneal dialysis. *European Journal of Clinical microbiology and Infectious Diseases*, **7**, 368–73.

11. Veech, R.L. (1988). The untoward effects of the anions of dialysis fluids. *Kidney International*, **7**, 587–97.

12. Topley, N. (1998). Membrane longevity in peritoneal dialysis, impact of infection and bio-compatible solutions. *Advances in Renal Replacement Therapy*, **5**, 179–84.

13. Mahiout, A. and Brunkhorst, R. (1995). Pyruvate anions meutralize peritoneal dialysate toxicity. *Nephrology Dialysis Transplantation*, **10**, 391–4.

14. Feriani, M., Dissegna, D., La Greca, G., and Passlick-Deetjen, J. (1993). Short term clinical study with a bicarbonate-containing peritoneal dialysis solution. *Peritoneal Dialysis International*, **13**, 296–301.

15. Yatsidis, H. (1993). A new stable bicarbonate dialysis solution for peritoneal dialysis, preliminary report. *Peritoneal Dialysis International*, **11**, 224–7.

16. Cancarini, G.C., Brunori, G., Camerini, C., Brasa, S., Manili, L., and Maiorca, R. (1986). Renal function recovery and maintenance of residual diuresis in CAPD and hemodialysis. *Peritoneal Dialysis Bulletin*, **7**, 77–9.

17. Twardowsky, Z.J. (1989). Clinical value of standardized equilibration tests in CAPD patients. *Blood Purification*, **7**, 95–108.

18. Burkart, J.M. (1995). Effect of peritoneal dialysis prescription and peritoneal membrane transport characteristics on nutritional status. *Peritoneal Dialysis International*, **15**, (Suppl.), S20–35.

19. Gotch, F.A. (1994). Prescription criteria in peritoneal dialysis. *Peritoneal Dialysis International*, **14**, (Suppl. 3), S83–87.

20. Keshaviah, P.R., Nolph, K.D., and Van Stone, J.C. (1989). The peak concentration hypothesis, urea kinetics approach comparing the adequacy of CAPD and hemodialysis. *Peritoneal Dialysis International*, **9**, 257–60.

21. NKF-DOQI (National Kidney Foundation. Dialysis Outcomes Quality Initiative) (1997). *Clinical Practice Guidelines for Peritoneal Dialysis Adequacy*. National Kidney Foundation, New York.

22. Watson, P.E., Watson, I.D., and Batt, R.D. (1980). Total body water volumes for males and females estimated from simple anthropometric measurements. *American Journal of Clinical Nutrition*, **33**, 27–39.

23. Du Bois, D. and Du Bois, E.F. (1916). A formula to estimate the approximate surface area from height and weight. *Archives of Internal Medicine*, **17**, 863–71.

24. Tzamaloukas, A.H. and Murata, G.H. (1996). Estimating urea volume in amputs on peritoneal dialysis by modified anthropometric formulae. *Advances in Peritoneal Dialysis*, **12**, 143–6.

25. Chen, H.H., Shetty, A., Afthentopoulos, I.E., and Oreopoulos, D.G. (1995). Discrepancy between weekly Kt/V and weekly creatinine clearance in patients on CAPD. *Advances in Peritoneal Dialysis*, **11**, 83–7.
26. Maiorca, R., Cantaluppi, A., Cancarini, G.C., Broccoli, R., Graziani, G. *et al.* (1983). Prospective controlled trial of a Y connector and disinfectant to prevent peritonitis in continuous peritoneal dialysis. *Lancet*, **8351**, 642–4.
27. Cancarini, G.C., Catizone, L., Fellin, G., Feriani, M., and Quarello, F. (1995). Peritonitis prevention in CAPD. A flushing versus flushing plus in line disinfection comparison. *Peritoneal Dialysis International*, **15**, (Suppl. 1), S51.
28. Durand, P.Y., Chanliau, J., Gamberoni, J., and Kessler, M. (1994). APD, Clinical measurement of the maximal acceptable intra-peritoneal volume. *Advances in Peritoneal Dialysis*, **10**, 63–7.
29. Arkouche, W., Delawari, E., My, H., Laville, M., Abdullah, E., and Traeger, J. (1993). Quantification of adequacy of peritoneal dialysis. *Peritoneal Dialysis International*, **13**, (Suppl. 2), S215–18.
30. Tattersall, J.E., Doyle, S., Greenwood, R.N., and Farrington, K. (1993). Kinetic modelling and underdialysis in CAPD patients. *Nephrology Dialysis Transplantation*, **8**, S35–38.
31. Canada-USA (CANUSA). Peritoneal Dialysis Study Group (1996). Adequacy of dialysis and nutrition in continuous peritoneal dialysis, association with clinical outcome. *Journal of the American Society of Nephrology*, **7**, 198–207.
32. Maiorca, R., Brunori, G., Zubani, R., Cancarini, G.C., Manili, L., Camerini, C. *et al.* (1995). Predictive value of dialysis adequacy and nutritional indices for mortality and morbidity in CAPD and HD patients. A longitudinal study. *Nephrology Dialysis Transplantation*, **10**, 2295–305.
33. Maiorca, R., Cancarini, G.C., Brunori, G., Zubani, R., Camerini, C., Manili, L. *et al.* (1996). Comparison of long-term survival between hemodialysis and peritoneal dialysis. *Advances in Peritoneal Dialysis*, **12**, 79–88.
34. Blake, P., Burkart, J.M., Churchill, D.N., Daugirdas, J., Depner, T., Hamburger, B.J. *et al.* (1996). Recommended clinical practice for maximizing peritoneal clearances. *Peritoneal Dialysis International*, **6**, (Suppl. 5), 448–56.
35. Twardowski, Z.J., Provant, B.F., Nolph, K.D., Khanna, R., Schmidt, L.M., and Salatowich, R.J. (1990). Chronic nightly peritoneal dialysis (NTPD). *Transaction of the American Society for Artificial Internal Organs*, **36**, 584–8.
36. Balaskas, E.V., Izatt, S., Chu, M., and Oreopoulos, D.G. (1993). Tidal volume peritoneal dialysis versus intermittent peritoneal dialysis. *Advances in Peritoneal Dialysis*, **9**, 105–9.
37. Twardowski, Z.J. (1988). Peritoneal Dialysis Glossary II. *Peritoneal Dialysis International*, **18**, 15–7.
38. Viglino, G., Neri, L., Gandolfo, C., and Cavalli, P.L. (1998). Calculations of Kt/V and creatinine clearance in APD. *Advances in Peritoneal Dialysis*, **14**, 68–71.
39. NKF. DOQI National Kidney Foundation Dialysis Outcomes Quality Initiative (1997). Clinical practice guidelines in hemodialysis and peritoneal dialysis adequacy. *American Journal of Kidney Diseases*, **30**, (Suppl. 2), S1-S132.
40. Piraino, B., Blender, F., and Bernardini, J.A. (1994). A comparison of clearances between tidal peritoneal dialysis and intermittent peritoneal dialysis. *Peritoneal Dialysis International*, **14**, 145–8.
41. Tzalamoukas, A.H. and Murata, G.H. (1999). Peritoneal dialysis patients with large body size, can it deliver adequate clearances? *Peritoneal Dialysis International*, **19**, 409–14.

42. Chertow, G.H., Burke, S.K., Dillon, M.A., and Slatopolsky, E. (1999). Long-term effects of sevelamer hydrochloride on the calcium-phosphate product and lipid profile of hemodialysis patients. *Nephrology Dialysis Transplantation*, **14**, 2907–14.

43. Opatmy, K.J.R., Opatma, S., Sefrna, F., and Wirth, J. (1999). The anemia in continuous peritoneal dialysis is related to Kt/V index. *Artificial Organs*, **23**, 65–9.

44. Di Paolo, N. and Sacchi, G. (1989). Peritoneal vascular changes in continuous ambulatory peritoneal dialysis, an in vivo model for the study of diabetic microangiopathy. *Peritoneal Dialysis International*, **9**, 41–5.

45. Afthentopoulos, I.E., Passadakis, P., Oreopoulos, D.G., and Bargman, J. (1998). Sclerosing peritonitis in continuous ambulatory dialysis patients, one center's experience and review of the literature. *Advances in Renal Replacement Therapy*, **5**, 157–67.

46. Twardowski, Z.J. and Khanna, R. (1994). Peritoneal dialysis access and exit site care. In *Textbook of Peritoneal Dialysis* (ed. R. Gokal and K.D. Nolph), pp. 271–314. Kluwer, Dordrecht.

47. Advisory Committee on Peritonitis Management of the International Society for Peritoneal Dialysis (1996). Peritoneal dialysis related peritonitis. Treatment recommandations (1996) up-date. *Peritoneal Dialysis International*, **16**, 557–73.

48. Maiorca, R., Cancarini, G.C., Zubani, R., Camerini, C., Manili, L., Brunori, G. *et al.* (1996). CAPD viability, a long-term comparison with hemodialysis. *Peritoneal Dialysis International*, **16**, 276–87.

49. Oreopoulous, D.G. (1999). The optimization of continuous ambulatory peritoneal dialysis. *Kidney International*, **55**, 1131–49.

50. Heimburger, O., Wanieski, J., Werinsky, A., Tranaeus, A., and Lindholm, B. (1990). Peritoneal transport in CAPD patients and permanent loss of ultrafiltration capacity. *Kidney International*, **38**, 495–506.

51. Di Paolo, N., Buoncristiani, U., Capotondo, L., Rossi, P., Bernini, M., Pucci, A.M. *et al.* (1996). Phosphatidycholine and peritoneal transport during peritoneal dialysis determine prognosis in continuous ambulatory peritoneal dialysis patients. *Nephron*, **44**, 365–70.

52. Fung, L., Pollock, C.A., Caterson, R.J., Hamony, J.F., Waugh, D.A., and Ibels, L.S. (1996). Dialysis adequacy and nutrition determine prognosis in continuous peritoneal dialysis patients. *Journal of the American Society of Nephrology*, **7**, 737–44.

53. Bergström, J., Heimberger, O., and Lindholm, B. (1998). Calculation of the protein equivalent of total nitrogen appearance, which formula should be used? *Peritoneal Dialysis International*, **18**, 467–73.

54. Nolph, K.D., Moore, H.L., Provant, B., Meyer, M., Twardowski, Z.J., Khanna, R. *et al.* (1993). Cross-sectional assessment of weekly urea and creatinine clearance and indices of nutrition in continuous peritoneal dialysis patients. *Peritoneal Dialysis International*, **13**, 178–83.

55. Malhotra, D., Tzamaloukas, A.H., Murata, G.H., Fox, L., Goldman, R.S., and Avasthi, P.S. (1996). Serum albumin in continuous ambulatory peritoneal dialysis, its predictions and relationship to urea clerance. *Kidney International*, **50**, 243–9.

56. Blake, P.G., Lindsay, R.M., Spanner, E., Heidenheim, P., Baird, P., Allison, M. *et al.* (1993). Factors modifying the relationship between Kt/V urea and normalized protein catabolic rate (PCRN) in CAPD. *Journal of the American Society of Nephrology*, **4**, 398.

57. Enia, G., Sicuso, C., Alati, G., and Zoccali, C. (1993). Subjective global assessment of nutrition in dialysis patients. *Nephrology Dialysis Transplantation*, **8**, 1094–8.

58. Young, G.A., Kopple, J.D., Lindholm, B., Vonesh, E.F., De Vecchi, A., Scalamogna, A. *et al.* (1991). Nutritional assessment of continuous ambulatory peritoneal dialysis patients, an international study. *American Journal of Kidney Diseases*, **17**, 462–71.

59. Cancarini, G., Costantino, E., Brunori, G., Manili, L., Camerini, C., Spitti, C. *et al.* (1992). Nutritional status in long-term CAPD patients. *Advances in Peritoneal Dialysis*, **8**, 84–7.

60. Ronco, C., Conz, P., Bosch, J.P., Loew, S.Q., and La Greca, G. (1994). Assessment of adequacy in peritoneal dialysis. *Advances in Renal Replacement Therapy*, **1**, 15–23.

61. Mitch, W.E., Jurkovitz, C., and England, B.K. (1993). Mechanisms that cause protein and amino-acid catabolism in uremia. *American Journal of Kidney Diseases*, **21**, 91–5.

62. Stein, A., Baker, F., Larrat, C., Bennett, S., Harris, K., Feehally, J. *et al.* (1994). Correction of metabolic acidosis and the protein catabolic rate in PD patients. *Peritoneal Dialysis International*, **14**, 187–96.

63. Jones, M., Kalil, R., Blake, P., Martis, L., and Oreopoulous, D.G. (1997). Modification of an amino-acid solution for peritoneal dialysis to reduce the risk of acidemia. *Peritoneal Dialysis International*, **17**, 66–7.

64. Avram, M.M., Goldwasser, P., Burrell, D.F., Antignani, B.S., Fein, P.A., and Mittman, N. (1992). The uremic dyslipidemia. A cross sectional and longitudinal study. *American Journal of Kidney Diseases*, **20**, 324–35.

65. Wheeler, D.C. (1996). Abnormalities of lipoprotein metabolism in CAPD patients. *Kidney International*, **50**, (Suppl. 50), S41–46.

3
Kidney transplantation
Ulrich Frei

Introduction: kidney transplantation as integral part of ESRD treatment

Since the first successful kidney transplants in twins more than 40 years ago, kidney transplantation has become an integral part in the treatment of end-stage renal disease (ESRD) in most of the developed countries around the world. Several important steps have been necessary to expand kidney transplantation from an experimental procedure into a widely practiced therapeutic option in such a way that it has become the most successful modality of renal replacement therapy.

From very early on an efficacious surgical technique was established and only minor developments have been made concerning the anastomoses of the renal vessels and the implantation of the ureter into the urinary bladder. Also of importance was the development of preservation solutions to extend the storage time, allowing kidney exchange over distances possible. The aim of these different preservation solutions was to keep the organ integrity intact during the cold ischemia time.

A second important achievement was the detection, serologic differentiation, and implementation of HLA (human leukocyte antigen) typing into organ allocation and exchange by J. van Rood (1). In particular, in the European setting, HLA matching has improved transplant outcomes significantly. A third achievement was the introduction of effective and powerful immunosuppressive drugs. Starting with corticosteroids and azathioprine, more recently cyclosporine, poly- and monoclonal anti-T-cell sera and a number of new drugs such as tacrolimus, mycophenolate mofetil (MMF), sirolimus, and anti-CD25 humanized antibodies have been added. Of particular importance was the development of improved detection and diagnostic methods of viral diseases such cytomegalovirus (CMV) infection and the introduction of efficient antiviral drug therapy. The improvement of antibiotic and antifungal therapy, and the introduction of effective prophylaxis and treatment of gastric bleeding (an early threat in high-steroid immunosuppression), had greatly positive impacts. New diagnostic tools, in particular ultrasound and Doppler flow imaging, have eased the differential diagnosis of graft functional impairment. Putting these development of the last twenty years together, kidney transplantation did improve with respect to short-term outcome in graft survival, reduction of rejection episodes, and improvement of long-term outcome, combined with a dramatic reduction in patient mortality. This occurred in spite of an extension of the limits to indications of transplantation with respect to age, underlying renal and concomitant diseases.

However, to become really an integral part in the treatment of ESRD, kidney transplantation had to be extended in numbers. The availability of transplantable organs is still the most important limiting factor for a wider use of renal transplantation. Nowadays, in most countries, the prerequisites for an organized organ-transplantation system have been introduced, such as transplant legislation, organ-procurement agencies, national and international organ exchange, and donor hospital programs, but so far with limited success. Unfortunately, only very few countries achieve a situation by which the new registrations and the annual transplants performed reach a balance. In most others, there is still only a steady growth of the waiting-lists!

Present status: kidney transplantation world-wide

Kidney transplantation is an integral part of the treatment of ESRD. This is true for most of the industrialized countries but also a number of developing countries are trying to implement transplant programs. A recent overview has been published by the USA Renal Data System (USRDS); other data sources are national, regional, and scientific registries such as the Collaborative Transplant Study (CTS) and published center reports (see Fig. 3.1).

To evaluate the contribution of renal transplantation to the global treatment of ESRD in different countries, one has to consider three different viewpoints, which at first glance will give conflicting results.

The first issue is the number of renal transplants performed per million population (pmp) annually. This gives the best insight in to organ availability in the respective country. By far the best data are reported for Spain with 47 transplants pmp. Second best is the USA with 46 transplants pmp. Most of the countries have numbers

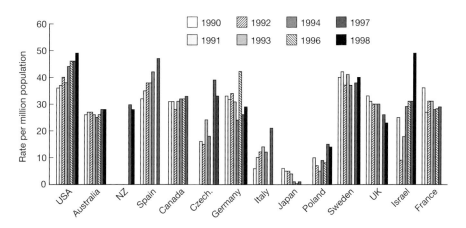

Fig. 3.1   International comparison of transplant activities (taken from the *USRDS Report* 2000).

between 25 and 35 pmp, e.g. Ireland 32 pmp. Poland has only 13 pmp, and Japan, due to legal and religious reasons, has only 1 transplant pmp.

The second parameter to be considered is the proportion (%) of ESRD patients with a functioning kidney graft. This information provides surprisingly different results if compared to the number of transplants performed annually. In Ireland 73%, Sweden 54%, and the Netherlands 50% of the total ESRD population has a functioning graft, whereas the USA (28%), Germany (23%) and Poland have much lower figures.

These figures need to be put into perspective by comparing the absolute numbers of patients having a functioning kidney graft in the selected countries compared to the total prevalent population. The highest figures are reported for Sweden (347 pmp; total prevalence of RRT patients or TPRRT = 643 pmp), Spain (334 pmp; TPRRT = 759 pmp), and the USA (334 pmp; TPRRT = 1131). Ireland has 301 pmp (TPRRT = 412) and Germany and France have only 161 and 153 pmp (TPRRT = 683 and 634, respectively). Poland, who showed a high proportion of grafted patients, has only small absolute numbers (64 pmp; TPRRT = 223).

The impact of transplantation on the ESRD treatment in different countries can be summarized or ranked in the following way: there are countries with a high total prevalence of ESRD, which are able to provide a transplant to a great proportion of them (e.g. Spain, Austria, Sweden, Norway, and Belgium). The USA, having a very high total prevalence, are performing well with respect to donation and transplant figures, but the proportion of patients actually alive with a transplant is rather low. In sharp contrast is Japan, with the highest prevalence of ESRD patients in the world and a transplant program so far not worth mentioning. Another group of countries, such as Germany, France, and Italy, have high total prevalence rates but only around 25% of them transplanted. This difference may be caused by the easy availability of other treatment modalities. There is another group of countries with a comparable lower total prevalence rate such as UK, Ireland, and the Netherlands. In these countries, the proportion is high but the absolute numbers are lower than in other developed countries, perhaps due to financial constraints or gatekeeper policies. There are a number of countries that are now developing their ESRD-treatment programs including transplantation (such as Poland). Some countries like Austria, Spain, or Belgium are able to meet their demands by cadaveric donor transplantation only.

For whom is kidney transplantation the optimal strategy of treatment of ESRD?

When and for whom to consider a transplant

The policies for assignment to the transplant waiting-list differ from country to country, and from institution to institution. They have changed over the years, with a tendency to widen the acceptance criteria. In general, patients who tend not to be accepted are older, more often female, diabetic, and carriers of viral disease such as hepatitis C (2).

In some countries, consensus conferences or medical associations have issued rules or guidelines to support decision-making. In view of the very long waiting-lists in most countries, there is no evidence that acceptance rates are low or influenced by non-medical criteria, although specific individual patients may be unfairly treated (3).

The question as to whether a patient can be considered as a transplant candidate is ideally addressed before commencing dialysis. The decision-making tree should start when the creatinine clearance of the patient drops below 20 ml/min. At this time-point the possibility of transplantation should be evaluated. This includes the question of whether there is a potential live donor. In most countries, pre-emptive transplantation—i.e. transplantation before commencing dialysis—is an accepted possibility, although the limited availability of cadaver donors make this a real alternative to dialysis only in the case of a live donation. Following initial experience with children, there are now data available in adults that indicate no higher risk of rejection and compare favorably with the outcome of dialysis patients (4). There is no difference between pre-emptive live or cadaveric grafts with respect to number of rejections and short-term outcome. If pre-emptive transplantation is possible, the patient avoids the burden of dialysis and the costs of dialysis are spared. Nevertheless, the number of pre-emptive transplants remains rather low (almost <5%).

Who should be transplanted? Who not?

Kidney transplantation today offers an improved chance of survival in carefully selected recipient populations when compared to dialysis. There are no firm data in the literature showing the percentage of a given ESRD population suitable for placement on a waiting-list. This proportion is greatly affected by age, type of underlying renal diseases, the distribution of concomitant diseases in the ESRD population, and of course the degree of availability of transplantation. Norway has shown by far the most extended acceptance policy, also in higher age groups. More than 70% of the Norwegian ESRD population is considered transplantable (5). A rough estimate is given by the size of the waiting-list in different countries. In the USA, 20.2% of the dialysis population is registered on the waiting-list, in Germany 25% (6). If one considers that in these two countries the mean age of the dialysis population is between 60 and 65 years, approximately 50% of the ESRD patients younger than 65 years are registered on the waiting-list.

The decision-making process for acceptance on the waiting-list is based on the goal aimed at achieving reasonable low patient-mortality rates (<5%) and high graft-success rates (>85–90%) at 1 year post-grafting. The criteria applied are based on registry data and experience with comparable risk groups (major surgery). If the risk of death after a transplant significantly exceeds the risk of continuing dialysis, or if the risk of loosing the graft exceeds significantly the risk of the whole (comparable) transplant population, then a transplant is not advised. However, the attitude applied rests more on consensus conferences and personal experience than on prospectively obtained evidence.

Kidney transplantation for children

Special attention has to be paid to the selection and preparation of pediatric recipients. According to the policy of the majority of pediatric centers, transplantation before or without dialysis is the preferred option. The main reason is to allow children an adequate growth and development. The donor source consists of a high percentage of live-donated kidneys by the parents. If there is no possibility for a live-donated kidney, children have a priority in all organ-allocation systems. Kidney transplantation in children of very young age yields inferior results if compared to adults aged 20–45 years, due to technical problems, higher rate of rejections, recurrence of renal disease, and sometimes non-compliance (See also Chapter 5).

How should the recipient be evaluated and prepared?

Risk evaluation—individual, population

The main goals of the evaluation are to check for potential contra-indications and establish which risk factors are present. Risk factors include, in particular, the underlying renal disease, the number and severity of concomitant diseases, immunological risk factors, and the patient's individual personality. The evaluation has to be carried out with the intention of improving the quality of life and to extend the lifespan.

There are only very few absolute contra-indications for renal transplantation today. Active uncontrolled cancer carries a higher risk of spreading metastasis while under immunosuppressive therapy, and therefore a higher risk of death. According to the experience from the Cincinnati Cancer Registry, some safety rules have been introduced concerning the sufficient waiting time between the date at which the malignancy was considered as 'cured' and transplantation, depending on the site and type of cancer (7).

A more politically than medically complicated matter concerns HIV-positive patients submitted to immunosuppressive therapy. There is a high risk of drug interaction with anti-retroviral therapy and an increased risk for septic complications (8). Early experience with inadvertently used kidneys from HIV-positive donors demonstrated early death of the recipients (9). There is, so far, no proof that anti-retroviral therapy will improve the prognosis of HIV-positive graft recipients. Most centers in the USA deny HIV-positive patients access to the waiting-list (10).

In addition, kidney transplantation is contra-indicated in patients with active infectious disease such as tuberculosis, osteomyelitis, septicemia, and other serious infections.

For patients with a short life-expectancy related to extra-renal diseases or complications, renal transplantation does not offer any advantage and may rather accelerate death.

Recipient selection work-up

Although there is no common policy in Europe for recipient selection (11), an attempt was made by the European Renal Association to compile best-practice guidelines (12). The risk evaluation starts with the patient's history. Whenever possible, the underlying renal disease should be precisely identified. The correct diagnosis is important because of possible recurrence, of extra-renal manifestations of the disease and the need for ongoing drug therapy such as for vasculitis. A general medical history should be taken with respect to previous cardiovascular events, arterial occlusive disease, duration of hypertension, infections (in particular viral infections such as hepatitis B and C), gastro-intestinal disorders, and diseases of the lower urinary tract, in particular for obstructions, reflux, and large-size polycystic kidneys. In females, the gynecological history should be taken. Attention should be paid to the mental status of the patient. Drug addiction, non-compliance, and psychiatric disorders may increase the risk of graft loss and needs particularly thorough evaluation.

Evaluation of the cardiovascular system

Convincing evidence is available that proves the impact of cardiovascular risk factors on patient survival after kidney transplantation. Investigations have been performed to select the best available method for cardiovascular work-up in transplant candidates. Echocardiography, although not prospectively tested, seems to be of pivotal importance to screen for cardiac abnormalities such as valvular disease, cardiomyopathy, pericardial disease, and impaired cardiac wall movement after myocardial infarction. Methods of exercise-testing to detect coronary artery disease turned out to be of limited value because of the impaired exercise capacity of dialysis patients. This applies both for exercise ECG and for thallium myocardial imaging. Exercise-testing has only been proven useful in patients with normal exercise capacity. Dobutamine stress-testing by echocardiography is considered a useful method although it is to some extent observer-dependant (13). Prospective use of coronary angiography detected a high number of lesions not yet found by non-invasive measures. The liberal use of coronary angiography in any suspicious case is therefore recommended (14). More difficult to answer is the question of how to deal with detected coronary lesions and stenoses. So far, the most often used policy is to treat uremic patients the same way as non-uremic patients. There is evidence available about a high restenosis rate in angioplasty compared with coronary bypass grafts (15). Data on coronary artery stenting are thus far limited (16).

The increasing age of the patient population gives peripheral vascular occlusive disease a high rank for morbidity in transplant patients. Of particular importance is the situation of the pelvic vessel axis (17). Due to accelerated arteriosclerosis, extensively calcified common iliac arteries have been found that make donor-graft anastomoses sometimes acrobatic. Not only in diabetics is the risk of leg amputations high. Special attention has to be paid to vascular occlusive disease of the carotid arteries (18).

Although not extensively studied in the literature, diseases of the venous return, in particular of pelvic veins after thrombosis with and without previous access catheters, may cause a certain risk of technical failures and early graft thrombosis.

Evaluation of the respiratory tract

The most serious pulmonary risk for transplant recipients consists of viral and opportunistic infections. The preparation of the recipient should evaluate whether or not there was, or is, an exposition for specific infectious causes, such as tuberculosis or fungi. Pulmonary work-up should include spirometry. Special attention should be paid to smoking habits. Active smoking carries a risk of bronchopulmonary infection in the early post-operative period, as is the case for other major surgery. There are recent data that prove an effect of smoking (>25 pack-years) on graft outcome and mortality, an effect that disappears 5 years after quitting (19).

Evaluation of the gastro-intestinal tract

This should include the evaluation of the upper gastro-intestinal (GI) tract for a history of bleeding, ulcers, or gastritis completed by endoscopy. There are no good data as to whether *Helicobacter pylori* should be eradicated before transplant. A history of inflammatory bowel disease should be considered. Large bowel diverticulosis and diverticulitis are quite frequent in elderly patients or in those with polycystic kidney disease, who are thus at a high risk of rupture and local peritonitis (20).

All transplant candidates should be tested for the presence of hepatitis B or C infection. Positive patients need also to be tested for the amount of replication or for HCV-RNA (hepatitis C virus RNA) to document active infection. In patients with replicating viral disease, a liver biopsy is often mandatory to evaluate if chronic hepatitis is present to indicate virostatic therapy such as lamivudine or interferon in HCV patients (21).

After transplantation, liver disease is more frequent in HCV-positive than in HCV-negative patients. In the long run, this leads to significant liver complications. The patients have a higher risk of developing proteinuria and infections. Long-term patient and graft-survival rates are lower if compared to HCV-negative graft recipients. Mortality is higher, mainly as a result of liver disease and infections. Nevertheless, transplantation is the best option for the HCV-positive patient with end-stage renal disease (21).

Evaluation of the urogenital tract

Besides a careful ultrasound investigation of the urinary tract in patients with a history of infections, reflux, or malformation, urodynamic evaluation is sometimes necessary. To avoid persistent infection, instrumental investigations should be omitted in diabetics and patients with ADPKD. Patients with lower urinary tract abnormality are often considered high risk for renal transplantation. According to the recent literature, presence of an ileal conduit does not adversely affect graft survival. The commonest complication is persistent urinary tract infection, which accounts only very seldom for graft loss (22).

Malignancies

Recipient work-up should include history and physical examination for cancer or hemopathy and routine radiological and ultrasound investigations. This may include feces occult blood testing in all patients and mammography in women over 40 years of age. Regardless of age, women should have a pelvic examination and a pap smear. Men aged over 50 should be screened for prostate carcinoma, with PSA evaluation and prostate ultrasound. Special attention should be paid to patients with analgesic nephropathy, in whom a complete imaging of the urinary tract should be available for excluding the presence or suspicion of an urothelial tumor. Bilateral nephrectomy or nephro–ureterectomy might be necessary prior to transplantation. Another frequent cause of cancer in the native kidneys is acquired cystic disease (23). It is recommended that long-term dialysis patients who are candidates for transplantation, be screened at regular time intervals with kidney ultrasonography and/or computed tomography.

Whether patients with a previous history of cancer but without evidence of active disease should be considered suitable for transplantation, is a difficult decision.

According to the available literature, the risk of recurrence depends on the type of cancer and on the duration of the disease-free period between treatment of cancer and transplantation. In a large retrospective study, the risk of recurrence was found to be 53% if the transplant was performed within 2 years of apparent recovery from neoplasia, 34% if the time interval was between 25 and 60 months, and 13% if the period was 5 years. Recently, a differentiation has been made between tumors occurring before or after commencing dialysis. The latter may carry a significantly worse prognosis. With some exceptions, a minimum waiting period of 2 years between 'curative' treatment of a neoplasm with a favorable prognosis and undertaking renal TX is desirable. A waiting period of approximately 5 years is desirable for lymphomas, most carcinomas of the breast, prostate, colon or renal carcinomas larger than 5 cm. No waiting period is necessary for incidentally discovered carcinomas, *in situ* carcinomas and possibly tiny focal carcinomas (7).

Primary renal disease

There are several underlying renal diseases that may recur in transplanted kidneys. This is true for some types of glomerulonephritis, as well as for systemic diseases involving the kidneys such as vasculitides or metabolic diseases. The overall percentage of kidneys lost due to recurrences is less than 5% and account for less than 10% of graft losses after the first year. Among the primary glomerular diseases, focal segmental glomerulonephritis (FSGS), membranous nephropathy, membranoproliferative glomerulonephritis, and IgA nephritis are not contra-indications for transplantation, although there are graft losses due to recurrence. They are particularly frequent in patients with a rapidly progressive FSGS with nephrotic syndrome, which can recur acutely and cause the loss of the graft on the very first day of transplantation. The adequate time for transplantation and type of organ donor in these patients remain matters of debate (24, 25). In the case of an anti-glomerular-barement membrane nephritis, the transplant should be postponed until the antibodies have disappeared from the serum.

With respect to the recurrence rate of systemic diseases, some differentiations have to be made. SLE, Schoenlein-Hennoch's purpura, ANCA-positive vasculitis, hemolytic uremic syndrome (HUS), and amyloidosis are not contra-indications for renal transplantation (26–29). In idiopathic mixed cryoglubinemia, the concern is focused on the liver disease; whereas light chain deposit disease should be taken as a contra-indication. Because of the limited number of observations, definite guidelines cannot be given.

The recurrence of metabolic diseases needs special attention. Morphologic recurrence of diabetic nephropathy is the rule for graft but is very seldom the cause of graft loss.

In primary hyperoxaluria, only combined liver/kidney transplantation is recommended because the outcome after kidney-only transplants is very poor (30). Cystinosis and Fabry's disease are not contra-indications for renal transplantation (See Chapter 9).

Concomitant diseases—risk factors

Diabetes mellitus   End-stage renal disease due to diabetic nephropathy is of increasing importance in all Western countries, with the highest incidence of up to more than 40% of all new patients taken onto RRT (31). Within this population, most cases are due to type II diabetes mellitus, whereas those of type I (truly insulin-dependant) are relatively constant over the years. It has been proven that ESRD due to diabetes mellitus carries the highest risk for early death due to cardiovascular causes. The pathogenetic background consists of a mixture of hypertension, lipid disorders, accumulation of AGE substances, and autonomic neuropathy. All kinds of renal or combined transplantation have proved to yield a better patient survival compared to dialysis, although prospective studies are not available and the results are influenced by the negative selection process applied to those patients not deemed suitable for transplantation (32).

In spite of an increased risk of an earlier recipient loss than in non-diabetics, all attempts should be made to give diabetic patients a chance to get a graft as early as possible. Although renal transplantation alone in diabetics is not able to halt or improve extra-renal diabetic complications, such as retinopathy, neuropathy, macro- and micro-angiopathy, there is an overall improvement of life expectancy, as shown from the USA-Renal Data Registry (USRDS). Registry data also have shown an improved survival of transplant recipients after first myocardial infarction, if compared to dialysis patients (33). The number of amputations and amaurosis may, however, be increased (34).

Diabetic graft recipients should undergo an intensive evaluation of cardiovascular risk factors. Coronary artery disease, pelvic and peripheral vessels disease have to be investigated with all suitable means. Because most of the recipients have a low exercise capacity, adequate exercise ECG cannot be performed and should be replaced by pharmacological stress echocardiography (35). In most centers, the policy is to perform a coronary angiography in candidates for simultaneous kidney–pancreas transplantation (SPK) or living related donor (LRD) transplantation with, however, the (often high) risk of exposing the patient with advanced renal failure to iodinated contrast media. Pre-existing coronary artery disease carrying an increased risk of post-TX complication or death, coronary bypass surgery, or angioplasty, with or without or stenting, should be performed before registering the patient on the waiting-list.

Immunological risk

All patients assigned to a waiting-list have to undergo a serologic typing for class I and II, and a molecular typing for class II antigens as well. Blood has to be drawn at regular intervals to store serum for cross match purposes and to screen for HLA antibodies (12, 36).

Patients with previous graft losses due to rejections and HLA sensitization due to blood transfusions or pregnancies, carry a higher risk, as well as patients with HLA-homzygosity after graft losses (37).

Individual risk factors—age, compliance

Age is a natural risk factor for death! This holds true in renal transplantation too. Registry data have shown that elderly recipients have an improved life-expectancy if compared with age-matched patients from the waiting-list remaining on dialysis (32). Whether there is an upper age-limit for transplantation in the elderly has not been established. Successful transplantation is reported up to the age of 70. The numbers above 70 years of age are, however, small and do not play a significant demographic role, although some very successful cases have come to notice (See Chapter 7).

Maintaining surveillance during pre-transplantation waiting time

In view of the prolonged waiting times for cadaver donor transplantation in most of the countries, efforts must be made to keep the recipient information as recent as possible. Depending on age and clinical condition, an update of critical parameters, such as cardiac condition and vascular status, has to be made at 6–12 months time intervals.

How to accomplish this goal?

Donor source

The history of transplantation started with living related donors, first twins, later siblings, and parents. In the 1990s, living donation was extended to distant relatives, spouses, and friends, thereby violating the dogma of HLA compatibility for live donors. Criteria for the use of live donors are not accepted to the same extent in all countries. The percentage of living donation differs from up to 50% (Norway) to less than 3% (in Poland or Czech Republic) (38).

Organ donation from the deceased brain-dead donor started with trauma victims, later extended to non-traumatic causes such as stroke, intra-cerebral bleeding and post-ischemic damage. The donor shortage extended the organ harvesting to more aged, hypertensive, and complicated donors. During the last few years, a new category, the non-heart-beating donor, was added, although their use does not comply with legislation in all countries.

Live donation

Despite the improvement in immunosuppression and better graft and patient survival in cadaveric kidney transplantation, the use of living donors for kidney transplantation still results in a slightly superior graft and patient survival, and less morbidity, due to fewer rejection episodes, less immunosuppression, and better immediate graft function.

Furthermore, the number of cadaveric grafts available is far less than is needed in order to transplant the increasing number of uremic patients on the waiting-lists of almost all countries. Therefore, the need for kidneys from sources different from cadaveric donors is steadily rising and, consequently, the use of related and unrelated living donors has increased.

As for the evaluation and assignment to the waiting-list for live donation, guidelines and recommendations have been formulated based on consensus conferences and some documented evidence. The USA outcome standards of recommendation are that patient survival should be at least 95% 1 year after grafting and that more than 90% of the grafts from living kidney donors should be functioning at 1 year.

Related living kidney donors

Before going any further into the details of evaluation and advice, an ABO blood group of the donor and recipient should be obtained, because ABO compatibility is, with very few exceptions, the fundamental prerequisite for live donation. The first goal of evaluation is to ensure a safe procedure for the donor; to ensure that there will be a minimum of risk with anesthesia and surgical intervention. It must be ascertained that the donor is healthy and that there is no risk of transmitting any disease. It must also be clear that the unilateral nephrectomy will have no foreseeable negative effects on the long-term residual renal function of the donor. To discuss and decide on alternative surgical procedures, such as nephrectomy performed by open surgery or laparoscopic technique.

To ensure that the autonomy of the potential donor is protected, the physician carrying out the primary evaluation should ideally be independent of the recipient's medical team and should not be a member of the transplant team. Legislation in some countries makes an independent physician or psychologist conditional. In some instances, the decision of an independent review board is a prerequisite.

Evaluation

If blood groups are compatible, a complete medical history and physical examination should be done, together with further investigations, as presented in Table 3.1. The medical history should exclude the presence of any sign of renal disease, such as hypertension, nephrolithiasis, proteinuria ($>300 \, mg/d$), hematuria, edema, and renal parenchyma infections. Absolute glomerular filtration rate (GFR) at the time of donation seems to play a significant role. Donor GRF of $<80 \, ml/min$ presents an increased risk for graft loss (39). Furthermore, thorough investigations are aiming at detecting cardiovascular risk factors, diabetes mellitus, malignancy, and systemic diseases. Psychological problems or diseases, and medications taken, should be searched for. Finally, renal angiography is performed to exclude vascular lesion(s) and as a basis for the decision on which kidney should be retrieved.

A number of exclusion criteria of live kidney donation are presented in Table 3.2. Special emphasis should be made on the possible presence of hereditary renal diseases. Donors should be offered life-long follow-up, with check-up examinations at regular time-intervals—never less than once a year.

Informed consent

Before obtaining consent to evaluation and donation, the potential donor must be informed about several important points. Despite thorough pre-operative work-up, the mortality risk of healthy donors was estimated to be 0.03% and the risk of morbidity 0.23% in large studies reported from donor operations performed in the 1980s (40).

Table 3.1   Evaluation of the potential living kidney donor

First step: Compatibility

ABO blood typing; HLA-AB and -DR tissue typing; cross-match

Second step: medical suitability

General evaluation:

History and physical examination.

Blood pressure; optional 24-h ambulatory recording.

Electrocardiogram, echocardiography, chest radiograph, optional pulmonary function tests.

Complete blood count, platelet count, coagulation factors.

Chemistry: blood urea nitrogen, S-creatinine, sodium, potassium, bicarbonate, fasting blood glucose, calcium, phosphorus, albumin, total protein, uric acid, liver enzymes, bilirubin, fasting cholesterol, triglycerides, high- and low-density lipoproteins.

Cardiovascular evaluation (including stress testing by exercise or dobutamine echocardiography and/or scintigraphy) for donors older than 50 years or with a history of heavy smoking or with mild hypertension.

In females: pregnancy test, gynecological examination if > 40 years; in males: PSA when >50 years.

Renal assessment

Urinanalysis, microscopy of urinary sediment; urine culture.

24-h urine for creatinine clearance or a direct evaluation of the GFR by CrEDTA or iohexol clearance.

24-h urine total protein excretion; urine for micro-albuminuria—(optional).
Radionuclide determination of glomerular filtration rate—as a separate evaluation of the function of the two kidneys.
Ultrasound examination of the kidneys and the abdomen.

Renal arteriogram.

Third step: additional risk factors

Cytomegalovirus titres (CMV), hepatitis B surface antigen (HBsAg), hepatitis C antibody (HCV), human immunodeficiency virus antibody (HIV), Epstein–Barr virus titres (EBV), herpes simplex virus (HSV), varicella zoster virus (VZV), toxoplasma ab and syphilis.

The potential, but unlikely, risks of kidney donation include short-term surgical risks and theoretical, but extremely unlikely, long-term risks of impaired kidney function and hypertension. The long-term risk of kidney donation is very low. According to some studies, the 'living donor' has a longer life survival than the general population, possibly due to the 'positive selection' factor (41). Living organ donation may entail a loss of time and money, and possible insurance problems. Psychological risks are low and more often donation results in improved self-esteem (42).

Despite the most extensive pre-operative work-up a full guarantee of successful outcome of the transplant cannot be given. Early and late possible complications in renal transplantation, in particular for the recipient, should be mentioned (Table 3.3).

Table 3.2 Exclusion criteria for a potential living kidney donor

General medical exclusion criteria

ABO incompatible; cross-match positive

Cardiovascular disease; hypertension without good control (>than 1 drug)

Pulmonary insufficiency

Diabetes mellitus

Drug addiction/dependence

HIV-positive; hepatitis B antigen-positive; hepatitis C–positive to a negative recipient; other severe infections

Malignancy

Long-term use of nephrotoxic drugs

Age below 18 years

Renal exclusion criteria

Impaired GFR, if compared to normal range for age and size

Proteinuria of more than 300 mg/day

Microhematuria, if not an urologic evaluation and a possible kidney biopsy are normal

Multiple kidney stones

Multiple cysts; three or more arteries

Family history of autosomal dominant polycystic kidney disease (ADPKD), unless ultrasound or CT scan is normal and donor age is above 30 years

Bilateral fibromuscular dysplasia (exceptions have been reported)

A potential family donor should always be in the position to withdraw his or her consent. Great care should be taken during the information procedure to ensure that the kidney donation is truly voluntary and in no way coerced. In some countries, external review boards have been instituted to ensure these prerequisites. The potential kidney donor should receive direct personal information, as well as written information. The potential kidney donor should sign a statement allowing the transplant surgeon to perform the nephrectomy and acknowledging the appropriate verbal and written information.

Unrelated living kidney donors

Acceptability of donors

A living organ donation program requires great care to ensure that donation is totally altruistic, without coercion or reward. Permission from the local ethical committee has to be obtained in some countries, while in other countries it is necessary to obtain permission from the court. Clearly defined protocols of investigation and management are essential, and such transplants should not be carried out in centers where they constitute only an occasional event (43).

The use of highly motivated, but unrelated, living donors, such as spouses, unmarried life-long partners, step-parents, or even close friends, is becoming more widely accepted, and graft-survival rates obtained are comparable with those of living related kidney donors and superior to cadaver kidney grafts (44).

Cadaver donation

For kidney transplantation to become an integral part of ERSD treatment, a high and sufficient number of cadaver donors are necessary. This requires a combined effort from society, healthcare authorities, the medical profession, and transplant physicians. It is the responsibility of society to establish broad public readiness to donate organs. It is the responsibility of the healthcare authorities to provide the logistic background for available organs to be used for transplantation under any circumstances. It is the responsibility of the medical profession to support organ donation by identifying potential donors at their specific sites in the hospitals, and to inform and support relatives of potential donors. The organization of organ procurement and retrieval should be separated from the transplantation unit to avoid conflicts of interest and to increase the trust of the public. Finally, a transparent and understandable organ-allocation scheme is a prerequisite for the trust of the public, aimed at reducing to a minimum the still high opposition rate to cadaver-organ retrieval expressed by families in many countries.

Contra-indications

The ideal kidney donor is a previously healthy individual aged 10–55 years, brain dead due to trauma or intracerebral bleeding, with no active infection, and with excellent organ function. There are several absolute and relative contra-indications to donation, the former to avoid transmitting pre-existing disease to the recipient and the latter to prevent poor function of the transplanted organ.

Donation is thus contra-indicated in the case of a previous or current history of cancer, except non-invasive brain tumors, non-melanoma, non-metastasizing skin tumors, and *in situ* cervical cancer. HIV-positive serology, or a history of activities with high risk for HIV infection, are contra-indications. The same applies for uncontrolled or untreated septicemia or septicemia of unknown origin. Hepatitis B-positive antigenemia is a contra-indication for hepatitis B-negative recipients (where negativity is defined as HBsAg-negative or HBsAg antibody-negative). However, hepatitis B-positive antigenemia is not a contra-indication for HBsAg-positive recipients (45).

The lack of kidney donors implies a need to extend the limits of the relative contra-indications in order to accept kidneys with less than optimal function. Sub-optimal kidney grafts should not be given to young recipients but, preferably, to elderly patients with a shorter life-expectancy, who express a preference and provide informed consent for a sub-optimal donor kidney as an alternative to prolonged dialysis. In some countries, special programs are dedicated to such donors and recipients, such as the Eurotransplant senior program (ESP).

Donor's medical history

In most European countries, the proportion of donors with intra-cranial bleeding as cause of death has increased, together with donors' age. Cause of death (cerebral vascular disease or trauma) and current medication are key questions. The most detrimental disease in the donor is severe vascular disease, with a possible reduction of renal function as a consequence of arteriosclerosis and nephrosclerosis.

Renal function

The potential donor's history of creatinine (SCr) and the level at admission, indicate the baseline donor renal function. The acute situation of hypotension caused by dilatation of the vascular bed as a consequence of brain death, may lead to (frequently reversible) deterioration in donor renal function.

A reduced creatinine clearance (CrCl) in the range of 60 ml/min would indicate a sub-optimal donor predictive of an inferior graft function. Donor kidneys with functional levels below this range should not be used, or should be considered for transplantation as a pair in the same recipient with the objective of reaching acceptable results. Dual transplantation of kidneys is a novel procedure used to increase the transplanted nephron mass (46).

Donor age

Renal function decreases with increasing age. It is therefore not surprising that donor age is one of the strongest factors affecting outcome after renal transplantation (47, 48). Living donor renal transplantation with highly selected older donors aged over 70 is quite successful. It is therefore difficult to set an absolute age limit without the risk of loosing some grafts with good potential. When evaluating elderly potential donors, especially those aged over 70, it is very important that risk factors other than age are absent or minimal.

In the Scandinavian countries, the median donor age is approaching 60 years and occasionally donors over the age of 70 are accepted. Within Eurotransplant, donors over the age of 65 are now accepted but almost all are used for recipients over the age of 65 without any HLA-matching and with ischemia times as short as possible. This has been suggested elsewhere too (49).

Risk of infection

The potential donor should be tested for HIV, hepatitis B and C, and CMV. Hepatitis B-positive donors may be accepted for transplantation to seropositive recipients. Hepatitis C-positive donors may be accepted for seropositive recipients if the PCR for HCV is also positive (50).

The donor should also be tested for cytomegalovirus (CMV) serology. The high probability of transferring CMV *de novo* or inducing CMV recurrence has led to the selection of recipients with CMV compatibility, if possible. With recent improvements in CMV prophylaxis, the importance of CMV compatibility has been reduced.

Epstein-Barr virus (EBV) is also tested for, since there is a substantial risk for a lymphoproliferative disorder following a primary infection. This is a threat for pediatric recipients.

Bacterial infections are commonly seen during long periods in the intensive care unit. Appropriate antibiotic treatment should ideally be given before organ retrieval, and then subsequently to the recipient for approximately 3–5 days. It has been documented that the outcome of recipients and grafts from bacteremic donors are comparable to non-bacteremic donors (51).

Risk of cancer

A cancer may be transmitted to a recipient from a donor who has had a malignancy in the past. It may also be transmitted if a malignancy is found during the retrieval operation, or when intra-cranial malignancy is the cause of death. Autopsy should always be encouraged, following organ retrieval, to check for unsuspected diagnoses of malignancy.

Non-heart-beating donors

Due to severe donor shortage in several countries, programs have been developed to make use of the organs of patients who have died under resuscitation or other clinical circumstances. In these donors, with a confirmed complete circulatory arrest for a defined period of time (by definition: non-heart-beating donors), *in situ* cooling starts by transfemoral intra-aortic infusion of preservation fluid for 60 min or even more. During this time, consent of the relatives is obtained for organ harvesting. By this procedure, around 90% viable kidneys can be harvested. Some centers have re-introduced the kidney-preservation machine with pulsatile organ perfusion during the cold ischemia time. This allows testing for the viability of the organs (52).

Who should get the graft? The complicated issue of organ allocation

Allocation

Due to the organ shortage in almost all the countries with active transplant programs, organ allocation has become a topic of utmost importance. There are two levels of conflict. The first concerns the conflict between utility and justice. The second concerns the conflict between individual demands and the interests of centers or physicians (see also Chapter 10). Although there are different solutions from country to country, in essence the basic principles are to develop a system that is able to balance the most important viewpoints on utility and equity or justice. The basic ethical considerations have been well described (53). The principle of utility aims for the best use of the scarce resource by trying to achieve the longest function of a given graft. The principle of equity or justice takes into consideration the situation of the individual. Factors here are the intensity of suffering and disease, the time lapsed in waiting for an organ, the risk of early death without a transplant, the fairness against minorities. To balance both principles, organ-allocation algorithms have been developed. The most elegant approach has been described by Wuijciak and Opelz (54).

How to get and maintain optimal results?

Optimizing techniques and treatment protocols pre-, peri-, and post-operatively

The decision to dialyze a patient immediately before transplantation depends on several factors such as: timing of the last dialysis, clinical assessment of volume status by clinical examination, and serum electrolyte levels, particularly potassium.

Pre-operative dialysis is recommended for patients with heart failure or over-hydration to correct volume abnormalities. To avoid the danger of intra-operative or post-operative hyperkalemia, dialysis is recommended before transplantation in patients with serum potassium greater than 5.5–6.0 mEq/l. To dialyze routinely is not recommended.

Donor risk factors for delayed graft function include cold ischemia time, older-age donor, and hypotension. Recipient risk factors for delayed graft function include hypovolemia and hypotension during and after surgery. Prolonged cold ischemia time and hypovolemia have been considered as classical risk factors for the development of delayed graft function (55, 56).

Basic prophylactic immunosuppression

Prophylactic immunosuppression consisted of corticosteroids in combination with azathioprine from 1962 to 1983. This combination was called later 'conventional immunosuppressive treatment', which could yield up to 65% graft survival at 1 year.

Cyclosporine A was introduced in 1983. Comparisons between cyclosporine A plus steroids with conventional therapy showed a dramatic improvement in 1-year graft survival, but also a better patient survival at 1 year.

For more than a decade, cyclosporine A has been the gold standard for immuno-suppression in association with low dose azathioprine and corticosteroids in the so-called 'triple therapy'. This triple therapy was used by more than 90% of the transplant centers over Europe with or without 'induction therapy'. Protocols without azathioprine, or even with cyclosporine monotherapy, have also been used.

Patient mortality in renal transplantation has been dramatically reduced to a few per cent in the first year (usually less than 2%) and 15–20% at 10 years. Graft survival has improved by about 15–20% during the first year and this advantage is maintained during the first decade. The actuarial graft-survival figures commonly obtained are 80–85% at 1 year, 70–75% at 5 years, and 50–55% at 10 years. Renal and vascular toxicity of cyclosporine A could be reduced by close monitoring of trough levels of cyclosporine A in the recipients. In addition, it was possible to stop steroids after 1 year without significant harmful effects (57). It was even possible to stop azathioprine deliberately or for poor hematological tolerance, or because of viral liver disease (chronic active hepatitis due HBV or HCV). Thus a fair proportion of recipients are now treated with cyclosporine A monotherapy (58).

The persistent problems with cyclosporine-based treatment are functional vaso-constrictive toxicity, as demonstrated by the high frequency of arterial hypertension under cyclosporine A in about 70–90% of recipients, and renal toxicity, demonstrated by higher serum creatinine and less optimal renal function compared with conventional therapy. This toxicity is not always reflected in the trough levels and pharmacokinetic curves are often needed. The long-term loss of grafted kidneys due to chronic deterioration of renal function has not been significantly modified by cyclosporine A. The annual loss is about 4% of functioning kidneys, and is due to 'chronic rejection' or chronic allograft nephropathy, a combination of immunological and non-immunological causes (see below). However, the overall transplant results and the half-life have improved from year to year under cyclosporine A.

Since 1995/1996, new drugs such as mycophenolate mofetil (MMF) and tacrolimus (FK 506) have been introduced. These drugs demonstrate a reduced incidence of acute rejection in the first year, but as yet it is too early to show any significant prolongation of graft survival over the long-term. Different combinations have been proposed with lower doses of cyclosporine A to reduce vascular and renal toxicity. However, data on the medium- and long-term safety of such cyclosporine-sparing regimens, including their influence on the occurrence of viral infections and *de novo* malignancies, are not yet available and therefore firm recommendations cannot be made at this point in time (59).

Induction therapy

Background

Induction therapy is defined as prophylactic immunosuppression by use of biological agents, started at the time of surgery and given, in addition to maintenance immuno-suppression, for a few days or weeks to induce better acceptance of the allograft. The attempt to use antibodies directed against lymphocytes or subpopulations was started in the 1960s. In open trials, improvements were observed in early graft survival, although at that time product safety and reproducibility was very poor. Prospective randomized trials on induction therapy were not performed until the early 1980s (60). The main goal of induction therapy is to reduce the number and the severity of acute rejections during the first 3–6 months post-transplant. However, this reduction does not always produce improved 1–3 years graft survival rates (61). This goal became relative in view of advances made in the use of the available basic immunosuppressive therapy. Induction therapy coincided for a long time with the risk of over-immunosuppression, in particular CMV disease and post-transplant lymphoproliferative disorders (PTLD) (62).

Most of the polyclonal antibodies marketed are anti-thymocyte globulins (ATG), which have significant differences in terms of target epitopes on the surface of activated T-lymphocytes between different preparations, and show variability between batches. The only preparation of monoclonal antibodies currently used for induction therapy is a muromonab-CD3 called OKT3 with a highly specific target: the CD3 molecule of the T-cell receptor. The murine mAb induces internalization of T-cell receptors and blocks lymphocyte activation. The preparation is administered as a direct intravenous injection of 5 mg every day usually for 7–14 days. Lower doses of OKT3 have been used (2.5 mg/d) with equivalent results (63).

Recently, two new monoclonal antibodies directed against the CD25 (high affinity IL2-receptor) molecule have obtained licenses, both in the USA and Europe, and may facilitate a 'modern induction' therapy. Basiliximab is a chimeric human/murine ant body directed against the alpha chain of the interleukin-2 receptor, which is up-regulated in activated T lymphocytes. The treatment consists of two IV infusions of 20 mg, one before surgery and one on day 4 post-transplantation (64). Daclizumab is a fully humanized monoclonal antibody and is also directed against the alpha chain (also called Tac protein or 55 kd subunit or CD25) of the high-affinity IL2 receptor. The treatment consists of 5 IV infusions administered before surgery and sub sequently every 2 weeks (65).

Sensitized recipients and induction therapy

Although induction therapy was often recommended in sensitized patients and re-transplants, the number of studies addressing this question is scarce.

Delayed graft function (DGF) and induction therapy

A beneficial, but only recently proven, effect should be the use of induction therapy in patients with delayed graft function. The rationale rests on the finding that DGF is often not only caused by ischemic damage but by immunological injury as well. A controlled trial on this issue involved 52 patients with immediate function versus 31 patients with DGF treated with ATG. The number of rejections was clearly reduced in the DGF group with an excellent 1-year graft-survival rate (93%), albeit lower than in the subgroup with immediate function (98%) (66).

Rejection therapy

For the treatment of the first acute cellular rejection episode, high doses of intravenous methylprednisolone are recommended. This treatment is expected to reverse most acute rejection episodes (67). Although the use of ATG/ALG or OKT3 as first-line therapy is effective, their adverse-event profile and cost mean that the use of corticosteroids, as first-line therapy, is preferred, whereas ATG/ALG or OKT3 are recommended for the treatment of severe acute rejection episodes (Banff grade III), recurrent acute rejection episodes, steroid-resistant rejection episodes, or in patients with contra-indications to corticosteroids (68).

ALG/ATG is preferable to OKT3 for the treatment of acute rejection episodes. Although both preparations are effective in reversing such episodes, OKT3 has a slightly poorer adverse-event profile because of the first-dose effect.

In patients with recurrent rejection after anti-T-lymphocyte antibody treatment, it is recommended to modify baseline immunosuppression, e.g. to change from cyclosporine to tacrolimus. In one study of patients with refractory rejection while on CsA maintenance treatment, CsA was discontinued and replaced by tacrolimus. Graft function improved in 78% of patients, stabilized in 11%, and showed progressive deterioration in 11% after the change of treatment (69).

Assessment of rejection therapy outcome

It has been proposed that a successful response to therapy is defined as a relative serum creatinine concentration value that is less than 110% of the day 0 (or rejection) creatinine level, and returns to the day 0 creatinine or lower during the first 5 days of therapy (70). Therapy success is best reflected by relative changes in the serum creatinine concentration, rather than by absolute levels, probably because the latter depend more on the severity of the rejection and the time of diagnosis than on the efficacy of therapy.

The Efficacy Endpoints Database Group has defined corticosteroid-resistant rejection as an acute rejection episode that has been treated only with 250–1000 mg of methylprednisolone and where the serum creatinine concentration increases as early as the third day of therapy, and continues to rise unless treated with a different anti-rejection therapy. It is important to emphasize that the assessment of corticosteroid-resistance is a clinical one. Renal biopsies taken after initial corticosteroid treatment overestimate the incidence of corticosteroid resistance, as shown in a recent study in which patients with a steroid-responsive acute rejection episode displayed histopathological signs of acute rejection in 60% of biopsies taken 5 days after therapy and in 27% of biopsies taken 10 days after therapy (71).

Treatment of acute rejection episodes refractory to standard therapy

The initial approach in the treatment of steroid-resistant rejection episodes is to switch to anti-T-lymphocyte preparations. However, in a minority of patients, repeat therapy with anti-T-cell antibody preparations does not provide an optimal solution while they continue to experience rejection refractory to standard therapy with corticosteroids.

Both polyclonal and monoclonal anti-T-lymphocyte preparations are usually successful in reversing acute uncomplicated, as well as corticosteroid-resistant, acute rejection episodes. Retrospective comparisons of OKT3 with polyclonal rabbit ATG have suggested either that both preparations are equally effective (72), that polyclonal antisera are more effective (73), or that OKT3 monoclonal is more effective, especially in treating episodes of acute vascular rejection (74). There is a consensus that the use of OKT3 is associated with more side-effects, especially those related to the cytokine release syndrome.

Long-term care and outcome—avoiding re-transplants

Impaired transplant function frequently complicates the initial post-transplant period. The differential diagnosis is extensive, evolves over the first several post-transplant days, and is best understood in the context of the timing of its occurrence. Early non-function with little or no urine output during the intra-operative, or very early post-operative period, principally reflects pre-transplant events that have compromised the quality of the donor organ, pre-existing unrecognized recipient immunity against donor tissue, or complications of the transplant surgery itself. Decreases in renal function that begin later during the initial transplant hospitalization, typically on or after the third post-operative day, most commonly result from anamnestic or *de novo* immunological responses by the recipient against donor antigen, or from the nephrotoxic side-effects of some of the immunosuppressive medications themselves.

The differential diagnosis of early non-function

Hyperacute rejection occurs when a kidney is transplanted into a recipient with pre-formed cytotoxic antibodies against donor class I (or, more rarely, class II) HLA antigens. The advent of modern cross-matching techniques has greatly diminished the incidence of hyperacute rejection. Oliguria, following a period of initially adequate renal function, frequently occurs during the first 24h due to hypovolemia as a consequence of dehydration, especially among patients who are vigorously dialyzed prior to surgery, and to interstitial sequestration of fluids due to the surgery itself (75). Occasionally, there is no graft function because of kinking of the renal artery. If this is the case, the graft should be repositioned as early as possible.

Acute tubular necrosis (ATN) is the commonest cause of delayed graft function. ATN is caused by donor conditions (pre-existing hypertension, hypotension, hypo volemia, vasopressors), by ischemic injury during preservation time (cold ischemia times >24h), and by warm ischemia time in case of extended surgery and repeated cross-clamping. The viability should be monitored by color-coded ultrasound Doppler and, because of the higher risk of rejection, an early biopsy is recommended. ATN carries a risk for sub-optimal long-term function (76).

Hematuria is an expected consequence of ureteral implantation. It may lead to clot formation and obstruction of the obligatory in-dwelling urethral catheter. Catheter obstruction can increase intraluminal pressure within the bladder, thereby threatening the ureteral anastomosis. Declining urine production may also create a false impression of rejection or acute tubular necrosis.

Urological complications (ureteral necrosis, hematomas, lymphoceles) develop in 5–15% of transplanted kidneys and contribute significantly to post-transplant morbidity. On the other hand, advances in surgical technique have made early complications, due to failed vascular anastomoses, rare.

Accelerated rejection occurs within the first 2–5 post-transplant days, a time-frame that may be too brief to allow the development of *de novo* reactions to donor antigens. This form of rejection is postulated to represent an anamnestic response to donor antigens resulting from prior sensitization. Accelerated rejection may be mediated by cytotoxic T lymphocytes, antibodies, or both, and is often associated with vasculitis or T-lymphocyte infiltration of the renal vessels.

Differential diagnosis of graft dysfunction within the first weeks

Acute rejection

Acute-rejection episodes are the main cause of graft dysfunction in the first post-transplant year. Although rejection episodes may occur at any time, they are most commonly observed during the initial 6 post-transplant months.

The introduction of new immunosuppressive drugs, such as cyclosporine A micro-emulsion (CyA-ME), tacrolimus, mycophenolate mofetil, and genetically engineered human monoclonal antibodies, have significantly decreased the incidence of acute rejection in various randomized trials, and 1-year cumulative biopsy-proven rejection frequencies of 17% have been reported (77). It is important to realize that the patients who are entered into randomized trials, usually undergo selection and high-risk patients are often not included. Therefore, it remains to be seen what the acute rejection rates will actually amount to in unselected patient populations.

Nephrotoxicity of calcineurin inhibitors

Cyclosporine A and tacrolimus cause a dose-related afferent arteriolar vasoconstriction and a decrease in glomerular filtration rate. Thrombotic microangiopathy is the cause of renal-graft dysfunction in about 15% of renal-transplant patients on CyA-ME (78) and is characterized by fibrin thrombi, focal necrosis, and mesangiolysis in association with occlusive cellular proliferation of the arterioles. Only a minority of patients with thrombotic microangiopathy have systemic evidence of the hemolytic syndrome. Chronic cyclosporine A nephropathy is characterized by striped tubulo-interstitial fibrosis, with or without degenerative hyaline changes in the walls of afferent arterioles (79). Cyclosporine and tacrolimus appear to be equally nephrotoxic. In both the USA and the European multi-center trials, no difference in renal function between the treatment arms was seen (80). Calcineurin nephrotoxicity can occur concomitantly with acute cellular rejection and acute tubular necrosis.

Most transplant programs monitor cyclosporine A and tacrolimus by measuring blood trough concentrations on a regular basis. Such blood levels are useful but imprecise indicators of immunosuppression or drug toxicity. While whole-blood trough concentrations are often higher in patients suffering from toxicity than in patients suffering from rejection, they may not differ significantly from those of patients with stable function. Indeed, there is considerable overlap between groups, wide intra-patient and inter-patient variability in the area under the time–concentration curve (a measure of drug exposure), and the peak and trough blood concentrations generated by any given dosage of either agent.

Urinary tract infections

Urinary tract infections are common after transplantation (81). The frequency depends on the patient's pre-transplant urinary tract condition (82). Fever, enlargement of the transplanted kidney, and tenderness of the surrounding tissues may result from pyelonephritis. Elevations in plasma creatinine, as a result of a urinary tract infection, are usually modest and oliguria should not ensue. A new and important threat for the grafts is the increasing frequency of ureter and graft infection by polyoma viruses (83).

Differential diagnosis of late progressive graft deterioration

Kidney allografts need long-term surveillance because of several immunological and non-immunological factors that affect graft function and may lead to graft loss. As native kidneys, grafts experience a loss of GFR with time and ageing. However, in general, the slope of the reciprocal values of creatinine (1/creatinine) curve is much steeper than in native kidneys. Therefore, all attempts have to be made to keep the graft's function stable for as long as possible. For in-depth information, there is a consensus protocol for long-term surveillance written by the USA transplant physicians (84). The differential diagnosis of progressive graft deterioration is difficult because of the overlapping, or similar, symptoms and signs caused by different entities given in Table 3.3 (85).

Entities

The profile of chronic allograft nephropathy is a mixture of pre-existing graft damage originating in the age and/or illnesses of the donor (hypertension, diabetes mellitus, etc.), damages that have occurred during the transplantation (ischemia, toxicity), or due to the allo-immune reaction (acute rejection, subclinical acute rejection, chronic rejection) and damages from the treatment, such as toxicity of immunosuppressive drugs or persistence in the patient of hypertension, hyperlipidemia, macrovascular disease, or infection. After the first post-transplant year, recurrence of the original disease plays an additional role. (see Fig. 3.2)

Table 3.3 Risk factors for renal graft loss

Quality of the graft		Immunological factors Immune injury/stress	Load Post-transplant stress
Pre-transplant injuries	Peri-transplant injuries		
Age	Brain death	PRA	Size match
Hypertension	Type of brain death	HLA match	Hypertension
Vascular disease	ICU measures	Immunosuppression	Drug toxicity
Genetic factors	Harvesting	Acute rejection	Recurrent disease
Diabetes mellitus	Preservation (time) Reperfusion	Drug compliance	Lipid disorders Donor CMV positive Post-transplant diabetes mell.

Adopted from (ref. 85).

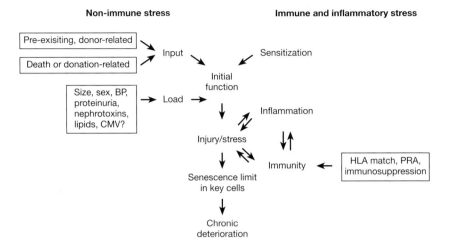

Fig. 3.2 Factors involved in kidney graft deterioration (taken from ref. 85).

Long-term patient survival: avoiding early death and morbidity

Mortality

Although the patients' survival has improved significantly there is still an unacceptable excess mortality in graft recipients compared with that of the general population. This increased risk is partially due to the past history of the patient, but renal transplantation and its treatment add additional factors, which may impair the life-expectancy of the recipient. According to data collected in several National and International Registries, almost 50% of the deaths are of cardiovascular causes, such as coronary artery disease with myocardial infarction, sudden death, and chronic heart failure. Infections rank as second cause of death, which include bacterial and viral diseases such as CMV and viral hepatitis. Of concern is that malignancies account for about 15% of recipients' deaths. The risk of developing some kind of malignancy after transplantation reaches 10–15% after 10 years and 25% after 20 years. Except for post-transplant lymphoproliferative disorders, and for skin malignancies, the risk of developing cancer is around three-fold that found in the non-transplanted population (86).

Prophylactic measures

Most of the therapeutic interventions implemented to reduce mortality are similar to those indicated to keep the graft function stable: to avoid or control all cardiovascular risk factors, such as hypertension, hyperlipidemia, diabetes mellitus, increased body mass index, and hyperparathyroidism. To keep these factors adequately controlled in the long run is much more difficult than merely transplanting a kidney.

To ease these attempts, adaptations of the negative impact of some drugs have to be considered, such as stopping steroids, avoiding calcineurin inhibitors, which may increase blood pressure and serum lipids. This may be of help but the mainstay is the sustained tight surveillance and permanent education of the patient.

Outcome information basis

The success and long-term graft and patient survival in kidney transplantation have significantly improved over the last two decades. Whereas in the 1980s the major improvement was to raise the 1-year graft and patient survival without influence on long-term outcome, now it turns out that the graft half-lives (the time that it takes to loose 50% of the grafts) do improve too. It is not easy to give unequivocal results, because data have to be very carefully analyzed on the basis of case mix, the number of elderly recipients, diabetics, and other influencing circumstances. Nowadays, well-performing information instruments are available. The data thus generated provide an optimal background for evidence-based decision-making and for informing patients objectively. Specific sites are listed in Table 3.4.

Economic impact of transplantation

Economic considerations

On first approach, kidney transplantation is the most cost-saving treatment modality for end-stage renal failure. However, the calculation and the factors involved in the cost of organ transplantation are much more diverse and complicated than generally expected. Kidney transplantation in a capitated environment, and in the times of managed care and DRGs, has to change previously used habits in order to reduce the

Table 3.4 Transplantation registries, organ exchange organisations and data bases

US Transplant Patient Data Source	http://www.patients.unos.org/tpd/
US Renal Registry	http://www.usrds.org/
UK Renal Registry	http://www.renalreg.com/
UK Transplantation Society	http://www.jr2.ox.ac.uk/bts/
Canadian Institute for Health Information	http://www.cihi.ca/eindex.htm
German Renal Registry	http://www.quasi-niere.de/world_d.htm
Swiss Transplant Organisation	http:// www.swisstransplant.org/
French Transplant Organisation	http:// www.france-transplant.com/
Australian and New Zealand Dialysis and Transplant Registry	http:// www.anzdata.org.au/
Collaborative Transplant Study	http://cts.med.uni-heidelberg.de/
Eurotransplant Foundation	http://www.transplant.org/

expenses by better standards and organizational measures. Key words, as 'the clinical transplant path', and intensified outpatient care, need consideration. Some special aspects of cost containment are addressed below.

Costs of pre-transplant work-up

The above-mentioned pre-transplant work-up is expensive—and if it turns out that the patient cannot be transplanted, it is spent uselessly. There have been suggestions, based on the experience of a great number of work-ups, to focus on the critical cardiovascular points before starting in-depth evaluation (87).

Hospital costs

Attempts have been made to reduce tremendously hospital costs and length of hospital stay. Whereas in most European countries the length of stay in hospital, post-transplantation, is between 12 and 21 days, the U.S. and Canada have achieved stays of less than 6 days. A prerequisite therefore is a well-organized out patient (intensified) care (88).

Costs of immunosuppression

The new immunosuppressive agents are more costly than standard immunosuppression or cyclosporine-based immunosuppression. Pharmaco–economic studies have shown that the reduction in the number of rejections and the reduction of the re-admittance rate, may balance these higher costs due to the reduction of the hospital re-admittance rate (89).

Costs of marginal grafts—critical donors

Special attention is required in the use of aged or marginal donor kidneys, which carry a much higher risk of delayed or impaired graft function resulting in prolonged hospitalization.

References

1. van Rood, J.J. (1969). Tissue typing and organ transplantation. *Lancet*, **1**, (7606), 1142–6.
2. McMillan, M.A. and Briggs, J.D. (1995). Survey of patient selection for cadaveric renal transplantation in the United Kingdom. *Nephrology Dialysis Transplantation*, **10**, (6), 855–8.
3. Curtoni, E.S., Magistroni, P., Fasano, M.E., Pratico, L., and Roggero, S. (1999). Waiting list for kidney transplant. Some patients wait too long. *Journal of Biological Regulators and Homeostatic Agents*, **13**, (1), 37–41.
4. Vats, A.N., Donaldson, L., Fine, R.N., and Chavers, B.M. (2000). Pretransplant dialysis status and outcome of renal transplantation in North American children: a NAPRTCS Study. North American Pediatric Renal Transplant Cooperative Study. *Transplantation*, **69**, (7), 1414–9.

5. Bentdal, O.H., Leivestad, T., Fauchald, P., Albrechtsen, D, Pfeffer, P., Lien, B., Foss, A., Oyen, O., Hartmann, A., Nordal, K., Sodal, G., Flatmark, A., Thorsby, E., and Brekke, I.B. (1998). The national kidney transplant program in Norway still results in unchanged waiting lists. *Clinical Transplants*, 221–8.

6. Frei, U. and Schober-Halstenberg, H.J. (1999). Annual Report of the German Renal Registry 1998. QuaSi-Niere Task Group for Quality Assurance in Renal Replacement Therapy. *Nephrology Dialysis Transplantation*, **14**, (5), 1085–90.

7. Penn, I. (1997). Evaluation of transplant candidates with pre-existing malignancies. *Annals of Transplantation*, **2**, (4), 14–7.

8. Brinkman, K., Huysmans, F., and Burger, D.M. (1998). Pharmacokinetic interaction between saquinavir and cyclosporine [letter]. *Annals of Internal Medicine*, **129**, (11), 914–5.

9. Schwarz, A., Offermann, G., Keller, F., Bennhold, I., L'age-Stehr, J., Krausem, P.H., and Mihatsch, M.J. (1993). The effect of cyclosporine on the progression of human immunodeficiency virus type 1 infection transmitted by transplantation–data on four cases and review of the literature [see comments]. *Transplantation*, **55**, (1), 95–103.

10. Spital, A. (1998). Should all human immunodeficiency virus-infected patients with end-stage renal disease be excluded from transplantation? The views of U.S. transplant centers. *Transplantation*, **65**, (9), 1187–91.

11. Fritsche, L., Vanrenterghem, Y., Nordal, K.P., Grinyo, J.M., Moreso, F., Budde, K., Kunz, R., Meyerrose, B., and Neumayer, H.H. (2000). Practice variations in the evaluation of adult candidates for cadaveric kidney transplantation: a survey of the European Transplant Centers. *Transplantation*, **70**, (10), 1492–7.

12. Berthoux, F., Abramowicz, D., Bradley, B.A., Ekberg, H., Frei, U., Morales, J.M., Olgaard, K., Paul, C.L., and Ponticelli, C. (2000). European Best Practice Guidelines for Renal Transplantation (First part), *Nephrology Dialysis Transplantation*, **15**, (Suppl. 7), 3–85.

13. Herzog, C.A., Marwick, T.H., Pheley, A.M., White, C.W., Rao, V.K., and Dick, C.D. (1999). Dobutamine stress echocardiography for the detection of significant coronary artery disease in renal transplant candidates. *American Journal of Kidney Diseases*, **33**, (6), 1080–90.

14. Braun, W.E. and Marwick, T.H. (1994). Coronary artery disease in renal transplant recipients. *Cleveland Clinic Journal of Medicine*, **61**, (5), 370–85.

15. Jahangiri, M., Wright, J., Edmondson, S., and Magee, P. (1997). Coronary artery bypass graft surgery in dialysis patients. *Heart*, **78**, 343–5.

16. Le Feuvre, C., Dambrin, G., Helft, G., Tabet, S., Beygui, F., Legendre, C., Peraldi, M.N., Vacheron, A., and Metzger, J.P. (2000). Comparison of clinical outcome following coronary stenting or balloon angioplasty in dialysis versus non-dialysis patients. *American Journal of Cardiology*, **85**, (11), 1365–8.

17. Galazka, Z., Szmidt, J., Nazarewski, S., Grochowiecki, T., Swiercz, P., Bojakowska, M. and Lao, M. (1999). Kidney transplantation in recipients with atherosclerotic iliac vessels. *Annals of Transplantation*, **4**, (2), 43–4.

18. Barbagallo, C.M., Pinto, A., Gallo, S., Parrinello, G., Caputo, F., Sparacino, V., Cefalu, A.B., Novo, S., Licata, G., Notarbartolo, A., and Averna, M.R. (1999). Carotid atherosclerosis in renal transplant recipients: relationships with cardiovascular risk factors and plasma lipoproteins. *Transplantation*, **67**, (3), 366–71.

19. Kasiske, B.L. and Klinger, D. (2000). Cigarette smoking in renal transplant recipients. *Journal of the American Society of Nephrology*, **11**, (4), 753–9.

20. Lederman, E.D., McCoy, G., Conti, D.J., and Lee, E.C. (2000). Diverticulitis and polycystic kidney disease. *The American Surgeon*, **66**, (2), 200–3.

21. Morales, J.M. and Campistol, J.M. (2000). Transplantation in the patient with hepatitis C. *Journal of the American Society of Nephrology*, **11**(7), 1343–53.
22. Akoh, J.A., Choon, T.C., Akyol, M.A., Kyle, K., and Briggs, J.D. (1999). Outcome of renal transplantation in patients with lower urinary tract abnormality. *Journal of the Royal College of Surgeons (Edinburgh)*, **44**, (2), 78–81.
23. Gulanikar, A.C., Daily, P.P., Kilambi, N.K., Hamrick-Turner, J.E., and Butkus, D.E. (1998). Prospective pretransplant ultrasound screening in 206 patients for acquired renal cysts and renal cell carcinoma. *Transplantation*, **66**, (12), 1669–72.
24. Dantal, J., Baatard, R., Hourmant, M., Cantarovich, D., Buzelin, F., and Soulillou, J.P. (1991). Recurrent nephrotic syndrome following renal transplantation in patients with focal glomerulosclerosis. A one-center study of plasma exchange effects. *Transplantation*, **52**, 827–31.
25. Frohnert, P.P., Donadio, J.V., Jr., Velosa, J.A., Holley, K.E., and Sterioff, S. (1997). The fate of renal transplants in patients with IgA nephropathy. *Clinical Transplants*, **11**, 127–33.
26. Agarwal, A., Mauer, S.M., Matas, A.J., and Nath, K.A. (1995). Recurrent hemolytic uremic syndrome in an adult renal allograft recipient: current concepts and management. *Journal of the American Society of Nephrology*, **6**, 1160–9.
27. Conlon, P.J., Brennan, D.C., Pfaf, W.W., Finn, W.F., Gehr, T., Bollinger, R.R., and Smith, S.R. (1996). Renal transplantation in adults with thrombotic thrombocytopenic purpura/haemolytic-uraemic syndrome. *Nephrology Dialysis Transplantation*, **11**, 1810–4.
28. Hiesse, C., Bastuji-Garin, S., Santelli, G., Moulin, B., Cantarovich, M., Lantz, O., Charpentier, B., and Fries, D. (1989). Recurrent essential mixed cryoglobulinemia in renal allografts. Report of two cases and review of the literature. *American Journal of Nephrology*, **9**, 150–4.
29. Singh, N., Gayowski, T., and Marino, I.R. (1996). Hemolytic uremic syndrome in solid-organ transplant recipients. *Transplantation International*, **9**, 68–75.
30. Jamieson, N.V. (1998). The results of combined liver/kidney transplantation for primary hyperoxaluria (PH1) 1984–1997. The European PH1 transplant registry report. European PH1 Transplantation Study Group. *Journal of Nephrology*, **11**, (Suppl. 1), 36–41.
31. Hirschl, M.M. (1995). The patient with type II diabetes and uraemia—to transplant or not to transplant [editorial]. *Nephrology Dialysis Transplantation*, **10**, (9), 1515–6.
32. Wolfe, R.A., Ashby, V.B., Milford, E.L., Ojo, A.O., Ettenger, R.E., Agodoa, L.Y., Held, P.J., and Port, F.K. (1999). Comparison of mortality in all patients on dialysis, patients on dialysis awaiting transplantation, and recipients of a first cadaveric transplant [see comments]. *The New England Journal of Medicine*, **341**, (23), 1725–30.
33. Herzog, C.A., Ma, J.Z., and Collins, A.J. (1998). Poor long-term survival after acute myocardial infarction among patients on long-term dialysis [see comments]. *The New England Journal of Medicine*, **339**, (12), 799–805.
34. Manske, C.L., Wilson, R.F., Wang, Y., and Thomas, W. (1997). Atherosclerotic vascular complications in diabetic transplant candidates. *American Journal of Kidney Diseases*, **29**, (4), 601–7.
35. Reis, G., Marcovitz, P.A., Leichtman, A.B., Merion, R.M., Fay, W.P., Werns, S.W., and Armstrong, W.F. (1995). Usefulness of dobutamine stress echocardiography in detecting coronary artery disease in end-stage renal disease. *American Journal of Cardiology*, **75**, (10), 707–10.
36. Kerman, R.H. (2000). Immunogenetics, histocompatibility, and crossmatching for kidney transplantation. In: Kahan, B.D., Ponticelli, C. eds. Principles and practice of renal transplantation. London: Martin Dunitz, 1–39.

37. Gebel, H.M. and Bray, R.A. (2000). Sensitization and sensitivity: defining the unsensitized patient. *Transplantation*, **69**, (7), 1370–4.

38. USRDS Annual Data Report 2000. http//www.usrds.org/adr.htm-7–8–2000.

39. Norden, G., Lennerling, A., and Nyberg, G. (2000). Low absolute glomerular filtration rate in the living kidney donor: a risk factor for graft loss [In Process Citation]. *Transplantation*, **70**, (9), 1360–2.

40. Johnson, E.M., Remucal, M.J., Gillingham, K.J., Dahms, R.A., Najarian, J.S., and Matas, A.J. (1997). Complications and risks of living donor nephrectomy. *Transplantation*, **64**, (8), 1124–8.

41. Fehrman-Ekholm, I., Elinder, C.G., Stenbeck, M., Tyden, G., and Groth, C.G. (1997). Kidney donors live longer. *Transplantation*, **64**, (7), 976–8.

42. Johnson, E.M., Anderson, J.K., Jacobs, C., Suh, G., Humar, A., Suhr, B.D., Kerr, S.R., and Matas, A.J. (1999). Long-term follow-up of living kidney donors: quality of life after donation. *Transplantation*, **67**, (5), 717–21.

43. Kasiske, B.L. and Bia, M.J. (1995). The evaluation and selection of living kidney donors. *American Journal of Kidney Disease*, **26**, 387–98.

44. Terasaki, P.I., Cecka, J.M., Gjertson, D.W., and Takemoto, S. (1995). High survival rates of kidney transplants from spousal and living unrelated donors [see comments]. *The New England Journal of Medicine*, **333**, 333–6.

45. Bedrossian, J., Akposso, K., Metivier, F., Moal, M.C., Pruna, A., and Idatte, J.M. (1993). Kidney transplantations with HBsAg+ donors. *Transplant Proceedings*, **25**, 1481–2.

46. Dietl, K.H., Wolters, H., Marschall, B., Senninger, N., and Heidenreich, S. (2000). Cadaveric 'two-in-one' kidney transplantation from marginal donors: experience of 26 cases after 3 years. *Transplantation*, **70**, (5), 790–4.

47. Gaber, L.W., Moore, L.W., Alloway, R.R., Amiri, M.H., Vera, S.R., and Gaber, A.O. (1995). Glomerulosclerosis as a determinant of posttransplant function of older donor renal allografts. *Transplantation*, **60**, 334–9.

48. Karpinski, J., Lajoie, G., Cattran, D., Fenton, S., Zaltzman, J., Cardella, C., and Cole, E. (1999). Outcome of kidney transplantation from high-risk donors is determined by both structure and function. *Transplantation*, **67**, (8), 1162–7.

49. Gjertson, D.W., Terasaki, P.I., Cecka, J.M., Takemoto, S., Cho, Y.W. (1997). Senior citizens pool for aged kidneys. *Transplantation Proceedings*, **29**, (1–2), 129.

50. Ali, M.K., Light, J.A., Barhyte, D.Y., Sasaki, T.M., Currier, C.B.J., Grandas, O., and Fowlkes, D. (1998). Donor hepatitis C virus status does not adversely affect short-term outcomes in HCV+ recipients in renal transplantation. *Transplantation*, **66**, (12), 1694–7.

51. Freeman, R.B., Giatras, I., Falagas, M.E., Supran, S., O'Connor, K., Bradley, J., Snydman, D.R., and Delmonico, F.L. (1999). Outcome of transplantation of organs procured from bacteremic donors. *Transplantation*, **68**, (8), 1107–11.

52. Balupuri, S., Buckley, P., Mohamed, M., Cornell, C., Mantle, D., Kirby, J., Manas, D.M., and Talbot, D. (2000). Assessment of non-heart-beating donor (NHBD) kidneys for viability on machine perfusion. *Clinical Chemistry and Laboratory Medicine*, **38**, (11), 1103–6.

53. Dossetor, J.B. (1988). Ethical issues in organ allocation. *Transplant Proceedings*, **20**, (Suppl. 1), 1053–58.

54. Wujciak, T. and Opelz, G. (1993). A proposal for improved cadaver kidney allocation. *Transplantation*, **56**, 1513–7.

55. Lee, C.M., Carter, J.T., Randall, H.B., Hiose, R., Stock, P.G., Melzer, J.S., Dafoe, D.C., Freise, C.E., and Alfrey, E.J. (2000). The effect of age and prolonged cold ischemia times on the national allocation of cadaveric renal allografts. *Journal of Surgical Research*, **91**, (1), 83–8.

56. Shoskes, D.A. and Halloran, P.F. (1996). Delayed graft function in renal transplantation: etiology, management and long-term significance. *Journal of Urology*, **155**, (6), 1831–40.
57. Ponticelli, C. and Opelz, G. (1995). Are corticosteroids really necessary in renal transplantation? *Nephrology Dialysis Transplantation*, **10**, (9), 1587–91.
58. Ponticelli, C., Tarantino, A., Segoloni, G.P., Cambi, V., Rizzo, G., Altieri, P., Mastrangelo, F., Castagneto, M., Salvadori, M., Valente, U., Cossu, M., Frederico, S., Pisani, F., Montagnino, G., Messina, M., Arisi, L., Carmellini, M., Piredda, G. and Corbetta, G. (1997). A randomized study comparing cyclosporine alone vs double and triple therapy in renal transplants. *Transplantation Proceedings*, **29**, 290–1.
59. Denton, M.D., Magee, C.C., and Sayegh, M.H. (1999). Immunosuppressive strategies in transplantation. *Lancet*, **353**, 1083–91.
60. Schroeder, T.J., Moore, L.W., Gaber, L.W., Gaber, A.O., and First, M.R. (1999). The US multicenter double-blind, randomized, phase III trial of thymoglobulin versus atgam in the treatment of acute graft rejection episodes following renal transplantation: rationale for study design. *Transplantation Proceedings*, **31**, (Suppl. 3B), 1S–6S.
61. Szczech, L.A. and Feldman, H.I. (1999). Effect of anti-lymphocyte antibody induction therapy on renal allograft survival. *Transplantation Proceedings c*, **31**, (Suppl. 3B), 9S–11S.
62. Opelz, G. and Henderson, R. (1993). Incidence of non-Hodgkin lymphoma in kidney and heart transplant recipients. *Lancet*, **342**, 1514–6.
63. Oh, H.K., Provenzano, R., Tayeb, J., Satmary, N., and Jones, B. (1998). Two low-dose OKT3 induction regimens following renal transplantation—clinical experience at a single center. *Clinical Transplants*, **12**, (4), 343–7.
64. Nashan, B., Moore, R., Amlot, P., Schmidt, A.G., Abeywickrama, K., and Soulillou, J.P. (1997). Randomised trial of basiliximab versus placebo for control of acute cellular rejection in renal allograft recipients. CHIB 201 International Study Group [published erratum appears in *Lancet* (1997), Nov 15, **350**, (9089), 1484]. *Lancet*, **350**, 1193–8.
65. Ekberg, H., Backman, L., Tufveson, G., Tyden, G., Nashan, B., and Vincenti, F. (2000). Daclizumab prevents acute rejection and improves patient survival post transplantation: 1 year pooled analysis. *Transplantation International*, **13**, (2), 151–9.
66. Lange, H., Muller, T.F., Ebel, H., Kuhlmann, U., Grebe, S.O., Heymanns, J., Feiber, H., and Reidmiller, H. (1999). Immediate and long-term results of ATG induction therapy for delayed graft function compared to conventional therapy for immediate graft function. *Transplantation International*, **12**, (1), 2–9.
67. Mazzucchi, E., Lucon, A.M., Nahas, W.C., Neto, E.D., Saldanha, L.B., Sabbaga, E., Ianhez, L.E., and Arap, S. (1999). Histological outcome of acute cellular rejection in kidney transplantation after treatment with methylprednisolone. *Transplantation*, **67**, (3), 430–4.
68. Kamath, S., Dean, D., Peddi, V.R., Schroeder, T.J., Alexander, J.W., Cavallo, T., and First, M.R. (1997). Efficacy of OKT3 as primary therapy for histologically confirmed acute renal allograft rejection. *Transplantation*, **64**, (10), 1428–32.
69. Woodle, E.S., Cronin, D., Newell, K.A., Millis, J.M., Bruce, D.S., Piper, J.B., Haas, M., Josephson, M.A., and Thistlethwaite, J.R. (1996). Tacrolimus therapy for refractory acute renal allograft rejection: definition of the histologic response by protocol biopsies. *Transplantation*, **62**, (7), 906–10.
70. Guttmann, R.D., Soulillou, J.P., Moore, L.W., First, M.R., Gaber, A.O., Pouletty, P., and Schroeder, T.J. (1998). Proposed consensus for definitions and endpoints for clinical trials of acute kidney transplant rejection. *American Journal of Kidney Diseases*, **31**, (6, Suppl. 1), S40–S46.

71. Gaber, L.W., Moore, L.W., Gaber, A.O., Tesi, R.J., Meyer, J. and Schroeder, T.J. (1999). Correlation of histology to clinical rejection reversal: a thymoglobulin multicenter trial report. *Kidney International*, **55**, (6), 2415–22.

72. Waiser, J., Budde, K., Schreiber, M., Bohler, T., Lobermann, L.A., and Neumayer, H.H. (1998). Antibody therapy in steroid-resistant rejection. *Transplantation Proceedings*, **30**, (5), 1778–9.

73. Uslu, A., Tokat, Y., Ok, E., Unsal, A., Ilkgul, O., and Kaplan, H. (1997). ATG versus OKT3 in the treatment of steroid-resistant rejection following living-related donor renal transplantation. *Transplantation Proceedings*, **29**, (7), 2805–6.

74. Schroeder, T.J., Weiss, M.A., Smith, R.D., Stephens, G.W., and First, M.R. (1991). The efficacy of OKT3 in vascular rejection. *Transplantation*, **51**, (2), 312–5.

75. Carlier, M., Squifflet, J.P., Pirson, Y., Gribomont, B., and Alexandre, G.P. (1982). Maximal hydration during anesthesia increases pulmonary arterial pressures and improves early function of human renal transplants. *Transplantation*, **34**, 201–4.

76. Boom, H., Mallat, M.J., de Fijter, J.W., Zwinderman, A.H., and Paul, L.C. (2000). Delayed graft function influences renal function, but not survival. *Kidney International*, **58**, (2), 859–66.

77. Halloran, P., Mathew, T., Tomlanovich, S., Groth, C., Hooftman, L., and Barker, C. (1997). Mycophenolate mofetil in renal allograft recipients: a pooled efficacy analysis of three randomized, double-blind, clinical studies in prevention of rejection. The International Mycophenolate Mofetil Renal Transplant Study Groups [published erratum appears in *Transplantation* (1997), Feb 27, **63**, (4), 618]. *Transplantation*, **63**, (1), 39–47.

78. Zarifian, A., Meleg-Smith, S., O'donovan, R., Tesi, R.J., and Batuman, V. (1999). Cyclosporine-associated thrombotic microangiopathy in renal allografts. *Kidney International*, **55**, (6), 2457–66.

79. Mihatsch, M.J., Ryffel, B., and Gudat, F. (1995). The differential diagnosis between rejection and cyclosporine toxicity. *Kidney International*, **52**, (Suppl.), S63–S69.

80. Mayer, A.D., Dmitrewski, J., Squifflet, J.P., Besse, T., Grabensee, B., Klein, B., Eigler, F.W., Heemann, U., Pichlmayer, R., Behrend, M., Vanrenterghem, Y., Donck, J., van Hooff, J., Christiaans, M., Moraks, J.M., Andres, A., Johnson, R.W., Short, L., Buchholz, B., Rehmert, N., Land, W., Schleibner, S., Forsythe, J.L., Talbot, D., and Pohanka, E. (1997). Multicenter randomized trial comparing tacrolimus (FK506) and cyclosporine in the prevention of renal allograft rejection: a report of the European Tacrolimus Multicenter Renal Study Group. *Transplantation*, **64**, (3), 436–43.

81. Takai, K., Aoki, A., Suga, A., Tollemar, J., Wilczek, H.E., Naito, K., and Groth, C.G. (1998). Urinary tract infections following renal transplantation. *Transplantation Proceedings*, **30**, (7), 3140–1.

82. Crowe, A., Cairns, H.S., Wood, S., Rudge, C.J., Woodhouse, C.R., and Neild, G.H. (1998). Renal transplantation following renal failure due to urological disorders. *Nephrology Dialysis Transplantation*, **13**, (8), 2065–9.

83. Binet, I., Nickeleit, V., Hirsch, H.H., Prince, O., Dalquen, P., Gudat, F., Mihatsch, M.J., and Thiel, G. (1999). Polyomavirus disease under new immunosuppressive drugs, a cause of renal graft dysfunction and graft loss. *Transplantation*, **67**, (6), 918–22.

84. Kasiske, B.L., Vazquez, M.A., Harmon, W.E., Brown, R.S., Danovitch, G.M., Gaston, R.S., Roth, D., Scandling, J.D.J., and Singer, G.G. (2000). Recommendations for the outpatient surveillance of renal transplant recipients. American Society of Transplantation [In Process Citation]. *Journal of the American Society of Nephrology*, **11**, (Suppl 15), S1–S86.

85. Halloran, P.F., Melk, A., and Barth, C. (1999). Rethinking chronic allograft nephropathy: the concept of accelerated senescence. *Journal of the American Society of Nephrology*, **10**, (1), 167–81.

86. Frei, U., Bode, U., Repp, H., Schindler, R., Brunkhorst, R., Vogt, P., Hauss, J. and Pichlmayr, R. (1993). Malignancies under cyclosporine after kidney transplantation: analysis of a 10-year period. *Transplantation Proceedings*, **25**, 1394–6.

87. Holley, J.L., Monaghan, J., Byer, B., and Bronsther, O. (1998). An examination of the renal transplant evaluation process focusing on cost and the reasons for patient exclusion. *American Journal of Kidney Disease*, **32**, (4), 567–74.

88. Carter, S. (1999). A cost analysis for transplantation and options post-Medicare. *Nephrology News Issues*, **13**, (11), 86–8.

89. Keown, P. (1999). Analysis of cost-effectiveness and cost-utility for immunosuppressive protocols in renal transplantation. *Transplantation Proceedings*, **31**, (1–2), 1140–1.

4
Multi-organ transplantation
Ulrich Frei

Introduction

In most patients, renal transplantation has to deal with a primary disease of the kidney. However, there are a number of clinical situations in which kidney failure is either a consequence of an extra-renal systemic disease or the cause for the failure of an other organ. The latter may happen simultaneously or sequentially. Therefore, there is a need for a simultaneous multi-organ transplant or the transplantation of different organs in sequence. In these cases, the rarely easy decision has to be made whether it is justified to use two precious organs, which might save the lives of two recipients, for one case with a sometimes open success. When reviewing the literature, it is obvious that multi-organ transplants have never been evaluated in a prospective manner, except for combined kidney–pancreas transplantation in some rare instances. Most available data consist of collected case histories. Nevertheless, it is now possible to draw some conclusions and to give advice on how to deal with these rare circumstances.

At present, an impressive number of multi-organ transplants have been reported. The most frequently combined transplants performed are a simultaneous kidney and pancreas transplant. This is due to the almost sole indication that is juvenile diabetes. Pancreas transplant after a successful kidney transplant is less commonly done.

The combination of a liver transplant with a kidney transplant is the second most often performed multi-organ procedure. In contrast to the pancreas situation, there is a wide range of different causes and circumstances. For example, there are hereditary diseases involving both organs, such as adult polycystic kidney and liver diseases or primary hyperoxaluria. There are liver diseases with renal consequences as hepatitis C or B. There are consequences of treatment complications in both directions, as infection by a viral hepatitis during renal replacement therapy (RRT) and renal failure in liver transplant recipients as a consequence of peri-operative renal damage and calcineurin inhibitor nephrotoxicity.

A growing number of heart recipients are in need of a sequential kidney transplant because of renal failure due to the use of nephrotoxic drugs.

A few single case reports describe a combined kidney and lung transplant, which has been performed in patients with cystic fibrosis.

The diabetic with ESRD: kidney and pancreas transplantation

Tight control of serum glucose reduces diabetic complications in diabetes type I (1). Although remarkable progress is currently being made in the field of islet transplantation (2), pancreas transplantation (PTX) is presently still the most effective measure for achieving long-lasting normoglycemia. However, this method is reserved to type I diabetics with severe progression of diabetic complications despite intensive insulin therapy.

According to the International Pancreas Transplant Registry (IPTR), a total of more than 14000 PTX have been reported world-wide, and the actual number of PTX exceeds 1500/year (3).

Type of PTX

Simultaneous pancreas and kidney transplantation (SPK)

In most cases, the pancreas and kidney are derived from the same donor. The major advantage of this procedure is the immunological identity of pancreas and kidney. Pre-emptive SPK is recommended in USA transplant centers at a creatinine clearance of less than 40 ml/min (4) or a serum creatinine >3 mg/dl (5), to minimize diabetes-associated complications, reduce diabetes-associated long-term treatment costs, and to prevent the preparations for dialysis and the dialysis therapy itself. In the Eurotransplant region, centers evaluate their diabetics for RRT at a creatinine clearance <30 ml/min and place them on the waiting-list with high priority when the creatinine clearance is <20 ml/min.

Pancreas transplantation after kidney transplantation (PAK)

This option is offered either to SPK patients with stable kidney transplants—creatinine clearance above 40 ml/min—after the failure of the pancreas transplant or to type I diabetics with a stable previous kidney transplant. Contra-indications for SPK are listed in Table 4.1 and do not differ widely from contra-indications to that of kidney alone transplantation.

Surgical techniques and complications

The introduction of the bladder-drainage technique by Sollinger (6), which preserves a safe drainage of the aggressive pancreas secretion, was a major step forward. However, complications are pain, bleeding, and strictures of the urethra, and bicarbonate losses of 10 g/day as well. Some patients need a conversion operation. The incidence of conversion-associated surgical complications is 15%. Progress in immunosuppressive therapy reduces the incidence of rejection and is followed by more stability in the course of PTX. This facilitated the re-introduction of the enteric drainage, which was applied to 60% of all PTX patients in the USA in 1998.

Hyperinsulinism is frequently observed after PTX. The systemic release of insulin via the iliac vein may be one factor explaining this phenomenon, as there is no

Table 4.1   Contra-indications for pancreas transplantation

C-peptide positive diabetes mellitus (relative)

Chronic non-treatable cardiac disease

Malignancy with tumor-free interval <2 years

Advanced macroangiopathy

Incompliance or psychic disorder, which does not guarantee adequate peri- and/or post-operative treatment

first-pass effect of insulin through the liver. Draining the venous effluent of the pancreas transplant via the superior mesenteric or portal vein (portal venous drainage) was reported as yielding comparable blood glucose control but lower insulin levels, and possible advantages in metabolic control over systemic venous drainage (7). Outcome of patients and transplants, and incidence of acute surgical complications in patients with portal venous vs. systemic venous drainage, are comparable.

Most complications after PTX (frequency 30–40%) are anastomotic leaks following bladder or enteric drainage, wound and intraperitoneal infections, graft pancreatitis, graft thrombosis, and urological problems directly related to the bladder drainage technique (see above).

Diagnosis of rejection

According to current data (transplantation period 1996–97) from the IPTR, pancreas graft loss due to rejection is observed in 2% of SPK, 7% of PAK (pancreas after kidney), and 9% of PTA (pancreas transplant alone) patients transplanted in the USA within the first year, and increases continuously thereafter over the years. Technical failure accounts for 8% of pancreas graft failures within the first year after PTX (1). Loss of pancreas graft due to death with functioning graft amounts to 6% after a mean follow-up of 3.8 years (8). Diagnosis of pancreas rejection may be a difficult problem; it is facilitated in most SPK patients, because rejection of the kidney usually occurs simultaneously with that of the pancreas graft. In these patients, the rise of the serum creatinine and/or the result of the kidney transplant biopsy might be an indicator— not only for kidney but also for pancreas rejection. However, in patients with PAK, diagnosis of rejection is more complicated. Monitoring of serum lipase/amylase is the only possibility to follow for pancreas transplant rejection. In bladder-drained patients, measurement of urinary amylase and or lipase is more specific than that of serum lipase and amylase (9, 10).

The 'gold standard method' for the diagnosis of pancreas transplant rejection is the biopsy, which can be performed via different accesses: percutaneous, laparascopic, cystoscopic in bladder drained patients, or duodenoscopic/intestinoscopic in enteric drained patients A grading scheme for acute and chronic pancreas allograft rejection is proposed by Drachenberg (11).

Maintenance immunosuppression

Prophylactic immunosuppression

In most studies, patients with kidney transplantation alone show lower rejection rates than PTX patients, possibly due to a higher immunogenicity of the pancreas transplant (10). With the introduction of cyclosporine (CyA), the frequency of acute rejection episodes decreased markedly but was still 60–80% under maintenance therapy with CyA, azathioprine (AZA), and steroids (12).

Substitution of AZA by mycophenolate mofetil (MMF) reduced the rejection rates for SPK patients from 75 to 31% (AZA vs. MMF) for acute biopsy—proven kidney rejection (13). Because of these encouraging results, historical attempts to withdraw steroids in SPK patients (14) were revived with tacrolimus (TAC)/MMF-based steroid withdrawal protocols (15), documenting that prospectively planned steroid withdrawal was possible in 72% of patients within the first year after SPK.

At present, TAC/MMF-based immunosuppression is applied to the majority of SPK patients, and has significant benefit in PAK and PTA patients. One-year rejection rates of 20% are reported for SPK patients remaining on TAC/MMF immunosuppression (16).

Antibody induction

The high immunogenicity of the pancreas transplant might be the reason that almost two-thirds of all SPK, PAK, and PTA patients, treated in the USA, received anti-T-cell agents as induction therapy between 1996 and 1999. Pancreas graft-survival rates were not significantly different for SPK and PTA transplants, regardless of whether or not anti-T-cell agents were used. However, for PAK patients treated with CyA, there was a significant improvement of pancreas graft survival when anti-T-cell induction was applied (6). According to these data, induction therapy with polyclonal or monoclonal antibodies may delay the onset and reduce the severity of rejection episodes compared to patients without induction therapy (12).

Results from the IPTR registry

With regard to the periods of 1987–89 and 1996–2000, 1-year survival of patients, pancreas, and kidney transplants, has improved from 90%/74%/83%, respectively, to 95%/83%/88%, respectively, for SPK patients treated in the USA. Patient survival in PAK and PTA groups was comparable to the outcome of SPK patients (1). Results are even better in centers with long-term experience, high frequency of transplantations, and expertise in the selection of suitable transplant candidates (Table 4.2).

During the periods 1987–89 and 1996–2000, 1-year survival of the pancreas transplants from PAK and PTA patients treated in the USA improved from 56% and 50% to 73% and 70%, respectively. Current 1- and 3-year survival rates of pancreas transplants performed in the USA according to the type of transplantation are given in Table 4.3.

Table 4.2   One, 5, and 10 year patient, pancreas, and kidney survival in 500 patients with simultaneous pancreas and kidney transplantation, transplanted at the University of Wisconsin between 1986 and 1997 (5)

	Patient	Pancreas	Kidney
1 year	96%	88%	89%
5 years	89%	78%	80%
10 years	76%	67%	67%

Table 4.3   Pancreas graft survival at 1 and 3 years for the different types of cadveric pancreas transplantation in the USA (reported to the IPTR-registry from 1/1996 to 7/2000) (1)

	1 Year	3 Years	*n*
SPK	84%	77%	3370
PAK	73%	58%	572
PTA	70%	58%	254

SPK: combined pancreas and kidney transplant.
PAK: pancreas after kidney transplant.
PTA: pancreas transplantation alone.

Patient survival

Compared to non-diabetics, long-term survival of diabetics on dialysis therapy is worse and can be markedly improved by successful kidney transplantation (17–19). The question of whether SPK offers a greater survival benefit to diabetics with ESRD, compared with kidney transplantation alone, is still an open debate. Survival benefits for patients with kidney transplantation alone (20), as well as no difference between both groups, are reported (21). However, one prospective (22) or large retrospective studies (23–25) show that SPK is superior to cadaveric kidney transplantation alone in diabetics with regard to long-term patient survival. Furthermore, SPK recipients developing end-stage renal disease between the ages of 21 and 40, showed better observed/expected lifespans and lower annual mortality rates than diabetics in the same age range, receiving only a cadaveric or a living donated kidney.

Kidney survival

Kidney transplant survival in type I diabetics benefiting from cadaveric SPK is comparable to kidney graft survival of type I diabetics with cadaveric kidney transplantation alone (21, 23); especially when these data are censored for patients who die with a functioning graft (26). However, living donation may also have the same positive impact on kidney graft survival for the subgroup of diabetic patients, as in the non-diabetic graft recipients.

Although the rate of kidney graft loss due to recurrence of disease in diabetics with successful kidney transplantation alone is reported as only 2% (27), clear survival benefit for kidneys transplanted into diabetics with long-lasting function of the pancreas transplant should be expected. Overt albuminuria is less frequent in SPK patients compared with diabetics having undergone kidney transplantation alone (28). A successful PTX is associated with significantly less severe diabetic glomerular lesions in kidneys previously transplanted into diabetic patients (29). Furthermore, established lesions of diabetic nephropathy of the native kidney could be reversed after 10 years, after PTA in a biopsy proven study (30).

Other effects of pancreas transplantation

Metabolism

Successful pancreas transplantation restores normal fasting and, during exercise, blood glucose levels and biphasic insulin response to glucose stimulation (31–33). Normalization of glycosylated hemoglobin occurs within weeks to months and can last for more than 15 years (34).

Normoglycemia following PTX is maintained at the expense of hyperinsulinism, which might be caused by peripheral insulin resistance (35). Systemic, but also portal venous insulin delivery with diminished insulin clearance by the liver, immunosuppressive therapy, incomplete suppression of insulin secretion because of denervation of the transplanted pancreas, and peripheral and hepatic insulin resistance, are mechanisms that are involved in this phenomenon (36–38). Immunosuppressive therapy with the use of steroids is a major reason for insulin resistance and hyperinsulinemia. Furthermore, calcineurin inhibitors (e.g. CyA and TAC) can be diabetogenic. This diabetogenicity may be related to different reasons: decreased insulin secretion (39), toxic effects on the beta cells (40), and insulin resistance (41). The United Kingdom Prospective Diabetes Study (UKPDS), with a follow-up of 10 years, showed that normoglycemia outweighs the theoretical risks of hyperinsulinemia (42).

Cardiovascular system, macro-vascular disease, micro-circulation, and hypertension

With increasing success rates, more patient at risk are transferred to PTX. Cardiovascular risk factors are most frequently responsible for the death of PTX patients (5). Following a standardized algorithm, safe transplantation with good short-term results could be achieved in patients with coronary artery disease. However, despite consequent revascularization, long-term results after 3 years showed more cardiovascular events in the group of patients with pre-operative diagnosed coronary artery disease (29%) compared with the group exempt from pre-operative coronary artery disease (8%) (43). Progression of established macro-vascular disease, followed by increased numbers of limb amputations, and/or cerebrovascular and cardiovascular events, has been reported despite successful PTX (44, 45). The question of whether PTX can influence the progression of early asymptomatic vascular disease, is yet unsolved. Nevertheless, there might exist a positive effect of PTX on cardiac function.

Early improvement of echocardiographic parameters of cardiac function, and normalization of left ventricular geometry, were found in a small series of SPK with a follow-up of 2 years. In contrast, diabetics with kidney transplantation alone stabilized their cardiac function but did not improve it beyond pretransplant values (46). The positive effects on cardiac function might be in part related to improvements in microcirculation, which are not described for the heart but for peripheral and conjunctival micro-vessels (47). Furthermore, lowering of the blood pressure after successful PTX is found (48) especially in patients treated with bladder drainage (49, 50).

Neuropathy

Diabetics with moderate neuropathy and successful PTX have longer survival times than diabetics without PTX or with early failure of PTX. In diabetics with severe neuropathy, there is no clear difference between these three groups (51). Recovery from diabetic neuropathy is frequently described for motor and sensory nerve conduction (52). Slight improvement of neurologic clinical signs, and of autonomic nervous function, can occur over the years (53). A relationship between improvement of autonomic neuropathy and survival benefits has been observed in a small collective (22). From the clinical point of view, most patients recover within short periods of time from painful polyneuropathy and restless legs after successful PTX, but can have long-lasting problems with diabetic gastro-enteropathy and/or bone disease, which can be in part related to neuropathy. Orthostatic hypotension may persist for which only limited therapeutic options are available (54).

Retinopathy

In multiple studies, it could be shown that the majority of PTX patients suffered from proliferative retinopathy at the time of transplantation. For this reason, most of these patients were treated with pan-retinal laser coagulation. This might explain why the majority of studies found a stabilization of diabetic retinopathy following PTX, which did not differ from the course of diabetic retinopathy in patients treated with kidney transplantation alone (55).

PTX as optimal strategy in diabetics with ESRD

PTX, especially SPK, is a procedure with excellent clinical results. However, post-operative morbidity remains high. The progress of immunosuppressive therapy is focused on drugs with low diabetogenicity and nephrotoxicity. The surgical techniques are well-established. The enteric drainage of the exocrine, and the portal venous drainage of the endocrine pancreas secretion, approximate the physiologic condition. It remains unclear at present if this procedure is associated with metabolic benefits that are of clinical relevance. The bladder-drainage technique is associated with improvement of hypertension and, since blood pressure is strongly associated with patient survival, this technique may be of advantage in patients with severe hypertension. SPK patients also benefit from the ability to monitor concentration of urinary enzymes for the diagnosis of pancreas rejection. Because of the survival benefit, even compared to type I diabetics who received a living donated kidney, SPK is the optimal strategy for treatment of end-stage renal disease for patients who are between 21 and 45 years of age at start of renal replacement therapy (56).

Liver and kidney transplantation

Liver and kidney transplantation is second to simultaneous pancreas and kidney transplantation as the most often-performed multi-organ procedure, currently numbering by the hundreds. So far, no systematic approach has been made to establish the indications and usefulness of this combined transplant procedure under different circumstances. The best-investigated single entity is combined liver and kidney transplantation in primary hyperoxaluria (PH, see Chapter 9). From several single-center reports published on combined liver and kidney transplantation performed for various different indications, it emerges that the procedure yields impressive successes, with the exception of terminal liver failure due to viral hepatitis, in dialysis patients (57–59).

The uremic patient with a failing liver

According to the prevalence of hepatitis B (HBV) and C (HCV) in a given hemodialysis population, the question arises whether or not to offer such patients a combined kidney and liver transplant. Because of the usually very long evolutions of hepatitis C, liver failure due to acquired hepatitis B represents the most frequent indication for a (combined) transplant. Two essential questions should be raised before putting such patients on a waiting list.

First, as with non-uremic liver recipients, the issue has to be clarified as to whether there is a need and a possibility of lowering, or even eradicating, replicative viral disease by pharmacotherapy. This is essential if the use of interferons is part of the treatment protocol because it is often observed that the use of interferons after a transplant may induce rejection.

The second important question is the condition of the recipient. As in liver transplantation in general, but particularly with combined liver and kidney transplantation, the condition of the recipient (as described by his Child-Pugh score) is strongly correlated with outcome. Critically ill intensive care unit (ICU) patients are very likely not to survive the procedure due to peri-operative complications such as prolonged ventilation, infections, and bleeding.

Therefore, if a patient on RRT is suffering from chronic liver disease, the question of whether they should undergo a combined transplant should be discussed at an early stage and he or she should be referred to a transplant unit with solid experience in combined transplantation (60).

The patient with liver and kidney disease

Although this group is small in numbers, it is the most interesting and demanding. It includes two different entities: first, patients with inherited diseases; and, second, those with viral liver disease complicated by autoimmune disease.

In only very rare circumstances are the liver and the kidney affected by the same pathogenetic and inherited mechanism. This is true for some forms of polycystic kidney and concomitant liver disease. Cystic malformations, as well as hepatic fibrosis and bile duct abnormalities (Caroli-Syndrome), have been found in juvenile polycystic kidney disease, as well as in the adult type. Nephronophtisis and the medullary cystic complex are sometimes associated with liver abnormalities. In rare cases, renal amyloidosis is the consequence of long-standing bile-duct infections in Caroli's disease (61–67).

In primary hyperoxaluria type I and II, an inherited metabolic defect in the oxalate metabolism located in the liver causes an oxalate storage disease with recurrent renal stones and extra renal manifestations, leading to death if not corrected. If a liver transplant is performed very early on then, as long as no renal impairment exists, no kidney transplant is necessary. In most cases, primary hyperoxaluria is only detected late when renal stones and impairment of renal function are present.

End-stage renal failure develops then within a short period (even with a profile of acute renal failure) and deleterious oxalate deposits may heavily damage blood vessels, bones, eyes, heart, and skin. In these cases, an urgent combined transplant of liver and kidney is recommended, together with very aggressive oxalate removal by daily dialysis as long as the transplanted kidney is not functioning optimally. Kidney transplantation in primary hyperoxaluria has an unacceptable high failure rate and is only recommended in very selected circumstances (68–71).

Some other rare metabolic disorders may also affect liver and kidney, such as methylmalonic acidemia (72) or glycogen storage disease with consecutive focal segmental glomerulosclerosis (FSGN) (73) or α1-antitrypsin deficiency and glomerular disease (74).

Chronic viral liver disease, mostly due to hepatitis C but also, very rarely, due to Hepatitis B virus HBV, is sometimes associated with the development of autoimmune disease, such as cyroglobulinemia, vasculitis, and extra-capillary glomerulonephritis (75).

The liver-graft recipient with renal failure

As well-observed in kidney transplantation, an entity is now encountered with increasing frequency after liver transplantation, which resembles chronic allograft nephropathy in the liver recipients own kidneys. Contributing factors are kidney damage during the peri-operative course with development of acute renal failure and exposure to episodes of high inflammation, chronic calcineurin inhibitor toxicity (76), *de novo* hypertension, and metabolic disorders such as hyperlipidemia or post-transplant diabetes mellitus.

The patient with hepato-renal syndrome

Hepato-renal syndrome, i.e. functional renal impairment due to chronic and severe liver failure, is not an indication for a combined liver and kidney transplant. Several observations have proven that hepato-renal syndrome is reversible after a successful isolated liver transplant, irrespective of the time spent in an ICU with hepato-renal syndrome requiring RRT (77).

Heart and kidney transplantation

The uremic with heart failure

There are a few case series, and a number of case reports, of patients treated by RRT who have undergone a combined heart and kidney transplantation because of cardiomyopathy (hypertensive or idiopathic) or ischemic heart disease in young age (78–80). There are some patients with end-stage heart disease and non-reversible renal disease, and some with end-stage renal disease and severe cardiac disease, un-amenable to other treatment. In a series of six cases the 2-year survival rate was 67% with fair to good kidney and heart functions (81). It is clear that this outcome is documented for very selected cases and by experienced multi-organ transplant specialists.

The patient with heart and kidney failure

Diseases affecting heart and kidney by an identical pathogenetic mechanism are rare. One of them might be amyloidosis of the heart and the kidney (82). There are no reports available about a combined transplant due to this indication.

The heart recipient with renal failure

Very early after the revival of cardiac transplantation in the early 1980s, renal damage due to the toxicity of calcineurin inhibitors became obvious (83). It turned out that beside calcineurin-inhibitor toxicity, hypertension and metabolic disorders may add additional risks (84). An independent risk factor is the age of the recipient (85). With increasing long-term survival of cardiac recipients, a growing number of them have to be submitted to RRT (86, 87). Whereas no reliable data are available, the percentage of patients requiring RRT in cardiac transplant survivors after 10 years may approach 8–10% (88). In patients with good cardiac function and no other contraindications, a renal transplant might be performed with successful outcome (89).

Lung and kidney transplantation

Lung disease and kidney failure

There are only very few cases of lung disease and kidney failure, which have not yet been published in the literature. Between 1990 and 1998, four cases of a combined lung and kidney transplant have been reported to the UNOS registry. This author is aware of two cases reported to Eurotransplant, both of them with cystic fibrosis as underlying disease, and consecutive renal amyloidosis in one case and focal segmental glomerulosclerosis in the other. Both of them survived for several years after transplant.

The lung transplant recipient with kidney failure

As after heart transplantation, there is a growing number of patients developing ESRD after lung transplantation following in generally the same pathogenetic mechanisms. In particular, in patients lung transplanted for cystic fibrosis, secondary oxalosis might be an additional risk factor for the kidneys (90).

References

1. Anonymous (1996). Lifetime benefits and costs of intensive therapy as practiced in the diabetes control and complications trial. The Diabetes Control and Complications Trial Research Group. *Journal of the American Medical Association*, **276**, (17), 1409–15.
2. Shapiro, A.M., Lakey, J.R., Ryan, E.A., Korbutt, G.S., Toth, E., Warnock, G.L., Kneteman, N.M., and Rajotte, R.V. (2000). Islet transplantation in seven patients with type 1 diabetes mellitus using a glucocorticoid-free immunosuppressive regimen [see comments]. *The New England Journal of Medicine*, **343**, (4), 230–8.
3. Anonymous (2000). Actual summary of data concerning patient-, graft- and donor characteristics, risk factors and outcome as well as immunosuppression, surgical details and number of transplants which are reported to the registry. *International Pancreas Transplantation Registry Newsletter*, **12**, 4–23.
4. Stratta, R.J., Larsen, J.L., and Cushing, K. (1995). Pancreas transplantation for diabetes mellitus. *Annual Review of Medicine*, **46**, 281–98.
5. Sollinger, H.W., Odorico, J.S., Knechtle, S.J., D'Alessandro, A.M., Kalayoglu, M., and Pirsch, J.D. (1998). Experience with 500 simultaneous pancreas-kidney transplants. *Annals Surgery*, **228**, (3), 284–96.
6. Cook, K., Sollinger, H.W., Warner, T., Kamps, D., and Belzer, F.O. (1983). Pancreaticocystostomy: an alternative method for exocrine drainage of segmental pancreatic allografts. *Transplantation*, **35**, (6), 634–6.
7. Gaber, A.O., Shokouh-Amiri, M.H., Hathaway, D.K., Hammontree, L., Kitabchi, A.E., Gaber, L.W., Saad, M.F., and Britt, L.G. (1995). Results of pancreas transplantation with portal venous and enteric drainage. *Annals Surgery*, **221**, (6), 613–22.
8. Stratta, R.J. (1998). Analysis of mortality after pancreas transplantation. *Transplantation Proceedings*, **30**, (2), 283.
9. Benedetti, E., Najarian, J.S., Gruessner, A.C., Nakhleh, R.E., Troppmann, C., Hakim, N.S., Pirenne, J., Sutherland, D.E., and Gruessner, R.W. (1995). Correlation between cystoscopic biopsy results and hypoamylasuria in bladder-drained pancreas transplants. *Surgery*, **118**, (5), 864–72.
10. Hricik, D.E. (2000). Kidney-pancreas transplantation for diabetic nephropathy. *Seminars in Nephrology*, **20**, (2), 188–98.
11. Drachenberg, C.B., Papadimitriou, J.C., Klassen, D.K., Weir, M.R., Cangro, C.B., Fink, J.C., and Bartlett, S.T. (1999). Chronic pancreas allograft rejection: morphologic evidence of progression in needle biopsies and proposal of a grading scheme. *Transplantation Proceedings*, **31**, (1–2), 614.
12. Stratta, R.J. (1999). Review of immunosuppressive usage in pancreas transplantation. *Clinical Transplantation*, **13**, (1, Pt 1), 1–12.

13. Odorico, J.S., Pirsch, J.D., Knechtle, S.J., D'Alessandro, A.M., and Sollinger, H.W. (1998). A study comparing mycophenolate mofetil to azathioprine in simultaneous pancreas-kidney transplantation. *Transplantation*, **66**, (12), 1751–9.

14. Cantarovich, D., Palneau, J., Couderc, J.P., Murat, A., Hourmant, M., Boatard, R., Dantal, J., Karam, G., Bouchot, O., and Soulillou, J.P. (1991). Maintenance immunosuppression without corticosteroids following combined pancreas and kidney transplantation. *Transplantation Proceedings*, **23**, (4), 2224–5.

15. Kahl, A., Bechstein, W.O., Lorenz, F., Steinberg, J., Pohle, C., Kampf, D., Mullar, A., Settmacher, U., Neuhaus, P., and Frei, U. (2001). Long-term prednisolone withdrawal after pancreas and kidney transplantation in patients treated with ATG, tacrolimus, and mycophenolate mofetil. *Transplantation Proceedings*, **33**, (1–2), 1694–5.

16. Kaufman, D.B., Leventhal, J.R., Stuart, J., Abecassis, M.M., Fryer, J.P., and Stuart, F.P. (1999). Mycophenolate mofetil and tacrolimus as primary maintenance immunosuppression in simultaneous pancreas-kidney transplantation, initial experience in 50 consecutive cases. *Transplantation*, **67**, (4), 586–93.

17. Friedman, E.A. (1995). Management choices in diabetic end-stage renal disease. *Nephrology Dialysis Transplantation*, **10**, (Suppl. 7), 61–9.

18. Port, F.K., Wolfe, R.A., Mauger, E.A., Berling, D.P., and Jiang, K. (1993). Comparison of survival probabilities for dialysis patients vs cadaveric renal transplant recipients [see comments]. *Journal of the American Medical Association*, **270**, (11), 1339–43.

19. Wolfe, R.A., Ashby, V.B., Milford, E.L., Ojo, A.O., Ettenger, R.E., Agodoa, L.Y., Held, P.J., and Port, F.K. (1999). Comparison of mortality in all patients on dialysis, patients on dialysis awaiting transplantation, and recipients of a first cadaveric transplant [see comments]. *The New England Journal of Medicine*, **341**, (23), 1725–30.

20. Manske, C.L., Wang, Y., and Thomas, W. (1995). Mortality of cadaveric kidney transplantation versus combined kidney–pancreas transplantation in diabetic patients [see comments]. *Lancet*, **346**, (8991–8992), 1658–62.

21. Lee, C.M., Scandling, J.D., Krieger, N.R., Dafoe, D.C., and Alfrey, E.J. (1997). Outcomes in diabetic patients after simultaneous pancreas-kidney versus kidney alone transplantation. *Transplantation*, **64**, (9), 1288–94.

22. Tyden, G., Bolinder, J., Solders, G., Brattstrom, C., Tibell, A., and Groth, C.G. (1999). Improved survival in patients with insulin-dependent diabetes mellitus and end-stage diabetic nephropathy 10 years after combined pancreas and kidney transplantation. *Transplantation*, **67**, (5), 645–8.

23. Smets, Y.F., Westendorp, R.G., van der Pijl, J.W., de Charro, F.T., Ringers, J., de Fijter, J.W., and Lemkes, H.H. (1999). Effect of simultaneous pancreas-kidney transplantation on mortality of patients with type-1 diabetes mellitus and end-stage renal failure. *Lancet*, **353**, (9168), 1915–19.

24. Becker, B.N., Brazy, P.C., Becker, Y.T., Odorico, J.S., Pintar, T.J., Collins, B.H., Pirsch, J.D., Leverson, G.E., Heisey, D.M., and Sollinger, H.W. (2000). Simultaneous pancreas-kidney transplantation reduces excess mortality in type 1 diabetic patients with end-stage renal disease. *Kidney International*, **57**, (5), 2129–35.

25. Rayhill, S.C., D'Alessandro, A.M., Odorico, J.S., Knechtle, S.J., Pirsch, J.D., Heisey, D.M., Kirk, A.D., Van der Werf, W., and Sollinger, H.W. (2000). Simultaneous pancreas-kidney transplantation and living related donor renal transplantation in patients with diabetes: is there a difference in survival? *Annals Surgery*, **231**, (3), 417–23.

26. Douzdjian, V., Rice, J.C., Gugliuzza, K.K., Fish, J.C., and Carson, R.W. (1996). Renal allograft and patient outcome after transplantation: pancreas-kidney versus kidney-alone

transplants in type 1 diabetic patients versus kidney-alone transplants in nondiabetic patients. *American Journal of Kidney Diseases*, **27**, (1), 106–16.

27. Basadonna, G., Matas, A.J., and Najarian, J.S. (1992). Kidney transplantation in diabetic patients: the University of Minnesota experience. *Kidney International Suppl*, **38**, S193–S196.

28. el-Gebely, S., Hathaway, D.K., Elmer, D.S., Gaber, L.W., Acchiardo, S., and Gaber, A.O. (1995). An analysis of renal function in pancreas-kidney and diabetic kidney-alone recipients at two years following transplantation. *Transplantation*, **59**, 1410–15.

29. Bilous, R.W., Mauer, S.M., Sutherland, D.E., Najarian, J.S., Goetz, F.C., and Steffes, M.W. (1989). The effects of pancreas transplantation on the glomerular structure of renal allografts in patients with insulin-dependent diabetes. *The New England Journal of Medicine*, **321**, 80–5.

30. Fioretto, P., Steffes, M.W., Sutherland, D.E., Goetz, F.C., and Mauer, M. (1998). Reversal of lesions of diabetic nephropathy after pancreas transplantation [see comments]. *The New England Journal of Medicine*, **339**, (2), 69–75.

31. Robertson, R.P., Sutherland, D.E., Kendall, D.M., Teuscher, A.U., Gruessner, R.W., and Gruessner, A. (1996). Metabolic characterization of long-term successful pancreas transplants in type I diabetes. *Journal Investigative Medicine*, **44**, (9), 549–55.

32. Redmon, J.B., Kubo, S.H., and Robertson, R.P. (1995). Glucose, insulin, and glucagon levels during exercise in pancreas transplant recipients. *Diabetes Care*, **18**, (4), 457–62.

33. Secchi, A., Martinenghi, S., Caldera, R., La Rocca, E., Di, C.V., and Pozza, G. (1991). First peak insulin release after intravenous glucose and arginine is maintained for up to 3 years after segmental pancreas transplantation. *Diabetologia*, **34**, (Suppl. 1), S53–S56.

34. Robertson, R.P., Sutherland, D.E., and Lanz, K.J. (1999). Normoglycemia and preserved insulin secretory reserve in diabetic patients 10–18 years after pancreas transplantation. *Diabetes*, **48**, (9), 1737–40.

35. Nankivell, B.J., Chapman, J.R., Bovington, K.J., Spicer, S.T., O'Connell, P.J., and Allen, R.D. (1996). Clinical determinants of glucose homeostasis after pancreas transplantation. *Transplantation*, **61**, (12), 1705–11.

36. Gaber, A.O., Shokouh-Amiri, M.H., Hathaway, D.K., Hammontree, L., Kitabchi, A.E., Gaber, L.W., Saad, M.F., and Britt, L.G. (1995). Results of pancreas transplantation with portal venous and enteric drainage. *Annals Surgery*, **221**, 613–14.

37. Caödara, R., La Rocca, E., Maffi, P., and Secchi, A. (1999). Effects of pancreas transplantation on late complications of diabetes and metabolic effects of pancreas and islet transplantation. *Journal of Pediatric Endocrinology & Metabolism*, **12**, (Suppl. 3), 777–87.

38. Bruce, D.S., Newell, K.A., Woodle, E.S., Cronin, D.C., Grewal, H.P., Millis, J.M., Ruebe, M., Josephson, M.A., and Thistlethwaite, J.R.J. (1998). Synchronous pancreas-kidney transplantation with portal venous and enteric exocrine drainage: outcome in 70 consecutive cases. *Transplant Proceedings*, **30**, (2), 270–1.

39. Teuscher, A.U., Seaquist, E.R., and Robertson, R.P. (1994). Diminished insulin secretory reserve in diabetic pancreas transplant and nondiabetic kidney transplant recipients. *Diabetes*, **43**, (4), 593–8.

40. Drachenberg, C.B., Klassen, D.K., Weir, M.R., Wiland, A., Fink, J.C., Bartlett, S.T., Cangro, C.B., Blahut, S., and Papadimitriou, J.C. (1999). Islet cell damage associated with tacrolimus and cyclosporine: morphological features in pancreas allograft biopsies and clinical correlation. *Transplantation*, **68**, (3), 396–402.

41. Berweck, S., Kahl, A., Bechstein, W., Platz, K., Muller, U., Neuhaus, P., and Frei, U. (1998). Clinical use of the euglycemic hyperinsulinemic clamp for diagnosis of tacrolimus-induced insulin resistance after combined pancreas-kidney transplantation. *Transplantation Proceedings*, **30**, (5), 1944–5.

42. Stratton, I.M., Adler, A.I., Neil, H.A., Matthews, D.R., Manley, S.E., Cull, C.A., Hadden, D., Turner, R.C., and Holman, R.R. (2000). Association of glycaemia with macrovascular and microvascular complications of type 2 diabetes (UKPDS 35), prospective observational study [see comments]. *British Medical Journal*, **321**, (7258), 405–12.

43. Schweitzer, E.J., Anderson, L., Kuo, P.C., Johnson, L.B., Klassen, D.K., Hoehn-Saric, E., Weir, M.R., and Bartlett, S.T. (1997). Safe pancreas transplantation in patients with coronary artery disease. *Transplantation*, **63**, (9), 1294–9.

44. Nankivell, B.J., Lau, S.G., Chapman, J.R., O'Connell, P.J., Fletcher, J.P., and Allen, R.D. (2000). Progression of macrovascular disease after transplantation [see comments]. *Transplantation*, **69**, (4), 574–81.

45. Morrisey, P.E., Shaffer, D., Monaco, A.P., Conway, P., and Madras, P.N. (1997). Peripheral vascular disease after kidney–pancreas transplantation in diabetic patients with end-stage renal disease. *Archives Surgery*, **132**, (4), 358–61.

46. Wicks, M.N., Hathaway, D.K., Shokouh-Amiri, M.H., Elmer, D.S., Mcculley, R., Burlew, B., and Gaber, A.O. (1998). Sustained improvement in cardiac function 24 months following pancreas-kidney transplant. *Transplant Proceedings*, **30**, (2), 333–4.

47. Cheung, A.T., Perez, R.V., and Chen, P.C. (1999). Improvements in diabetic microangiopathy after successful simultaneous pancreas-kidney transplantation: a computer-assisted intravital microscopy study on the conjunctival microcirculation. *Transplantation*, **68**, (7), 927–32.

48. La Rocca, E., Gobbi, C., Ciurlino, D., Di, C.V., Pozza, G., and Secchi, A. (1998). Improvement of glucose/insulin metabolism reduces hypertension in insulin-dependent diabetes mellitus recipients of kidney-pancreas transplantation. *Transplantation*, **65**, (3), 390–3.

49. Lorenz, F., Kahl, A., Pohle, C., Kampf, D., Bechstein, W., Mueller, A., Neuhaus, P., and Frei, U. (1999). Bladder drained pancreas improves arterial hypertension in patients with simultaneous pancreas and kidney transplantation (SPK). *Transplantation*, **67**, (7), S173A.

50. Hricik, D.E., Chareandee, C., Knauss, T.C., and Schulak, J.A. (2000). Hypertension after pancreas-kidney transplantation: role of bladder versus enteric pancreatic drainage. *Transplantation*, **70**, (3), 494–6.

51. Navarro, X., Kennedy, W.R., Aeppli, D., and Sutherland, D.E. (1996). Neuropathy and mortality in diabetes: influence of pancreas transplantation. *Muscle Nerve*, **19**, (8), 1009–16.

52. Navarro, X., Sutherland, D.E., and Kennedy, W.R. (1997). Long-term effects of pancreatic transplantation on diabetic neuropathy [see comments]. *Annals Neurology*, **42**, (5), 727–36.

53. Cashion, A.K., Hathaway, D.K., Milstead, E.J., Reed, L., and Gaber, A.O. (1999). Changes in patterns of 24-hr heart rate variability after kidney and kidney–pancreas transplant. *Transplantation*, **68**, (12), 1846–50.

54. Hurst, G.C., Somerville, K.T., Alloway, R.R., Gaber, A.O., and Stratta, R.J. (2000). Preliminary experience with midodrine in kidney/pancreas transplant patients with orthostatic hypotension. *Clinical Transplantation*, **14**, (1), 42–7.

55. Wang, Q., Klein, R., Moss, S.E., Klein, B.E., Hoyer, C., Burke, K., and Sollinger, H.W. (1994). The influence of combined kidney–pancreas transplantation on the progression of diabetic retinopathy. A case series. *Ophthalmology*, **101**, (6), 1071–6.

56. Kahl, A., Bechstein, W.O., and Frei, U. (2001). Trends and perspectives in pancreas and simultaneous pancreas and kidney transplantation. *Current Opinion Urology*, **11**, (2), 165–74.

57. Katznelson, S. and Cecka, J.M. (1996). The liver neither protects the kidney from rejection nor improves kidney graft survival after combined liver and kidney transplantation from the same donor. *Transplantation*, **61**, (9), 1403–5.

58. Kliem, V., Ringe, B., Frei, U., and Pichlmayr, R. (1995). Single-center experience of combined liver and kidney transplantation. *Clinical Transplantation*, **9**, 39–44.

59. Lang, M., Kahl, A., Bechstein, W.O., Neumann, U., Settmacher, U., Frei, U., and Neuhaus, P. (1998). Combined liver–kidney transplantation: long-term follow-up in 18 patients. *Transplantation Proceedings*, **30**, (5), 1865–7.

60. Hiesse, C., Samuel, D., Bensadoun, H., Blanchet, P., Castaing, D., Adam, R., Chraibi, A., Charpentier, B., and Bismuth, H. (1995). Combined liver and kidney transplantation in patients with chronic nephritis associated with end-stage liver disease. *Nephrology Dialysis Transplantation*, **10**, (Suppl. 6), 129–33.

61. Pirenne, J., Aerts, R., Yoong, K., Gunson, B., Koshiba, T., Fourneau, I., Mayer, D., Buckels, J., Mirza, D., Roskams, T., Elias, E., Nevens, F., Fevery, J., and McMaster, P. (2001). Liver transplantation for polycystic liver disease. *Liver Transplantation*, **7**, (3), 238–45.

62. Chui, A.K., Koorey, D., Pathania, O.P., Rao, A.R., McCaughan, G.W., and Sheil, A.G. (2000). Polycystic disease: a rare indication for combined liver and kidney transplantation. *Hong Kong Medical Journal*, **6**, (1), 116–18.

63. Jung, G., Benz-Bohm, G., Kugel, H., Keller, K.M., and Querfeld, U. (1999). MR cholangiography in children with autosomal recessive polycystic kidney disease. *Pediatric Radiology*, **29**, (6), 463–6.

64. Jeyarajah, D.R., Gonwa, T.A., Testa, G., Abbasoglu, O., Goldstein, R., Husberg, B.S., Levy, M.F., and Klintmalm,G.B. (1998). Liver and kidney transplantation for polycystic disease. *Transplantation*, **66**, (4), 529–32.

65. Swenson, K., Seu, P., Kinkhabwala, M., Maggard, M., Martin, P., Goss, J., and Busuttil, R. (1998). Liver transplantation for adult polycystic liver disease. *Hepatology*, **28**, (2), 412–15.

66. Lang, H., von Woellwarth, J., Oldhafer, K.J., Behrend, M., Schlitt, H.J., Nashan, B., and Pichlmayr, R. (1997). Liver transplantation in patients with polycystic liver disease. *Transplantation Proceedings*, **29**, (7), 2832–3.

67. Washburn, W.K., Johnson, L.B., Lewis, W.D., and Jenkins, R.L. (1996). Liver transplantation for adult polycystic liver disease. *Liver Transplantation and Surgery*, **2**, (1), 17–22.

68. Saborio, P. and Scheinman, J.I. (1999). Transplantation for primary hyperoxaluria in the United States. *Kidney International*, **56**, (3), 1094–100.

69. Scheinman, J.I. (1998). Recent data on results of isolated kidney or combined kidney/liver transplantation in the U.S.A. for primary hyperoxaluria. *Journal of Nephrology*, **11**, (Suppl. 1), 42–5.

70. Kemper, M.J., Nolkemper, D., Rogiers, X., Timmermann, K., Sturm, E., Malago, M., Broelsch, C.E., Burdelski, M., and Muller-Wiefel, D.E. (1998). Preemptive liver transplantation in primary hyperoxaluria type 1: timing and preliminary results. *Journal Nephrology*, **11**, (Suppl. 1), 46–8.

71. Scheinman, J.I. and Saborio, P. (1997). Optimal management of renal failure in primary hyperoxaluria in infancy, and the use of combined kidney/liver transplantation [editorial; comment]. *Pediatric Transplantation*, **1**, (1), 4–7.

72. van 't, H., Loff, W.G., Dixon, M., Taylor, J., Mistry, P., Rolles, K., Rees, L., and Leonard, J.V. (1998). Combined liver-kidney transplantation in methylmalonic acidemia. *Journal of Pediatrics*, **132**, (6), 1043–4.

73. Faivre, L., Houssin, D., Valayer, J., Brouard, J., Hadchouel, M., and Bernard, O. (1999). Long-term outcome of liver transplantation in patients with glycogen storage disease type Ia. *Journal of Inherited Metabolic Disease*, **22**, (6), 723–32.

74. Elzouki, A.N., Lindgren, S., Nilsson, S., Veress, B., and Eriksson, S. (1997). Severe alpha1-antitrypsin deficiency (PiZ homozygosity) with membranoproliferative glomerulonephritis and nephrotic syndrome, reversible after orthotopic liver transplantation. *Journal of Hepatology*, **26**, (6), 1403–7.

75. Abrahamian, G.A., Cosimi, A.B., Farrell, M.L., Schoenfeld, D.A., Chung, R.T., and Pascual, M. (2000). Prevalence of hepatitis C virus-associated mixed cryoglobulinemia after liver transplantation. *Liver Transplantation*, **6**, (2), 185–90.

76. Finn, W.F. (1999). FK506 nephrotoxicity. *Renal Failure*, **21**, (3–4), 319–29.

77. Jeyarajah, D.R., Gonwa, T.A., McBride, M., Testa, G., Abbasoglu, O., Husberg, B.S., Levy, M.F., Goldstein, R.M., and Klintmalm, G.B. (1997). Hepatorenal syndrome combined liver kidney transplants versus isolated liver transplant. *Transplantation*, **64**, (12), 1760–5.

78. Colucci, V., Quaini, E., Magnani, P., Colombo, T., De Carlis, L., Grassi, M., Merli, M., and Pellegrini, A. (1997). Combined heart and kidney transplantation: an effective therapeutic option—report of six cases. *European Journal of Cardiothoracic Surgery*, **12**, 654–8.

79. Savdie, E., Keogh, A.M., Macdonald, P.S., Spratt, P.M., Graham, A.M., Golovsky, D., Stricker, P.D., Spicer, T., Hayes, J.M., Crozier, J., and *et al.* (1994). Simultaneous transplantation of the heart and kidney [published erratum appears in *Aust N Z J Med*, 1994; Dec. 24 (6): following 762]. *Australian and New Zealand Journal of Medicine*, **24**, 554–60.

80. Jurmann, M.J., Herrmann, G., Frimpong-Boateng, K., Frei, U., Ringe, B., Wahlers, T., Fieguth, H.G., Coppola, R., Heigel, B., and Haverich, A. (1988). [Combined heart and kidney transplantation in terminal myocardial and renal insufficiency]. *Deutsche Medizinische Wochenschrift*, **113**, 1757–60.

81. Col, V.J., Jacquet, L., Squifflet, J.P., Goenen, M., Noirhomme, P., Goffin, E., and Pirson, Y. (1998). Combined heart–kidney transplantation: report on six cases. *Nephrology Dialysis Transplantation*, **13**, (3), 723–7.

82. Fernandez, A.L., Herreros, J.M., Monzonis, A.M., and Panizo, A. (1997). Heart transplantation for Finnish type familial systemic amyloidosis. *Scandinavian Cardiovascular Journal*, **31**, (6), 357–9.

83. Myers, B.D., Ross, J., Newton, L., Luetscher, J., and Perlroth, M. (1984). Cyclosporine-associated chronic nephropathy. *The New England Journal of Medicine*, **311**, 699–705.

84. Sehgal, V., Radhakrishnan, J., Appel, G.B., Valeri, A., and Cohen, D.J. (1995). Progressive renal insufficiency following cardiac transplantation: cyclosporine, lipids, and hypertension. *The American Journal of Kidney Disease*, **6**, (1), 193–201.

85. Lindelow, B., Bergh, C.H., Herlitz, H., and Waagstein, F. (2000). Predictors and evolution of renal function during 9 years following heart transplantation. *Journal of American Society of Nephrology*, **11**, (5), 951–7.

86. Goldstein, D.J., Zuech, N., Sehgal, V., Weinberg, A.D., Drusin, R., and Cohen, D. (1997). Cyclosporine-associated end-stage nephropathy after cardiac transplantation: incidence and progression. *Transplantation*, **63**, (5), 664–8.

87. van Gelder, T., Balk, A.H., Zietse, R., Hesse, C., Mochtar, B., and Weimar, W. (1998). Renal insufficiency after heart transplantation: a case-control study. *Nephrology Dialysis Transplantation*, **13**, (9), 2322–6.

88. Herlitz, H. and Lindelow, B. (2000). Renal failure following cardiac transplantation. *Nephrology Dialysis Transplantation*, **15**, (3), 311–14.

89. Kuo, P.C., Luikart, H., Busse Henry, S., Hunt, S.A., Valantine, H.A., Stinson, E.B., Oyer, P.E., Scandling, J.D., Alfrey, E.J., and Dafoe, D.C. (1995). Clinical outcome of interval cadaveric renal transplantation in cardiac allograft recipients. *Clinical Transplantation*, **9**, 92–7.

90. Schindler, R., Radke, C., Paul, K., and Frei, U. (2001). Renal problems after lung transplantation of cystic fibrosis patients. *Nephrology Dialysis Transplantation*, **16**, (7), 1324–8.

5

Optimal care of the pediatric patients with end-stage renal disease

Michel Broyer

Pediatric patients should not be considered as adults but of small size. Of course, the physician must take into account the size of children but the goal, when taking care of these patients, is to achieve normal growth and development in order to bring children and adolescents to adulthood in the best possible status.

Today, in this age-group, dialysis is not considered an optimal approach, since it often seriously affects the overall quality of life. All efforts are now made to succeed pre-emptive transplantation before the time dialysis may be needed, or before the functional end of a first or second graft.

Thus, the trend in Scandinavia, the UK, and North America, is to avoid any form of dialysis, and in 30–75% of patients the first-line treatment when reaching end-stage renal disease is a kidney transplant.

There are, nevertheless, a number of children who still require dialysis, either as first treatment or after failure of a graft. For these patients, an optimal procedure must be applied, which will be described in this chapter, from the recommendations already available in the literature (1–3), data from registries (4–6), and personal experience.

Incidence and prevalence of renal failure in children

The figures available come from non-exhaustive registries and certainly represent an under-estimation; they also depend on the age limit considered as pediatric. The most recent and detailed data were reported in North America. For the period 1995–97, there were 15 new pediatric patients reaching end-stage renal failure (ESRD), under 19 years of age, per year and per million child population (pmcp), reaching 9, 7, 14 and 28 pmcp for the age groups 0–4, 5–9, 10–14, and 15–19 years, respectively (6). The mean sex ratio male/female for these new patients was 0.55. The last data available from the EDTA-registry, for the year 1992, are probably less informative due to under-reporting. The number of new patients entering ESRD under 15 years of age in 1992 varied from 3 pmcp in Spain and Italy, to 4 pmcp in Germany and the UK, 6 pmcp in France and Israel, and 7 pmcp in the Netherlands; 14% were under 2 years, 15% between 2 and 5 years (4).

The total number of children living thanks to renal replacement therapy—dialysis or transplantation—with the same reservations due to under-reporting, was estimated as 37–42 pmcp in France (7) and in Canada, 34 pmcp in the USA (8), and 53 pmcp in the UK (9). More valid are estimations of the proportion of children within the total number of patients on RRT: children under 15 years of age represented 0.8% of all patients treated in the USA for ESRD in the year 1995–97 (6), and this proportion was exactly doubled when considering the cut-off for pediatric age as 19 years. Similar figures are coming from European studies. Some data suggest that the incidence of ESRD in children was decreasing during the last years. For example, an exhaustive study in a limited geographical area in France reported a decrease of the incidence in children under 15 years from 9.1 pmcp to 7.5 pmcp for the period 1981–85 to 1986–90. The figures given by the USRDS are more difficult to interpret. The absolute number of children lunder 15 starting RRT was 425 in the period 1988–91 (10) and 565 in the period 1995–97 (6), but the proportion of patients under 15 years in the total number of patients starting RRT in the same period decreased from 0.82% to 0.70%.

Causes of ESRD in children

The causes of ESRD are different in children and in adults, and also probably according to geographical area. The three main categories are:

(1) structural abnormalities, including uropathies, hypoplasia, dysplasia, etc.;
(2) glomerulonephropathies;
(3) hereditary or genetically determined diseases.

The proportions of these three main groups of causes were quite different in the EDTA registry and in the USRDS reports. Structural abnormalities represented 36% in the EDTA registry and only 19% in the USRDS reports; glomerulonephropathies were predominant in the USRDS (40%) versus 30% in the EDTA; hereditary diseases represented 16% in the EDTA and 11% in the USRDS. There was a trend in the EDTA towards the decrease in glomerulonephropathies found in the USRDS reports, since there were 47% of ESRD due to this cause in the 1994 report for the period 1985–91 versus 40% in the 1999 report for the period 1993–97. The difference between American and European data may be at least partly explained by the high proportion of African Americans in the USRDS and the higher number of glomerulonephropathies in this population (51% versus 35% in Caucasians).

Indication to start renal replacement therapy

In children, dialysis was classically begun when creatinine clearance declined to 5 ml/mn/1.73 m^2. This level corresponds to a plasma creatinine around 400 μmol/l in infants, 500–600 in children under 20 kg body weight (BW), and 700–800 in older children and adolescents. These figures are not the only criteria to be considered but also such clinical symptoms as lethargy, fatigue, drowsiness, and gastro-intestinal disorders, including severe anorexia. Hypertension related to fluid and sodium overload, especially in glomerulopathies despite restriction of fluid intake, usually leads to a decision to start dialysis whatever the level of GFR. In fact, dialysis treatment is started at a creatinine clearance of around 10 ml/mn/1.73m^2 in order to maintain the best growth possibilities and to avoid acute complications such as pericarditis, seizures, and so on.

Finally, when aiming to perform pre-emptive transplantation, it is better to start the process when GFR reaches 15ml/mn/1.73m^2, except in the case of very slow degradation rate (<5ml/mn/year) for which 10ml/mn/1.73m^2 may be a possible limit.

Overall treatment strategy

As is the case for adult patients, apart from transplantation, two modalities must be available for treating children at the time of ESRD: hemodialysis (HD) and peritoneal dialysis (PD). Neither of these techniques has been shown to be superior in pediatric patients, and in the long-run, some patients may need both as an alternative to the other. Ideally, the selection of the modality must be made according to the individual case taking into account the age of the patient and the preference of the family after receiving full information. PD is recommended for infants and young children, but is less acceptable in adolescents because of the change in body image related to the catheter. Both modalities may be provided in a center or at home, but usually HD is performed in a center and PD at home after training in the hospital. PD can be performed as CAPD with manual handling; in fact it is currently applied as automated therapy with a cycler. This technique is probably the best for protecting day-to-day life and school attendance, the patient being treated during the night. In addition, automated PD allows higher doses of dialysis than CAPD. Hemodialysis must be available for children in specialized pediatric centers, with the possibility, if needed for any reason, for being performed at home after adequate training. In any case, as already mentioned, transplantation is by far the best modality for children and adolescents, and the time on dialysis must be limited in most cases to the time required for preparing, organizing, and waiting for a graft. There are some cases for whom the decision to transplant may be postponed, for example, in a short-stature adolescent growing with a catch-up on dialysis under rhGH treatment, because transplantation may be followed by a lower growth velocity and finally poor adult height. Another situation for postponing transplantation is the case of rapidly progressive primary or secondary glomerulonephritis, in order to avoid immediate recurrence on the graft. After graft failure, due to massive recurrence of focal sclerosis, there is a very high risk of a similar recurrence and a repeat graft is not recommended.

Organization of services and facilities required for children

It has been advocated that a limited number of specialized child centers should be established to cope with their problems, rather than treat the occasional child who presents with chronic renal failure in a local adult center. Treatment of children in adult centers often results in complications due to inappropriate dialysis techniques; moreover, treatment of children on an adult ward may create additional psychological problems in both populations. Due to the relatively small number of children starting dialysis each year, one pediatric center per million child population per country was considered sufficient to provide treatment for all children with ESRD. But to avoid long-distance travel, more centers have been created in some countries. Pediatric units, which should be separated from adult treatment areas, are usually small (less than 20 patients on dialysis) with a relatively high staff-to-patient ratio. They have to be run by a pediatric nephrologist fully trained in both specialities. Nurses in such units must be experienced with both children and dialysis. Several facilities not required for adult patients are needed in a specialized pediatric unit, including a full-time dietician, social worker, teacher, play therapist, and a psychologist. A dietician is all the more mandatory as dietary prescriptions are of major importance in children. One out of seven deaths reported in the pediatrics EDTA registry of children on dialysis in the early period was caused by hyperkalemia and cardiovascular overload, both complications related to dietary non-compliance. A teacher should be attached to the hospital team to provide tutoring during dialysis and to establish a direct liaison between the hospital and the school in order to achieve the best possible educational program for each child. Instruction during dialysis also emphasizes the importance of a proper educational program. The role of the social worker and psychologist are obvious for helping families to cope with all the problems and stress generated by dialysis. As a matter of fact, psychological distress and depression, the main causes of non-compliance (11), are often observed and justify close monitoring and intervention when necessary. Pediatric surgery and urology, and the support of a general pediatric unit, are also required.

A specialized pediatric unit must be capable of offering all modes of treatment for ESRD, not only hospital hemodialysis but also continuous ambulatory peritoneal dialysis (CAPD), or automated PD (APD) and home hemodialysis. Above all, kidney transplantation has to be planned for the child as soon as possible. When a specialized pediatric unit is not available in the vicinity for a child with ESRD, it is recommended that dialysis should at least be started in the nearest specialized center and thereafter continued at a regular clinical assessment in this unit as the child undergoes maintenance dialysis in a non-specialized center.

The pediatric dialysis ward must be designed to be a pleasant and open place. Nothing is more dreadful for a child, and also for the parents watching, than to enter a closed room for repeated treatment three times a week; it generates phantasmagoric fears. The freedom given for anyone to visit or accompany a child during the dialysis session—without interfering with care or the teaching program—is important for de-dramatizing this quite frightening treatment. Despite the risk of having too many people in the dialysis room, such dialysis units are not in fact overcrowded, since parents rapidly understand that their presence is most often not really useful.

Regular hemodialysis in children

The basic principle and procedures of hemodialysis in children are the same as in adults. However, the equipment must be adapted to pediatric patients in order to avoid complications.

Vascular access

This is a major problem in pediatric patients. External arteriovenous shunts were extensively used in the past, but no longer nowadays. The best long-term access for hemodialysis in children is certainly an arteriovenous fistula, created as early in advance as possible, 3–6 months before planned use. This must be done by a specially trained surgeon under an operating microscope and after imaging of the limb-venous network. The fistula is usually created in the non-dominant arm, between the radial artery at the wrist and cephalic vein, with a side (artery) to end (vein) anastomosis (12, 13). This procedure may be applied with success, even in infants weighing 4–5 kg. Sometimes a deep vein is used and a second operation is needed for superficialization. This vascular access is certainly the best and has the longest half-life and the lowest rate of complications. Occasional stenosis can be managed by percutaneous angioplasty (14). If the forearm vessels are not suitable for fistula creation, a saphenous vein autograft may be inserted in a loop configuration in the forearm (15), with the risk of large dilatation and aneurysm formation after long use. An artificial vessel (Goretex®, etc.) may also be inserted in the forearm, but the half-life of this material is limited by its tendency to thrombosis. In the event of exhaustion of vessels in both arms, creation of a vascular access in the thigh between the superficial femoral artery and the proximal saphenous vein is possible, as well as subcuteaneous insertion of an artificial vessel. In this site, the risks of infection are greater and in small children this may cause hemodynamic problems at the time of grafting on the iliac artery. Consequently this type of access must be considered as the last choice.

A temporary vascular access can be provided by a soft silastic catheter (Hickman) positioned into the right atrium through the subclavian or jugular vein, and fixed subcutaneously with a Dacron cuff. Depending on the size of the patient, catheters with different internal diameters are used, e.g. 8F caliber, 18-cm length in infants, or 12F caliber, 28-cm length in teenagers; double and single lumen catheters are available above the 10F caliber. The patency of this catheter is obtained by injection of heparinized saline (2000 iu/ml) at the end of dialysis sessions, acting as a lock, with a cap placed at the external end. This approach may be life-saving in a child or an infant who cannot be treated by PD while awaiting the development of a fistula. It is also used if a short period of dialysis is programmed in case of graft from a related living donor; but, generally speaking, it must be avoided, since in a large proportion of cases this kind of catheter is associated, after a variable time, with infection and/or secondary thrombosis of large deep veins (16). This threat is dreadful in young patients, with a life-long expectancy in renal failure. Despite this drawback this technique is currently very popular in North America for hemodialysis of young children (17).

Dialyzer and blood-lines

The dialyzer and blood-lines should be carefully adapted to the size of the child. Two parameters must be taken into account: the extra-corporal blood volume, and the efficiency of the dialyzer. The volume of the extra-corporal blood circuit should never exceed 10% of patient blood volume, estimated to be 80 ml/kg BW. Calculation of the volume of the dialyzer blood compartment should include the change associated with negative pressure for ultrafiltration, usually mentioned by the manufacturer. There are special pediatric blood-lines with an internal volume as low as 20 ml. It should be kept in mind that blood flow is proportionately restricted. Table 5.1 gives a list of dialyzers with a membrane surface area $< 1 \, m^2$ especially used in children.

In order to avoid a desequilibrium syndrome related to excessive efficiency of dialysis, the dialyzer should be chosen to avoid high urea dialysance. The choice of the dialyzer may be based, in a first approximation, on a ratio of dialyzer surface area to patient surface area of about 0.75. The urea dialysance should not exceed 3 ml/mn/kg BW during the first dialysis session, and may be estimated from the information given by the manufacturer and the blood flow.

Hemodialysis machine/monitor

Pediatric dialysis should be performed with monitors allowing a high degree of safety, in addition to a highly accurate measurement of ultrafiltration and a large array of technical possibilities including a well-calibrated, precise blood pump, bicarbonate dialysis (absolutely mandatory in children for the limitation of side-effects) (1), variable sodium concentration, single-needle dialysis, and the possibility of hemodiafiltration.

The dialysis session

After the creation of an arteriovenous (AV) fistula in an upper limb, some precautions must be taken: blood sampling and blood pressure measurements with an inflatable cuff must be avoided on this limb. One of the major drawbacks of hemodialysis in children is the pain associated with needle puncture. It is now a routine procedure to have the parents or staff systematically apply at the site(s) of puncture topic anesthesia with EMLA$^®$ cream or a patch set 1–2 h before the puncture. This procedure must be used at the first dialysis session and continued subsequently.

Psychological preparation for the procedure is important. A visit to the dialysis unit should be arranged to show the child other children working with the teacher or playing games, and it should be explained that every effort will be made to avoid causing pain.

Needle puncture must be performed by experienced personnel; single needle is often the only possibility in small children and provides acceptable blood flow.

The first session deserves special attention because of the risk of desequilibrium syndrome in the event of a too rapid drop in blood urea. This may be prevented by the choice of dialyzer and by setting blood flow to maintain the urea dialysance at below 3 ml/mn/kg. Mannitol (20%) 1 g/kg BW is given by an intravenous (IV) pump: one-third during the first hour and two-thirds at a constant rate for the remaining time. Valproate is recommended if blood urea is over 30 mmol/l. The next two or three sessions may be conducted similarly. According to the tolerance and the individual needs, mannitol and valproate are leveled off, while urea dialysance may be progressively increased to 5 or 6 ml/mn/kg.

Table 5.1 Some commercially available dialyzers for children with a surface area $< 1 m^2$

Dialyzers	Membrane type	Surface (m^2)	Priming volume (ml)	U.F. coefficient (ml/hmmHg)	Urea clearance (ml/min)	Sterilization
100 HG Cobe	Hemophane	0.2	18	2	82	Gamma
Pro 100 Gambro	Polycarbonate	0.3	25	2.2	71	ETO
Surflux 30 L Nipro	Polysulfone	0.4	30	1.7	78–120	steam
F3 Fresenius	Triacetate	0.35	25	3	118	Gamma
Pro 200 Gambro	Polycarbonate	0.50	43	3.5	114	ETO
CA50 G Baxter	Cell. diacetate	0.50	38	1.8	110	Gamma
B305A Meditor	PMMA	0.50	35	3.8	137	Gamma
Filtral 6	PAN	0.55	48	15	136	ETO
200 HG Cobe	Hemophane	0.60	34	3.5		Gamma
Fu Fresenius	Polysulfone	0.70	44	2.8	155	steam
CA70G Baxter	Cell. diacetate	0.70		3.4	153	Gamma
Filtral 8	PAN	0.70	53	19	148	ETO
Sureflux 70 G Nipro	Triacetate	0.70	45	5	169	Gamma
B3 08A Meditor	PMMA	0.80	49	5.9	163	Gamma
300 HG Cobe	Hemophane	0.80	44	4.5		Gamma
CA 90 G Baxter	Diacetate	0.90		4.2	161	Gamma
NC 0985G Sorin	Synth. mod. cell	0.90		2.9	164	Gamma
400 HG Cobe	Hemophane	0.90		5.9	169	Gamma
Dicea 90G Baxter	Cell. diacetate	0.90		6.8	173	Gamma

PMMA: polymethylmetacrylate.
PAN: polyacrylonitrile.
SMC: synthetic modified cellulose.

Dietary compliance is a major factor in tolerance of the hemodialysis session. This point is developed later on in this chapter

Prescription and adequacy

The best criteria for adequacy of dialysis in children should be clinical, that is to say, normal growth velocity, good nutritional status, and acceptable school or vocational training performance. It is known by experience that these aims can indeed be achieved with the maximum dose of dialysis, but this interfers with social constraints, quality of life, and also cost. Consequently, it was proposed to use the surrogates that have been widely studied in adults, such as Kt/V for urea or other indexes that have not yet been completely validated in children. It seems that the minimal figure recommended in adults for KT/V, i.e. 1.3, would represent an under-estimation for children. For this index, it would be better to raise the limit to about 2 or even more. Note that the two-pool model for urea kinetic modeling is more appropriate in small children, the single pool resulting in an over-estimation (18). In addition, it was reported that due to a greater recirculation and solute sequestration in children, causing a large post-dialysis rebound, it would be better to use another index, the solute removal index (SRI). This is the ratio of the amount of solute removed to the solute content of the body at the beginning of the session, a weekly index being the sum of the three sessions of the week. According to Verrina *et al.* (19), it must be at least 1.7 in children. Whatever the index, the dose of dialysis must be evaluated in all pediatric patients at least monthly and the residual renal function every 6–12 months. The starting prescription is usually 2–3 h of dialysis three times a week, which must be adjusted regularly considering indexes, clinical parameters, and constraints.

Another problem of dialysis adequacy is the accurate appreciation of the true dry weight in a child whose body size is growing. The usual approach to this problem is to adjust progressively the post-dialytic weight according to the tolerance to a progressively increasing UF. This approach may be misleading, especially in case of hypertension, since anti-hypertensive drugs favor poor tolerance to UF, and thus the correct dry weight cannot be estimated. However, the assessment of dry weight of a child on dialysis is of major importance. Several methods may be used. The reference method is the measure of extracellular space by a marker such as inuline. Among the few studies performed in children on dialysis, Leroy *et al.* (20) found that inuline space was appropriate between 19 and 24% of body weight. Non-invasive methods, such as bioimpedancemetry, and the measure of the diameter of the inferior vena cava were reported to be useful. These two parameters have been shown to vary with total body water and are an easy means to assess dry weight. Reference intervals for different ages and sizes in normal children were recently published for both parameters (21).

Regular peritoneal dialysis

In children, peritoneal dialysis is currently more often used than HD in some areas such as North America. In the USRDS 1999 report (6), among children under 16 years,

60% were on PD and 40% on HD. Peritoneal dialysis is the modality of choice for patients less than 20 kg. Virtually all infants on dialysis receive PD, while adolescents equally receive PD and HD. The use of PD is less frequent in Europe, according to the last EDTA registry data, with only 35% of children less than 16 years treated by PD, and a large variation according to country, ranging from 82% in the UK, for example, to 8% in France (4).

Some contra-indications to PD make HD compulsory; for example, a history of multiple abdominal surgical procedures with secondary adhesions, colostomy, or ureterostomy. There are several types of PD: intermittent PD (IPD), continuous ambulatory peritoneal dialysis (CAPD), and automated peritoneal dialysis (APD) using an automatic cycler, usually during the night (see Chapter 2).

As in adults, chronic peritoneal dialysis is performed through a silastic catheter inserted into the peritoneal cavity in the operating room under general anesthesia and by a trained surgeon, even if it seems a simple operation. Attention must be paid that the size of the catheter fits the size of the abdomen. The catheter enters the skin on the lateral edge of the rectus abdominalis, rather than on the linea alba, and it is important that the general direction of the catheter given by the subcutaneous course is towards the Douglas dead end, the ideal place for the catheter tip. The peritoneal wound is closed by means of a purse string around the catheter, and only one cuff is sutured on to the skin to prevent bacterial contamination. In small children, it is recommended to perform at least a partial omentectomy in order to prevent the omental wrap of the catheter and its obstruction by omental fringes.

There are some pediatric specificities. In small children, the peritoneal surface area does not correlate with weight. Infants have more than twice the peritoneal surface area per unit weight compared to adults. As a consequence, peritoneal efficiency is higher, with increased glucose absorption associated with decreased osmotic gradient and reduced ultrafiltration, especially during long dwells. The dwell time must be shortened accordingly. Moreover, protein loss is higher in small children—it was reported as an average of 0.12 g/kg/day but sometimes reaches higher amounts.

Intermittent PD

Usually intermittent PD is performed on three consecutive days twice a week, with one or two days off in between. This correspond to 40–60 hours/week, with at each cycle of 1 h, 10–15 min infusion of around 1000 ml/m² of dialysate followed by a dwell time of 30 min and a drain time of 15–20 min. This method is rarely used except for some children during hospitalizations.

CAPD

In this technique, dialysis is performed during the day, and four or five exchanges are performed manually with bags of appropriate size. The abdomen remains empty during the night, but another exchange may cover the night. The clear advantages of this technique are its facility and its low cost, but it is more time-consuming for the parents and includes a higher number of connections/disconnections. In addition, it may hamper normal activity.

APD

APD consists of multiple exchanges during the night. Four or five exchanges are usually made by an automatic cycler delivering $1000-1200 \text{ml/m}^2$ or $30-50 \text{ml/kg}$ by cycle, every 2 h. Some patients may receive an additional cycle of $12-15$ h during the day. This technique provides complete freedom during the day and is less time-consuming, with only one connection/disconnection per day. It is also very flexible, allowing, for example, the volume of each exchange to be decreased in case of hernia or hydrothorax, while increasing the number of cycles; or, conversely, increasing the total dialysate volume, while increasing the number of exchanges. This modality is applied when the parents are not fully available during the day or when the child cannot attend school if receiving CAPD. Most children treated by PD in Europe are receiving APD.

PD dosage and adequacy

The PD prescription should be individualized, taking into account the residual renal function, the size of the patient (using body surface area rather than weight), and the peritoneal membrane characteristics. The initial prescription should be 1000ml/m^2 body surface area (BSA), increased to $1200-1500 \text{ml/m}^2$ BSA according to tolerance. Tolerance is usually assessed empirically but the measurement of intraperitoneal pressure with a simple device may add to patient comfort, thereby avoiding exceeding $10-12$ cm of water (22). It is more effective to increase the exchange volume than the number of exchanges in order to increase solute clearance. The membrane characteristics must be determined by a peritoneal equilibration test (PET), with a test volume of dialysate scaled to BSA, e.g. 1100ml/m^2, and several samplings of dialysate at 0, 120, and 240 min, and a blood sampling at 120 min in order to determine the patient's peritoneal membrane transfer capacity as high, average, or low (23). This information is useful for optimizing the dwell time.

Twenty-four hour collection of urine and dialysate fluid should be obtained regularly, especially after a peritonitis episode. The sum of residual renal creatinine clearance and creatinine dialysance must be at least $601/1.73 \text{m}^2/\text{week}$ and dialysis prescription adapted accordingly (24, 25).

As already discussed for children on hemodialysis, other indexes may be used to assess adequacy. A weekly Kt/V urea should be at least of 2.0 but the few pediatric data reported with this approach give rather higher figures (19).

Medical treatment of children on dialysis

Aside from waste purification by means of PD or HD, and nutritional prescriptions, children in ESRD must receive additional medical treatment in order to prevent/treat renal osteodystrophy/secondary hyperparathyroidism (HPT), correct anemia, control blood pressure, and improve growth velocity if necessary.

The prevention of renal osteodystrophy/secondary HPT

This must be started as soon as GFR decreases below $60\,\text{ml/mn}/1.73\,\text{m}^2$ and is pursued systematically after commencing dialysis. This prevention is based on the daily administration of one of the active vitamin D molecule derivatives. Molecules with alpha hydroxylation are recommended since their half-life is limited to a few hours, an important point in the event of overdosage. The daily dose of $(1-\alpha)$ OHD3 is 0.25–$0.5\,\mu\text{g}$ as prophylaxis or 1–$4\,\mu\text{g}$ as treatment, and of $1,25\,(\text{OH})_2\text{D3}$ is 0.12–$0.25\,\mu\text{g}$ as prophylaxis and 0.5–$2\,\mu\text{g}$ as treatment; the oral daily route is active, but it seems that IV or oral pulse calcitriol is more effective in case of obvious hyperparathyroidism (26).

Limitation of phosphorus intake is recommended, but difficult to achieve and not really effective, to maintain phosphatemia between 40 and $60\,\text{mg/l}$. Aluminium gels are now completely abandoned in children as phosphate binder, because of the high risk of brain damage. Calcium carbonate or acetate are currently used at a dose of 1–$10\,\text{g/day}$ administered during meals in order to bind food phosphate (27). Vitamin D and calcium prescriptions must be adjusted according to the systematic check of blood calcium and phosphorus concentrations every 2 weeks, alkaline phosphatases and PTH every 3 months. Bone X-rays are also useful once or twice a year in case of symptoms. PTH must be maintained between the highest limit of normal and two or three times this level in order to prevent adynamic bone disease, on the one hand, and persistant secondary hyperparathyroidism, on the other. Sometimes, due to non-compliance or lack of prevention, tertiary hyperparathyroidism may develop; vitamin D is then unable to decrease PTH and hypercalcemia is observed when increasing vitamin D. In this situation subtotal PTX is the only solution.

The correction of anemia

This is obtained in children, as in adults, by erythropoietin and iron. Almost all children are anemic at the end-stage of renal insufficiency, and erythropoietin is often initiated before starting dialysis (17). The particularity of children is to need a larger dose expressed per kg BW, especially in the youngest: 300–$400\,\text{U/kg BW/week}$ for those under 5 years of age, to 100–$150\,\text{U/kg BW/week}$ for those above 15 years; hyperparathyroidism may increase the need for higher doses. Subcutaneous injection is the most effective route, but can be painful and this may be prevented by topic anesthesia. The aim is to maintain the hematocrit level between 32% and 36% (24). Iron stores are often insufficient and iron must be given either orally (2–$5\,\text{mg/kg/day}$) or IV if the deficit is high. Routine monitoring of several iron-status parameters, ferritine as well as transferrin saturation coefficient, is necessary to adjust this treatment. Hypochromic red cell count is another way to detect iron deficit.

Hypertension

This must be controlled as closely as possible, blood pressure must be maintained within 2 SD from the mean of normal children. This is usually done with adequate

UF during dialysis and compliance to dietary sodium restriction. In the case of renal diseases, such as HUS and FSGS, hypertension must be treated by drugs such as an angiotensin-converting enzyme-inhibitor alone or in association with a beta blocker or a calcium-channel antagonist. In such patients, anti-hypertensive drugs may be responsible for dialysis hypotension, precluding the necessary UF. Then a vicious circle causes severe hypertension due to both hyperreninemia and ECF excess. Stopping anti-hypertensive drugs the day of dialysis may help alleviate the problem; bilateral nephrectomy may also be indicated.

Growth retardation

Growth retardation is a frequent complication of chronic renal failure. Correction of osteodystrophy, adequate nutrition, control of acidosis, and increased dialysis dose may improve growth velocity (28), but may not change the growth rate much. All these points must be carefully controlled for at least 6 months without a satisfactory result on growth before deciding to start daily treatment with rhGH. Of particular importance is the control of hyperparathyroidism. GH is administered subcutaneously at a dose of $4IU/m^2/day$ or $0.05mg/kg/day$. A number of studies have reported a clear increase in growth velocity up to 10cm/year the first year of this treatment (29), but the results are better in children on conservative treatment than on dialysis, and there is a waning effect with time.

Nutrition and diet

Careful dietary management is of utmost importance in children with ESRD. Anorexia is almost constant and naturally lowers the intake of energy and protein. Assessment of intakes by a dietitian is a part of the regular check-up. If necessary, energy supplements in the form of glucose polymer or maltodextrine are prescribed. Energy intake—at least 100% of recommended dietary allowance (RDA)—must be provided half-and-half by fat and carbohydrates. The ratio of polyunsaturated to saturated fatty acid should be 1.5 to 1. Nasogastric tube-feeding or gastrostomy, preferentially with a button, is often necessary in infants and young children to provide at least the minimum intakes for age (30); this seems mandatory for preventing the development of mental retardation in uremic babies (31, 32).

Dietary compliance is a major factor for improving tolerance of the hemodialysis session. Sodium restriction is very important. In case of non-compliance to this restriction there is excessive weight gain between hemodialysis sessions associated with a risk of visceral complications and poor tolerance to the required UF during the dialysis session. Reduction in protein intake, from usual habits, is prescribed in order to avoid too high a blood urea level at the start of the dialysis session, which is associated with headache and nausea during the session due to a desequilibrium syndrome. It is recommended that protein intake is adjusted in order to maintain the blood urea level under 30mmol/l before dialysis, and to provide at least 100–120% of RDA according to age. This also allows to limit phosphorous intake.

Dietary restrictions are very frustrating for children. Acceptance of dietary recommendations is much easier if, during the first hour on dialysis, the child is allowed to eat what he/she wants, such as chocolate or salty foods. This could be part of a trade between the child and the team, the permission for free eating during the first hour of the session being given only if there is evidence of satisfactory general dietary compliance

The problem of dietary restriction is less marked in case of treatment with PD, due to a daily purification, and in this case both the protein and the sodium intake may be greater. In addition, a significant amount of glucose is absorbed by the peritoneum and this must be taken into account when calculating the energy intake—all the more so in children of younger age (1.5–3 g/kg/day). A high protein intake, up to 180% of RDA, is even recommended in small children on PD (32).

Kidney transplantation

As already stated, kidney transplantation is the treatment of choice in children with ESRD. Consequently, the aim is to perform pre-emptive transplantation whenever possible. Although this principle is agreed upon by all pediatric nephrologists, transplantation is not always immediately possible. In the 1999 USRDS report (6), the treatment modality at 2 years following onset of ESRD was a functioning graft in 62% of children aged 0–9 years and 56% of children 10–19 years of age. The data from the EDTA (4) showed, in 1994, large differences between countries: 50% of children had a functioning graft after 1 year in the Nordic countries, while the 50% mark was reached by 2 years in the UK, 3 years in Germany, and 4 years in France. These data would certainly be different if updated, since new rules for kidney distribution were implemented in some countries giving a high level of priority to children. Pre-emptive transplantation was performed in 30–50% of children in the Nordic countries, but to a lesser extent in 1994 in other European countries.

Living related donor transplantation is widely accepted for pediatric patients, but the proportion of children receiving an LRD graft is very variable: 52% of children aged 0–9 years received an LRD graft in 1999 in the USA. This proportion is much higher in some single-center reports, reaching 80%, while it was as low as 16% in the last available EDTA report, again with large differences among countries.

Preparation for transplantation

The work-up protocol differs according to each center. Blood transfusions have been abandoned by most centers, but a recent publication reports a very high success rate of cadaver grafts after one or two blood transfusions given under cyclosporine treatment preventing sensitization (34). Evaluation and repair of the lower urinary tract is mandatory. A voiding cystography is part of the checklist. Immunizations must be updated, if necessary, especially against varicella, measles, rubeola, poliomyelitis, and hepatitis B. Serological status for CMV, EBV, HVC, and toxoplasmosis is useful to know. Positive HIV serology was considered as a contra-indication, but it may change with the new therapeutic approaches. It is also part of the checklist to look for coagulation abnormalities favoring thrombosis, such as factor V Leyden, mutation in the factor II gene, and hyperhomocystinemia.

Severe renal hypertension may require left nephrectomy during the preparation period, completed by right nephrectomy at the time of grafting. A similar approach may be applied to children with persisting massive proteinuria. In the case of nephrotic syndrome, due to the high risk of graft thrombosis, the best approach would be to perform a bilateral nephrectomy and to wait 3–4 weeks on peritoneal dialysis with albumin infusions in order to clear the coagulation disorders.

For children who have had seizures and received phenobarbital, hydantoine, or carbamazepine, it is recommended to try switching to other anti-convulsivant drugs such as valproic acid or clonazepam, which do not induce hepatic activation of microsomial catabolism of steroids and cyclosporine.

Preparation for transplantation also includes explaining in advance what will happen after grafting, the risk of failure, the need for a regular medical follow-up, and, above all, for daily medical treatment including immunosuppressive drugs and possibly steroids with their transient but sometimes important cosmetic and other side-effects.

It is mandatory that, after receiving all the adequate information, the child, if at an age of understanding, will positively volunteer to undergo transplantation.

Peri-operative management

In the case of cadaveric transplantation, the best HLA matching should be looked for, but this is contradictory with the short waiting time desired for this age group. In any case, a full mismatch must be refused as it is associated with poor results (35). The trend in the past was to preferentially use an adult cadaver kidney for children, due to the high incidence of graft thrombosis using a pediatric cadaver kidney. In fact, using a prophylactic protocol with low molecular weight heparin started before surgery and continued for 3 weeks, the risk of thrombosis is greatly decreased, allowing the use of pediatric donors (36). This protocol is recommended in any risk situation for thrombosis.

Conversely, the advantage of pediatric donors is to be associated with a progressive increase in GFR in the long-term, in proportion to growth in the youngest patients, which is not observed with an 'adult' graft (37).

Operative and post-operative management must be very careful in children. In particular, hemodynamic stability must be maintained at the time of declamping the graft artery. In patients with normal cardiac function, blood pressure and central venous pressure are sufficient to achieve this goal. Monitoring of pulmonary artery pressure by means of a Swan Ganz catheter is necessary in the case of abnormal cardiac function.

After surgery it is advised to maintain the child in an intensive care unit in order to insure the best hemodynamic conditions with fluid administration just below the threshold of overload; this can be achieved only with constant surveillance. Very young children sometimes have to be maintained on artificial ventilation when a large kidney is put in the abdomen, limiting the course of the diaphragm and respiratory movements.

Medical treatment and follow-up

Medical treatment after grafting is similar in children and in adult patients, except that drug doses are adapted according to body size. Immunosuppressive (IS) drugs have to be continued indefinitely and part of the follow-up is to monitor and encourage compliance to the prescription, since non-compliance is a major cause of graft failure, especially in adolescents. No protocol was shown to be definitely the best but some trends may be stressed. The role of corticosteroids in growth retardation is a clear indication to favor an IS protocol with the lowest corticosteroid dosage possible.

Several studies have shown a higher risk of rejection in children as compared to adult patients, and it is no surprise to see that in the large NAPRTCS registry, antibody induction was an independent factor for graft survival (38). Consequently, it could be recommended to start IS treatment with one of the available induction molecules: ATG, OKT3, or, with fewer side-effects, an anti IL2-receptor such as basiliximab or dacluzimab. Simultaneously, triple therapy is applied by most centers, including cyclosporine (Neoral), azathioprine, and corticosteroids. Prednisone is progressively tapered to a daily dose defined by the transplant unit as between 5 and 10 mg/m^2, and most patients may be switched to alternate day therapy receiving twice this daily dose every other day in the morning in order to improve growth velocity (39). Attempts to stop steroids, even in selected patients, were associated with a risk of rejection in half to two-thirds of cases. Some centers use tacrolimus instead of cyclosporine, and/or MMF instead of azathioprine, and it appears that these protocols would facilitate interrupting steroids

Other prescriptions in transplanted children include prophylactic drugs during the first weeks or months, such as gancyclovir, acyclovir, or valacyclovir for CMV, trimetoprime for pneumocystis carini, amphotericine for fungal infection, and anti-hypertensive agents. Prevention of corticosteroid effects on bone may be attempted with calcium and vitamin D oral supplements.

The follow-up of a child must be planned systematically in order not to miss any problems at their early stage, especially rejection. On the other hand, this follow-up should not interfere too much with school attendance and planned vacations.

This follow-up is mainly the responsibility of the transplant center where the graft was performed, but individual solutions must be found, involving a local physician and laboratory in order to avoid loss of time and money for patients not living in the vicinity.

The frequency of laboratory investigation, at first weekly, can be extended to every 2 weeks after 6 months, and to every 3 weeks or 1 month after 1 year, and to every 2 months after 3–5 years. Any change in IS protocol indicates more frequent monitoring.

Results and complications

The results of kidney transplantation have improved constantly from its inception. Patient survival should tend towards 100%, which is the case in some single-center reports. Results are different in large registries such as USRDS or NAPRTCS.

In NAPRTCS (40), including 4898 patients grafted since1987, actuarial patient survival was 96.5, 95.6, and 92.7 at 1, 2, and 5 years post-transplant, respectively, with higher figures for living donors. Graft survival again is generally better in single-center reports. Five-year graft survival was, for example, 93% in a cohort of 70 patients grafted with a cadaver kidney between 1990 and 1996 (34). In NAPRTCS, for patients grafted since 1987, graft survival was 90%, 87%, and 77% for living donors, and 80%, 74%, and 61% for cadaver donors at 1, 2, and 5 years, respectively.

A number of complications may occur after kidney transplantation. In the postoperative period, acute tubular necrosis may be observed and, when severe, may lead to a permanent reduction of nephron mass. Surgical complications, such as urinary leak, also can occur. Thrombosis of the graft renal artery or vein is a frequent cause of graft failure, mainly in the case of a pediatric cadaver donor less than 2 or 5 years of age.

Rejection is the main complication of transplantation. Consequently the main objective of follow-up is to detect rejection as early as possible. The classical symptoms of a rejection crisis include fever, graft tenderness, oliguria, and decrease in GFR. In fact, such symptoms are quite rare or even exeptional after the first month, and rejection is only marked by a slight increase in plasma creatinine, slight proteinuria, and sometimes hypertension and a lower hemoglobin level. Echography of the graft may detect an increase in the size of the graft and variable changes in echogenicity or in the Doppler ultrasound examination. In fact, transplant biopsy is needed to ascertain the diagnosis and direct treatment. A rejection crisis is usually treated by IV high-dose methylprednisolone ($1\,g/1.73\,m^2$), followed or not by a temporary increase of corticosteroids and/or by a switch from cyclosporine to tacrolimus in case of incompletely reversible rejection.

Chronic rejection is most often the sequela of an acute crisis but may also develop insidiously. Multivariate analysis of the correlates to chronic rejection found several independent factors. The most important is the history of acute rejection and the number of crises in both pediatric and adult series. GFR at 1 year, no antibody induction, insufficient dosage of cyclosporine (trough level $< 100\,ng/ml$ at 1 month), and African American origin, were also factors reported in pediatric studies. Considering this analysis, it would be of the highest importance to decrease the number of rejection episodes by using more effective protocols.

Recurrence of primary renal disease accounts for around 10% of graft losses in children. This is mainly due to the recurrence of nephrotic syndrome in patients who had FSGS. Recurrence is observed in 30% of these patients but also in the same proportion of cases of membranoproliferative glomerulonephritis. Recurrence seems rarer in case of IgA glomerulonephritis. Atypical HUS may recur, but usually not the typical post-diarrheic HUS.

Hypertension is a major concern in transplanted children, with a risk of encephalopathy. Consequently, blood pressure must be carefully checked and controlled adequately with anti-hypertensive agents. Calcium channel-blockers, such as nifedipine or nicardipine, are useful. Angiotensin-converting enzyme-inhibitors are also very effective and may be preferred in the long term but not during the initial phase, especially in the case of delayed graft function. In addition, they are contraindicated in the case of graft artery stenosis. Graft artery stenosis is becoming a rare cause of hypertension after transplantation and can most often be successfuly treated by transluminal angioplasty.

Infections are a permanent risk in children. In the early post-operative period, septicemia may develop, and the discovery of an organism grown from the preservation container or the aspiration drains must be immediately followed by the administration of a large spectrum antibiotic cocktail before the results of culture are available. Cytomegalovirus (CMV) seronegative patients, receiving a graft from a seropositive donor, are at risk of developing CMV disease. In this case, prophylactic treatment with gancyclovir, acyclovir, or valacyclovir was reported to be effective, but the best approach seems to be to start gancyclovir as soon as a positive CMV antigenemia appears. Careful follow-up of patients at risk—the EBV-negative patient receiving an EBV-positive graft—allows early diagnosis with the blood EBV PCR and often a complete reversibility after stopping or decreasing the dosage of IS drugs. Preventively, it is better not to give a second course of induction in patients at risk.

Complications related to steroids are also possible: gastro-duodenal hemorrhage, psychiatric disturbances, diabetes mellitus, and aseptic bone necrosis are becoming quite rare with the lower dosage currently used. Cushingoid appearance, acne, and osteoporosis are more frequent and depend on the dosage. Growth retardation is often observed but is very variable and also depends on GFR. The threshold-inhibiting dosage for growth is around $5\,mg/m^2/day$ and the alternate day mode of administration allows better growth.

Last, but not least, malignancies also are possible—mainly lymphoproliferative disease, which appears more frequent in patients with stronger immunosuppressive treatment.

Despite these possible complications, and assuming a careful follow-up by a specialized pediatric transplant center with a good compliance from the children and families, kidney transplantation represents the truly optimal approach for the treatment of end stage renal disease in children.

References

1. Renal Association (1995). Special arrangements for children with renal disease. In *Treatment for adult patients with renal failure. Recommended standards and audit measures.* Royal College of Phycisians, London. 30–31.
2. Agence Nationale d'Accreditation et d'Evaluation en Santé (1997). Recommandations pour la pratique clinique, indications de l'épuration extra renale dans l'insuffisance rénale chronique terminale. *Nephrologie*, **18**, 199–275.
3. Warady, B.A., Alexander, S.R., Watkins, S., Kohaut, E., and Harmon, W.E. (1999). Optimal care of the pediatric end-stage renal disease patient on dialysis. *American Journal of Kidney Diseases*, **33**, 567–83.
4. Valderrabano, F., Jones, E.H.P., and Mallick, N.P. (1995). Report on management of renal failure in Europe, XXIV, 1993. *Nephrology Dialysis Transplantation*, **10**, (Suppl. 5), 1–25.
5. Warady, B.A., Hebert, D., Sullivan, E.K., Alexander, S.R., and Tejani, A. (1997). Renal transplantation, chronic dialysis, and chronic renal insufficiency in children and adolescents.

The 1995 Annual Report of the North American Pediatric. Renal Transplant Cooperative Study. *Pediatric Nephrology*, **11**, 49–64.

6. US Renal Data System (1999). *1999 Annual Data Report*. National Institute of Health, National Institute of Diabetes and digestive and Kidney Diseases Bethesda MD, April 1999.

7. Deleau, J., Andre, J.L., Briancon, S., and Musse, J.P. (1994). Chronic renal failure in children, an epidemiological survey in Lorraine (France) 1975–1990. *Pediatric Nephrology*, **8**, 472–6.

8. Agodoa, L.Y. and Eggers, P.W. (1995). Renal replacement therapy in the United States, data from the US Renal Data System. *American Journal of Kidney Disease*, **25**, 119–33.

9. Goh, D., Evans, J.H., Houston, I.B., Mallick, N.P., Morton, M.J., Johnson, R.W. *et al.* (1994). The changing pattern of children's dialysis and transplantation over 20 years. *Clinical Nephrology*, **42**, 227–31.

10. US Renal Data System (1994). *1994 Annual Data Report*. National Institute of Health, National Institute of Diabetes and digestive and Kidney Diseases Bethesda MD.

11. Simoni, J.M., Asarnow, J.R., Munford, P.R., Koprowski, C.M., Belin, T.R., and Salusky, I. (1997). Psychological distress and treatment adherence among children on dialysis. *Pediatric Nephrology*, **11**, 604–6.

12. Bourquelot, P., Cussenot, O., Corbi, P., Pillion, G., Gagnadoux, M.F., Bensman, A. *et al.* (1990). Microsurgical creation and follow-up of arteriovenous fistulae for chronic hemodialysis in children. *Pediatric Nephrology*, **4**, 156–9.

13. Bagolan, P., Spagnoli, A., Ciprandi, G., Picca, S., Leozappa, G., Nahom, A. *et al.* (1998). A ten year experience of Brescia Cimino arteriovenous fistula in children, technical evolution and refinements. *Journal of Vascular Surgery*, **27**, 640–4.

14. Lahoche, A., Beregi, J.P., Kherbek, K., Willoteaux, S., Desmoucelle, F., and Foulard, M. (1997). Percutaneous angioplasty of arteriovenous (Brescia-Cimino) fistulae in children. *Pediatric Nephrology*, **11**, 468–72.

15. D'Apuzzo, U.C., Gruskin, C.M., Brennan, C.P., Stiles, Q.R., and Fire, R.N. (1973). Saphenous vein autograft arteriovenous fistula for extended dialysis in children. *Acta Pediatrica Scandinavica*, **62**, 28–32.

16. Sharma, A., Zilleruelo, G., Abitbol, C., Montane, B., and Strauss, J. (1999). Survival and complications of cuffed catheters in children on chronic hemodialysis. *Pediatric Nephrology*, **13**, 245–8.

17. Lerner, G.R., Warady, B.A., Sullivan, E.K., and Alexander, S.R. (1999). Chronic dialysis in children and adolescents. The 1996 annual report of the North American Pediatric Renal Transplant Cooperative Study. *Pediatric Nephrology*, **13**, 404–17.

18. Warady, B.A., Fivush, B., Andreoli, S.P., Kohaut, E., Salusky, I., Schlichting, L. *et al.* (1999). Longitudinal evaluation of transport kinetics in children receiving peritoneal dialysis. *Pediatric Nephrology*, **13**, 571–6.

19. Verrina, E., Brendolan, A., Gusmano, R., and Ronco, C. (1998). Chronic renal replacement therapy in children, which index is best for adequacy? *Kidney International*, **54**, 1690–6.

20. Leroy, D., Dechaux, M., Guest, G., Broyer, M., and Sachs, C. (1985). Extra cellular volume and blood pressure in 82 hemodialysed children. *Proceedings of the EDTA-ERA*, **22**, 847–50.

21. Dietel, T., Filler, G., Grenda, R., and Wolfish, N. (2000). Bioimpedance and inferior vena cava diameter for assessment of dialysis dry weight. *Pediatric Nephrology*, **14**, 903–7.

22. Fischbach, M., Terzic, J., Dangelser, C., Schneider, P., Roger, M.L., and Geisert, J. (1997). Improved dialysis dose by optimizing intraperitoneal volume prescription thanks to intraperitoneal pressure measurements in children. *Advance in Peritoneal Dialysis*, **13**, 271–3.

23. Warady, B.A., Alexander, S.R., Hossli, S., Vonesh, E., Geary, D., Watkins, S. *et al.* (1996). Peritoneal membrane transport function in children receiving long-term dialysis. *Journal of the American Society of Nephrology*, **7**, 2385–91.

24. Churchill, D.N., Taylor, D.W., and Keshaviah, P.R. (1996). Adequacy of dialysis and nutrition in continuous peritoneal dialysis. Association with clinical outcomes. *Journal of the American Society of Nephrology*, **7**, 198–207.

25. NFK-DOQI (1997). Clinical practice guidelines for peritoneal dialysis adequacy. *American Journal of Kidney Diseases*, **30**, (Suppl. 2), S67–S108.

26. Fukagawa, M., Okasaki, R., Takano, K., Kitaoka, M., Kaname, S., Ogata, E. *et al.* (1990). Regression of parathyroid hyperplasia by calcitriol-pulse therapy in patients on long term dialysis. *New England Journal of Medecine*, **323**, 421–2.

27. Wallot, M., Bonzel, K.E., Winter, A., Georger, B., Lettgen, B., and Bald, M. (1996). Calcium acetate versus calcium carbonate as oral phosphate binder in pediatric and adolescent hemodialysis patients. *Pediatric Nephrology*, **10**, 625–30.

28. Tom, A., McCauley, L., Bell, L., Rodd, C., Espinosa, P., Yu, G. *et al.* (1999). Growth during maintenance hemodialysis, impact of enhanced nutrition and clearance. *Journal of Pediatrics*, **134**, 464–71.

29. Berard, E., Crosnier, H., Six-Beneton, A., Chevallier, T., Cochat, P., and Broyer, M. (1998). Recombinant human growth hormone treatment of children on hemodialysis. French Society of Pediatric Nephrology. *Pediatric Nephrology*, **12**, 304–10.

30. Coleman, J.E., Watson, A.R., Rance, C.H., and Moore, E. (1998). Gastrostomy buttons for nutritional support on chronic dialysis. *Nephrology Dialysis Transplantation*, **13**, 2041–6.

31. Geary, D.F. and Haka-Ikse, K. (1989). Neurodevelopmental progress of young children with chronic renal disease. *Pediatrics*, **84**, 68–72.

32. Kohaut, E.C., Whelchel, J., Waldo, F.B., and Diethelm, A.G. (1987). Aggressive therapy of infants with renal failure from infancy. *Pediatric Nephrology*, **1**, 150–3.

33. Hölttä, T., Rönnholm, K., Jalanko, H., and Holmberg, C. (2000). Clinical outcome of pediatric patients on peritoneal dialysis under adequacy control. *Pediatric Nephrology*, **14**, 889–99.

34. Niaudet, P., Dudley, J., Charbit, M., Gagnadoux, M.F., MacLeay, K., and Broyer, M. (2000). Pretransplant blood transfusion with concomitant cyclosporine in pediatric transplantation. *Pediatric Nephrology*, **14**, 451–6.

35. Opelz, G., Wujciak, T., and Döhler, B. for the Collaborative Transplant Study (1999). *Transplantation Proceedings*, **31**, 717–20.

36. Broyer, M., Gagnadoux, M.F., Sierro, A., Fischer, A.M., and Niaudet, P. (1991). Preventive treatment of vascular thrombosis after kidney transplantation in children with low molecular weight heparin. *Transplantation Proceedings*, **23**, 1384–5.

37. Dechaux, M., Charbit, M., Cherif, N., Guest, G., Vargas-Poussou, R., Marechal, M.F. *et al.* (1997). Evolution de la filtration glomérulaire après transplantation rénale chez l'enfant. *Annales de Pédiatrie (Paris)*, **44**, 176–82.

38. Tejani, A.H., Stablein, D.M., Sullivan, E.K., Alexander, S.R., Fine, R.N., Harmon, W.E. *et al.* (1998). The impact of donor source, recipient age, pre-operative immunotherapy and induction therapy on early and late acute rejections in children, a report of the North American Pediatric Renal Transplant Cooperative Study (NAPRTCS). *Pediatric Transplantation*, **2**, 318–24.

39. Broyer, M., Guest, G., and Gagnadoux, M.F. (1992). Growth rate in children receiving alternate-day corticosteroid treatment after kidney transplantation. *Journal of Pediatrics*, **120**, 721–5.

40. Benfield, M.R., McDonald, R., Sullivan, E.K., Stablein, D.M., and Tejani, A. (1999). The 1997 Annual Renal Transplantation in Children Report of the North American Pediatric Renal Transplant Cooperative Study (NAPRTCS). *Pediatric Transplantation*, **3**, 152–67.

6

Pregnancy in women on renal replacement therapy

Claude Jacobs

The hormonal abnormalities that are commonly encountered in women with advanced/end-stage renal disease (ESRD) strongly interfere with conception and successful outcome of pregnancy. They are very incompletely—if at all—corrected with well-conducted dialysis treatment. Pregnancy is, thus, a rare event among women of childbearing age who undergo long-term hemodialysis (HD) or peritoneal dialysis (PD). In contrast, pregnancies are much more common among women whose renal function is restored thanks to a successful transplant, with, in most cases, an excellent outcome and a very low rate of short- or long-term complications in mothers and children.

Dialysis and pregnancy

The major factor that interferes with conception in advanced uremic/dialysis women is anovulation, which may exist even in those who are still menstruating (1). The hormonal derangements that cause or accompany anovulation are multiple and still incompletely understood (2). Women on dialysis have increased levels of luteinizing hormone (LH), a slight increase of follicle-stimulating hormone (FSH), and a rather low concentration of estradiol. The physiological mid-cycle surge of LH and FSH does not occur and the progesterone levels during the lutein phase of the menstrual cycle remain low, all of these factors resulting often in amenorrhea (3). Elevated concentrations of endorphins, prolactin, and, recently evidenced, of leptin, also contribute to infertility. Besides hormonal derangements, the psychological problems generated by the major impact on life-style imposed by the constraints of dialysis techniques, also have a strongly negative effect on the likelihood of conception, through reduction or even arrest of sexual activity, the lack of sexual desire resulting mainly from chronic fatigue, or a depressive state.

The improvements introduced in recent years, aiming at a less stressful management of dialysis treatments and a more liberal use of recombinant human erythropoeitin (rH-EPO) for correcting uremic anemia, have a very positive effect on dialysis patients. Improved libido is an important part of the overall improvement in well-being provided by successful correction of anemia with rH-EPO, with measurable effects such as return of regular menses and to much improved sexual activity, while the objective modifications of the hormonal status in terms of serum concentrations of sexual hormones (in particular prolactin) vary according to several investigators (4, 5). On the other hand, therapeutic trials with prolactin-antagonists such as bromocriptine or substitution regimens with progestional agents have proved unsuccessful in most cases.

Demographic profile

The true incidence of conceptions in dialysis patients is difficult to estimate; since most papers report only successful outcomes, losses of pregnancy prior to clinical confirmation are incompletely registered or reported. A positive diagnosis of pregnancy remains difficult in women on dialysis. Urine pregnancy tests are unreliable, moderate elevation of serum concentration of beta-human chorionic gonadrotopin (β-HCG) may be misleading, since it may be due only to its non-elimination by the failing kidney. Recently, a progression of anemia or a rapidly developing hyporesponsiveness to rH-EPO in women on dialysis has been shown as an early diagnostic clue to pregnancy (6). In practice, the positive diagnosis of pregnancy and stage of gestation rest mainly on the results of ultrasonography. Ultrasound investigation is currently the most reliable tool for estimation of gestational age and detection of fetal growth abnormalities at all stages of pregnancy, and should be performed at regular time-intervals, particularly during the last trimester of pregnancy (7).

Surveys conducted in recent years have yielded conception rates ranging from 0.3% per 100 patient-years in Belgium (8), up to 2–4% in HD women and 1.1% in women on PD among more than 6200 women aged less than 44 years treated in the USA between 1992 and 1995 (9). A nationwide study conducted in Japan evidenced a conception rate of approximately 3.4% in women treated with HD: 19 of the 74 pregnancies occured in patients on dialysis for more than 10 years and resulted in surviving infants in 9 cases (47.4%) (10). About 5% among 450 women treated with HD in Saudi Arabia between 1985 and 1990 became pregnant (11).

The frequency of conception is reported as being two to three times higher in hemodialysis than in peritoneal dialysis patients. The reason(s) for this difference remains thus far unclear (9). Pregnancy is most commonly reported in women who have been dialyzed for one year or less. However, like in Japan, quite a substantial percentage of pregnancies (20%) registered in the USA occured in women who had been on dialysis for more than 10 years (12). Family planning counseling is therefore advised for women on dialysis of reproductive age, and birth-control options should be presented to women who clearly declare that they are not willing to become pregnant (3). Oral contraceptives combining estrogen and progestin components are effective in dialyzed women, with the same reservations, limitations, and precautions to be taken as in non-uremic women, particularly regarding a satisfactory control of blood pressure. Progestin-only contraceptives can be prescribed to women who have contra-indications to estrogens. Intra-uterine devices may worsen menstrual bleeding, thus aggravating anemia and should be avoided in women on PD, since they may increase the risk of peritonitis. Barrier techniques (condoms, caps, etc.) are harmless but not consistantly successful. Male or female sterilization, as a definitive contraceptive method, can be considered in very rare specific cases.

For women who could consider becoming pregnant on dialysis, detailed information should be provided on the likelihood of successful outcome of pregnancy, as well as on maternal, fetal, and neonatal risks (7).

The outcome of pregnancies in women undergoing maintenance dialysis has improved in recent years. Among 120 cases of pregnancy in dialyzed women published between 1971 and 1998, reviewed by Giatras *et al.* (13), 71% of the 55 cases published after 1990 resulted in liveborn infants who survived, while only 57% did so before 1990. Birth of a live infant is reported in 60% of 15 cases reviewed in Belgium; the success rate being 80% when dialysis was initiated after the onset of pregnancy (4 of 5) but only 50% (5 of 10) when dialysis preceded the onset of pregnancy (8). Among 87 pregnancies reviewed by Canadian authors in 1998, the fetal survival was found to be similar for 62 patients on HD and 25 patients on PD, being 72% and 82%, respectively (14). In the nationwide survey conducted in the USA between 1992 and 1995 on pregnancies in dialyzed women, the infant survival rate was 40.2% in the 184 pregnancies that occured after start of dialysis, and 73.6% in the 57 women who started dialysis after conception, with no statistical difference between HD and PD patients in the latter subgroup (39.5 vs. 37%) (9).

Neonatal deaths in infants born of dialyzed women range between 7.5% in the large American series (9), 12% in the Japanese study (10), and reaches 20% in the Belgian study (8). Successful outcomes are favored by the maintenance of some residual renal function and increased delivery of dialysis during gestation, mainly by augmentation of the number of HD sessions up to four and even six per week, or increasing the daily fluid exchanges in PD patients.

Spontaneous abortions and stillbirths account for the majority of pregnancy losses. The majority of infants born to dialysis-treated women are preterm, with a gestational age at delivery in the 30.5–32.4 weeks' range and a birth weight averaging 1.6 kg. Congenital abnormalities are not reported as markedly more frequent than in the general population, but the risk of occurence of abnormalities and delay in development is increased by prematurity (15). Pregnancy does not increase the risk of death in dialysis women. In the large American series of 320 women, there were only two natural deaths: one 12 h post partum of unknown cause (with the infant surviving) and one other woman died of fulminant central nervous system flare of lupus associated with rapidly progressive end-stage renal failure (1).

Management of pregnancy in women on dialysis

The management of pregnancy in dialyzed women requires a close multidisciplinary cooperation involving nephrologists, obstetricians, nutrition specialists, and neonatologists. Many more cases have been published on pregnancies in women treated with HD than with PD. Although the long, slow, smooth, depurative process of PD can be a theoretical advantage over the more 'aggressive' HD procedure, both methods can actually be used safely in pregnant women. Among 149 pregnancies occuring in women after start of HD and 35 after start of PD, the percentages of surviving infants were 39.5% and 37.5%, respectively, with no difference in the frequency of prematurity and low-birth weight babies between the two dialysis techniques (9).

Optimal management of the pregnant woman on dialysis

The aim here is to offer the mother and infant, as physiological a course of pregnancy as possible, ending in an eventless delivery, at a time as close as possible to the normal term, resulting in a healthy infant of close to normal birthweight with no increase of neonatal complications or congenital abnormalities. The main guidelines to be followed for achieving these objectives have been widely validated by the medical community in charge of these patients in recent years (13, 16).

Among the pregnant women on dialysis, at least 25% of them conceive at an advanced stage of renal insuffisiency, prior to starting dialysis (9). In these women, a dialysis method should definitely be started if the serum creatinine is greater than 5–6 mg/dl or glomerular filtration rate (GFR) is less than 15 ml/min/1.73 m^2, even in the absence of clinical symptoms attributable to uremia (17). Management of hypertension is usually easier once dialysis is instituted and dietary intake can be liberalized, particularly the much needed appropriate protein supply.

The dose of dialysis in pregnant women

This has to be substantially increased versus non pregnant women of similar body weight and size, or versus their own prepregnancy dialysis regimen. Five or six HD sessions per week should thus be performed with small surface dialyzers and prolonged dialysis times for a total of about 20 h per week, in order to avoid the too rapid fluid and osmolar shifts that can cause harmful hypotensive episodes and acute electrolytic derangements (1, 17, 18). The commonest dialysis guideline is to maintain a predialysis blood urea nitrogen (BUN) concentration under 50 mg/dl. Keeping blood urea at a low level aims at reducing the incidence of polyhydrammios, the excessive production of amniotic fluid being caused by the solute diuresis imposed on the normal fetal kidney submitted to the high concentration of urea and other wastes present in the maternal uremic environment. The preservation of some residual renal function for as long a time as possible is most helpful for reducing the magnitude of interdialytic weight gain, thus rendering the course of dialysis sessions more comfortable and permitting an optimized control of fluid balance and nutritional status.

The changes from the conventional HD regimen require adjustments in the composition of the dialysis fluid in order to avoid alcalosis and hypokalemia, disturbances in calcium–phosphate balance, the latter having to take into account the fetal skeletal development. Efficient and safe anticoagulation of the HD extra-corporeal circuit can be provided with heparin, which does not cross the placental barrier and is not teratogenic in contrast to coumadin. Pregnant women treated with coumadin, for any given reason, should be switched to subcutaneous heparin to ensure appropriate anticoagulation.

Women treated with PD

In such women, the necessary increase of dialysis dose has to be obtained in the late stage of pregnancy by increasing the number of daily exchanges, with the volume of each exchange having to be reduced (19–21). Management and performance of PD are made easier and greater with the use of automatic cyclers, which permit the delivery of regimens customized to each individual case over 24h. The risk of peritonitis in PD-treated pregnant women is low, but peritonitis episodes may set off premature labor. Bloody dialysate outflow may indicate impending spontaneous abortion and women presenting with this symptom should be hospitalized for observation (17).

Whatever the dialysis technique, a re-evaluation of maternal dry weight has to be performed at short time-intervals, taking into account the fetal weight gain, which is estimated at 1–1.5 kg during the first trimester of pregnancy and one pound per week thereafter (13). Frequent ultrasound examinations are warranted for checking the fetal growth.

Elevation of blood pressure or aggravation of pre-existing hypertension

These are frequent in pregnant women on dialysis and have to be treated aggressively with anti-hypertensive medications, if the return to a carefully assessed dry weight is insufficient for obtaining an adequate control of blood pressure. The objective is to maintain a blood pressure below 140/90 mmHg throughout pregnancy without hypotensive episodes. α–Methyl–dopa remains, after more than 40 years of experience, the drug of preference because of its efficacy and very low incidence of serious side-effects. Despite much less experience accumulated with clonidine, this drug appears also safe for treating hypertension in pregnancy, with, however, a greater incidence of side-effects (drowsiness, thirst) and the potential risk of hypertensive rebound if it is stopped abruptly. The use of calcium channel-blockers should be limited to severe hypertension unresponsive to other drugs; they may potentiate the hypotensive effects and neuromuscular blockade of magnesium salts, which may be prescribed in case of pre-eclampsia. Beta blockers have to be used with great caution, since they may induce fetal growth restriction, neonatal bradycardia, hypoglycemia, and respiratory depression. Labetabol has not been associated with such complications and is thus preferred to beta blockers. Hydralazine is deemed devoid of side-effects; it is generally used in combination with another first-line anti-hypertensive agent, the same being valid for prazocin (1).

Actually, at the present time, only angiotensin-converting enzyme-inhibitors (ACE-I) and, by extension, angiotensin II receptor antagonists, remain firmly contra-indicated in pregnant women. A placental passage of ACE-I in the maternal–fetal direction has been demonstrated in an experimental placenta perfusion model (22). Complications associated with their use comprise oligohydraminos, resulting in pulmonary hypoplasia, with neonatal death due to respiratory failure, hypocalvaria, renal tubular hypoplasia, and patent ductus arteriosus (23). Although some surveys did not report the occurrence of abnormalities in women exposed to ACE-I during the first trimester of pregnancy only (24), a high incidence of fetal complications is documented with this class of medications, pledging for abstaining from their use at all trimesters of pregnancy (25).

Hypertensive emergencies may respond successfully with intravenous (IV) hydralazine or labetabol, oral nifedipine (26), or, in extreme cases, intravenous sodium nitroprusside. Recent observations have shown that oral nifedipine (10–20 mg at repeated intervals) has a blood pressure lowering effect comparable to that of IV hydralazine (1–3 mg/h) or IV labetabol (20 mg) (27). Very close monitoring of maternal blood pressure and fetal vital parameters are mandatory in these hazardous conditions. Uncontrollable hypertension in pre-eclamptic women may precipitate delivery as a life-saving procedure both for mother and infant. The efficacy of low-dose aspirin for preventing pre-eclampsia remains controversial (28); it is reported ineffective among women with underlying medical illness (29). Nevertheless experts in the field used to precribe 80 mg of aspirin daily from the second trimester of pregnancy onwards (1).

Uremic anemia

This usually worsens during pregnancy, the patients requiring an increase of the prepregnancy rH-EPO weekly doses to maintain a target hematocrit of 33–35% (hemoglobin: 11–12 g/dl). The absence of transfer of rH-EPO across the placenta has been evidenced in an experimental human placenta perfusion model (30). No case of teratogenicity associated with the use of rH-EPO was found during a Medline search performed on March 2001. Under careful follow-up, adequate doses of rH-EPO do not entail significant elevation of blood-pressure levels. The necessary iron supplementation required by rH-EPO therapy should be administered intravenously during the HD sessions and via very distal limb superficial veins (useless for HD vascular access) in PD patients, given the poor digestive absorption and tolerance of oral iron salts. Several rH-EPO regimens can be considered, either with low doses (20–40 mg) given at each dialysis session or a higher dose (100 mg) infused every week or fortnight, based on the results of iron status parameters and the efficacy of the correction of anemia with rH-EPO treatment. In the absence of more reliable indicators of adequacy of iron status, the transferrin saturation and serum ferritin concentration should be monitored at close time-intervals (every 4–6 weeks), the desired values of the two parameters being >20% and in the 200–300 μg/l range, respectively (31). Whether an increased percentage of hypochromic red cells (>10%) is as reliable an indicator of inadequate iron status in pregnant women as in non-pregnant patients, remains to be evaluated. In most pregnant women on dialysis for whom rH-EPO remains unavailable, blood transfusions are necessary for maintaining an hematocrit of at least 30%, thus increasing the risk of sensitizations that will render eventual future organ transplantation more difficult to perform.

Maintenance of a good nutritional status

This is of crucial importance for reducing the risk of fetal growth retardation and prematurity. Detailed nutrition guidelines for pregnant women with renal insufficiency prior to, or during, renal replacement therapy have been elaborated (32). Total caloric supply should be at least 35 kcal/kg/body weight. The dietary protein intake should amount to that prescribed to a non-pregnant woman plus additional needs entailed by pregnancy: 1.2 g/kg of pregravida body weight (BW) + 10 g daily for HD patients, and 1.40 g/kg/BW + 10 g + daily dialysate losses in women treated with PD (1). Serum albumin concentration is an imperfect indicator of protein nutitional status, but the only one that is easily measurable: a serum-albumin concentration lower than 3.5 g/dl is widely considered as a valid indicator of protein malnutrition. A poor nutritional status, unresponsive to well-understood dietary counseling, particularly if a weight gain of less than 6 kg is observed in the last half of pregnancy, should entail aggressive treatment including, if necessary, enteral or parenteral nutritional support (32). Supplementation of potassium and water-soluble vitamins is usually required, because of their increased removal due to an intensified dialysis regimen. Supplementation of folic acid is particularly important to reduce the occurrence of neural tube defects. An additional supply of calcium salts has to be adjusted according to the calcium content of the HD dialysis bath (or PD bags) and the amount of calcium taken as phosphate-binder, the total desirable daily calcium intake being around 2000 mg (1). Prescription of oral or IV vitamin D derivatives can be considered in individual cases under careful biological surveillance.

Obstetric management in women on dialysis

Premature birth is the major obstetric problem encountered in pregnancies of dialyzed women: it is frequently associated with polyhydramnios or results from an emergency cesarean section performed because of fetal distress or maternal complications. Premature uterine contractions are forerunners of premature delivery—they should be prevented and alleviated by prolonged bed-rest. Uterine contractions may be controlled to some extent by β-agonists, if the maternal blood pressure permits safely their use. The (inconstant) efficacy of indomethacin has to be balanced with the risk of serious neonatal complications, especially in infants born before the 30th week of gestation, such as anuria, necrotizing enterocolitis, intra-cranial hemorrhage, or patent ductus arteriosus (33, 34). Magnesium salts (sulfate) should be used with great caution to avoid toxic adverse effects such as respiratory depression, cardiac conduction derangements, or cardiac arrest. Monitoring of magnesium serum concentration is necessary; the upper limit not to be exceeded being in the 1.8–3 mmol/l range (35).

Optimal time for delivery

This remains debated: some experts advise an elective delivery at 36 weeks of gestation, if fetal lung maturity can be demonstrated, and not to prolong the pregnancy beyond 38 weeks of gestation (1). Vaginal delivery is the routine technique, cesarean section being performed only in case of obstetric complications. In women treated with PD, peritoneal drainage is performed before (extra-peritoneal) surgery, PD being resumed with small volumes of dialysate 24 h after surgery, or in the case of peritoneal leak, after 1 or 2 weeks of temporary HD treatment.

Renal transplantation and pregnancy

Whereas successful pregnancies remain very infrequent in women treated with HD or PD, they number by the thousands worldwide in renal transplant recipients (36–37). Restoration of fertility, libido, and sexual activity, usually goes together with that of the renal function provided by a well-functioning kidney transplant. Repeated pregnancies (up to six in the same mother) (38) and twin/triplet pregnancies with delivery of healthy babies, are well-documented in the literature (39). The true total incidence of pregnancies in transplanted women remains, however, unknown, since early miscarriages or non-successful pregnancies in general are not mentioned in the papers published on the subject. Given the necessarily small number of successful pregnancies that may be observed, even during a long timespan in each single transplant institution, demographic data, as well as valid information on clinical aspects and outcome for mothers and fetuses, primarily rest on data collected in specific surveys designed by large national/international registries devoted to patients treated with RRT (10, 37, 4–2). Analyses performed on the data collected in these surveys over the past 20 years are of key importance for addressing the specific issues related to the occurrence of pregnancy in a renal transplant patient:

1. Does pregnancy have a transient or permanent adverse effect on the transplanted organ and which risk factors have to be avoided, detected, and/or controlled to prevent a deterioration of graft function?
2. How should immunosuppressive drugs be prescribed and monitored during pregnancy?
3. What is the profile of maternal complications during pregnancy and at delivery?
4. What are the effects of renal transplantation and immunosuppressive regimens on neonatal outcome and later health-status in infants/children born to kidney recipients?

Regularly updated information on these issues allow guidelines to be elaborated and modified, aiming at rendering the course and the short- and long-term outcome of pregnancy safer in transplanted women.

Impact of pregnancy on renal graft function

An almost unanimously favorable opinion emerges from the numerous reports addressing this issue that have been published during the past 20 years, according to which, pregnancy *per se*, has no adverse effect on renal transplant function, and does not cause an accelerated deterioration of the grafted kidney following pregnancy, in the vast majority of patients, **provided that the following conditions are met**:

(1) prepregnancy, the women should have a stable renal function with a serum creatinine $< 130 \mu mol/l$;
(2) proteinuria should be $< 1 g/24 h$;
(3) blood pressure should be well-controlled ($< 140/90 mmHg$);
(4) there should be no evidence of graft rejection;
(5) maintenance immunosuppression should be stable and well-tolerated.

The usual increase of creatinine clearance observed during pregnancy in healthy women is reported similarly for transplanted patients, with a return to baseline values within 3 months post partum (43–46). The greatest increment in Glomerular Filtration Rate (GFR) is recorded in those patients whose graft function was best before conception (43).

Data compiled in large registries evidence that up to 15% of pregnant kidney recipients may, however, develop either a transient or permanent impairment of kidney function (47) and/or an increase in proteinuria (43, 44). The National Transplantation Pregnancy Registry, maintained in the USA, reported an 11.1% rejection rate and 7.5% graft loss rate at 2 years in 197 renal allograft recipients treated with cyclosporine during pregnancy. These data were, however, not compared with a control group of non-pregnant women (48). On the other hand, recent controlled studies performed in several facilities involving pregnant transplant patients matched with non-pregnant female controls, and also transplanted males, disclosed no impact of pregnancy on graft function or survival (49), and this up to 3 (46), and even 11–12, years post-pregnancy (45). Thus, overall, the risk of a significant, irreversible deterioration of a grafted kidney function resulting from pregnancy *per se*, in carefully counseled and well followed-up women with stable renal function, can reasonably be considered as very low. Prepregnancy proteinuria greater than 1 g/24 h associated or not with a serum creatinine concentration greater than 135 μmol/l, may reflect a chronic rejection process that should be clearly documented by renal biopsy: if present, the risk of graft deterioration or loss during or after pregnancy is greatly enhanced (1, 50). Most rejection episodes and changes in immunosuppressive therapy occur commonly during the first 2 years after transplantation, which renders pregnancy rather undesirable during this period in view of better preservation of graft function and optimal neonatal outcome (see below). Whilst a transplantation-to-conception interval of 2 years is the recommendation usually made to transplanted women (1), an interval greater than 5 years between such two events has been found as particularly favorable in a series of 17 pregnancies from 15 cyclosporine-treated recipients, whose prepregnancy serum creatinine of 115 μmol/l showed no significant change during or after pregnancy, and whose graft survival was 100% at 2 years following pregnancy (51).

Immunosuppressive (IS) drugs in pregnancy

The effects of IS drugs in pregnant women have to be analyzed according to their qualitative and quantitative efficacy for preserving the function of the graft, their influence on the gestational development of the fetus, and their consequences on the health status of the newborn and of the child later in life.

Corticosteroid (CS)

Steroids (mainly prednisone), remain an almost universally used component of immunosuppressive regimens used in organ transplantation. CS may aggravate maternal hypertension and trigger the occurrence of gestational diabetes mellitus. Prednisone crosses the placenta, the ratio of fetal–maternal blood concentration of its active metabolite prednisolone being approximately 1:10. CS may thus cause post-partum adrenal insufficiency in the newborn if the daily dose taken by the mother is higher than 15 mg. No increased risk of malformations in neonates has been attributed to CS, which is not specifically involved in intra-uterine growth retardation.

Overall, prednisone is categorized as a low-risk drug in pregnancy and high-dose CS therapy remains most commonly the first-line treatment of acute rejection in pregnant women. A supplementation of CS dosage is also commonly prescribed during labour, delivery, and during a few days post delivery (52).

Azathioprine (AZA)

A very large experience has been accumulated over the past 40 years with this historical IS therapy for organ transplantation. AZA and its main metabolite (6–mercaptopurine) also cross the placenta. Although AZA is teratogenic in animals, fetal malformations have been extremely rarely reported in humans. From the considerable experience also gained in the use of AZA in rheumatic diseases, it has been recently stated that this drug does not carry an increased risk for congenital malformations in exposed infants (53). However, leucopenia and thrombocytopenia have been reported in infants whose mothers had been submitted to AZA during pregnancy. This adverse effect can be minimized by maintaining in the mother a total leucocyte count of at least 7500/ml.

Cyclosporine (CSA)

The well-documented nephrotoxicity of CSA, the variety of its other side-effects, and the complexity of its pharmacokinetics (which also differ between the two currently available formulations), render a close monitoring of the dose prescribed to pregnant transplant recipients mandatory, together with a frequent verification of its potential adverse effects on the maternal kidney function and on the fetal growth. Several factors may interfere with the metabolism and blood concentrations of CSA during pregnancy: they may be raised by a fall in hematocrit (with a greater proportion of the drug remaining free in the plasma), or through an inhibition of the hepatic metabolism of CSA related to higher concentrations of estrogen and progesterone. On the other hand, the effects of increase in body weight and plasma volume, which enlarge the volume of distribution red cell mass and of CSA, tend to diminish the blood concentration of the drug. Several studies have thus shown a substantial decrease of blood levels of CSA in pregnant women compared to prepregnancy levels (54, 55). Conventionally measured trough CSA blood levels may not reflect the true exposure to the drug. Despite this drawback, and given the variability in CSA dose requirements during pregnancy, it is recommended that trough CSA levels be checked once or twice monthly during the last two trimesters of pregnancy, with adjustments being made for maintaining trough levels within the usual therapeutic range (52). If adequately monitored, CSA does not cause a significant deterioration of graft function during pregnancy: a small rise in post-partum maternal serum creatinine (+9.6 μmol/l) was reported in a recent series of 29 women, who had had no change in renal function during pregnancy (56)—a profile similar to that documented in the large cohort of patients analyzed in the US National Transplantation Pregnancy Registry (40). CSA crosses the placenta with fetal–maternal concentration ratios ranging from 1:3 to 1:1. No excess of congenital anomalies are reported in large series of newborns from CSA-treated mothers compared to offsprings of mothers not treated with CSA (1, 52). Shortening of gestational age and lower birthweight of neonates are mentioned in several series: the mean birthweight of neonates was thus 2190 g in the 29 pregnancies reported from Ireland (56). A low birthweight (less than 2500 g) was found in 50% of 197 pregnancies analyzed in the US registry, 54% of the live births were premature (less than 37 weeks of gestation), and pre-eclampsia complicated the course of pregnancy in 29% of the mothers. The US registry individualizes maternal drug-treated hypertension, diabetes, and serum creatinine greater than 15 mg/dl, as risk factors to newborns of CSA-treated female transplant recipients (48). Renal function develops normally in children exposed to CSA during the whole duration of pregnancy, as demonstrated by the results observed in a series of 12 infants investigated at 2.6 ± 1.8 years of age: average inulin clearance was $117 \pm 28 \, \text{ml/min}/1.73 \, \text{m}^2$, clearance of PAH $545 \pm 124 \, \text{ml/min}/1.73 \, \text{m}^2$. No disturbances of tubular functions were detected (57).

Tacrolimus (FK 506)

The mechanisms of the immunosuppressive action of tacrolimus are close to that of CSA: the drug has a similar degree of nephrotoxicity, potential exacerbation of maternal hypertension, and other side-effects such as incidence of diabetes mellitus, neurological or digestive symptoms. Clinical experience with tacrolimus is currently much greater in liver transplant recipients and this holds also true for pregnant women. Rather than from single-case (58) or small series reports (59), a more informative contribution is provided by a recent cumulative review of the course and outcome of 100 pregnancies in 84 women treated with tacrolimus between 1992 and 1998, among whom 66% were liver and 27% kidney recipients, respectively (60). None of the graft-rejection episodes occuring during pregnancy resulted in graft loss, mean gestation time was 35 weeks, 59% of the deliveries were premature, and the mean birthweight (2573 g) was proportional for the gestational age in 90% of cases. Hyperkalemia (which had been previously reported in smaller series of newborns) (59), hypoxia, and renal dysfunction were transient complications occuring in neonates, among whom four presented inconsistent malformations. The nature and rate of maternal and neonatal complications attributed to tacrilomus thus appear quite similar to that described with other immunosuppressive drugs.

Mycophenolate mofetil (MMF)

This more recent purine antagonist is credited for considerably reducing the incidence of acute rejection episodes in kidney-graft recipients compared to AZA-treated patients. MMF therapy is associated with mainly digestive side-effects (diarrhea, nausea, vomiting), leukopenia, and infections. Fetal malformations have been documented in animals at doses lower than those recommended for humans when corrected for body surface area (52, 61). As of February 2001, no information is available through a Medline search on the management and safety of MMF in pregnant renal transplant recipients.

Sirolimus (rapamycin)

The mechanisms of action of this immunossupressive drug, newly introduced into clinical organ transplantation, is distinct from that of calcineurin inhibitors (CSA and FK 506). Its main currently advocated advantage is its lack of nephrotoxicity. Several recent reviews on this drug mentioned no specific information on pharmacological, experimental, or clinical effects concerning pregnant animals or humans, or data on teratogenicity (61–63). Rapamycin is still in a developing phase and its prescription to pregnant transplant recipients cannot be recommended until further information becomes available.

Monoclonal antibodies

Muromonab-CD3 (OKT3) is a murine IgG monoclonal antibody mainly used in steroid-resistant acute allograft rejection, less frequently as an immunosuppressive induction agent. Because it causes severe side-effects, it is indeed employed most of the time as a rescue drug given to overcome critical situations. Experience with OKT3 in pregnant women is thus very limited: five of seven patients reported in the literature treated with OKT3 for acute-organ rejection, lost their graft due to irreversible rejection. There were, however, four successful pregnancy outcomes in this series, with no malformations in the neonate (52). OKT-3 readily crosses the placenta and from the hitherto limited experience a potential teratogenicity of the drug cannot be excluded. As of early 2001, there is no information available on the use in pregnant transplant patients of more recently developed monoclonal antibodies, such as daclizumab or basiliximab, which are prescribed in association with other IS regimens for prevention of acute rejection episodes.

Management of complications in pregnant renal transplant recipients

Alteration of renal function during pregnancy is an immediately perilous event, which requires quick diagnosis and appropriate treatment. The variety of IS drugs that has become available in recent years has widely diversified the IS regimens designed for transplant patients. Following the initial combination of CS + ASA, triple IS therapy made of CS+AZA+CSA became very popular during the last decade. More recently, several other combinations have been implemented or tested such as CS+MMF+ CSA, CS+FK506, CSA+RAPA+FK506, FK506+MMF+CS, and so on, with the double objective of reducing the frequency and gravity of acute/chronic organ rejection, and diminishing the adverse side-effects due to each of the compounds.

In the presence of a worsening renal function in a pregnant renal transplant recipient, an early accurate diagnosis is mandatory to distinguish between transplant rejection (due to insufficient immunosuppression) drug nephrotoxicity (overdosage), recurrence of underlying renal disease, or urinary tract obstruction. Ultrasound examination of the graft and, in some difficult cases, renal biopsy, may be indicated to evidence the cause of the impairment of renal function, which may lead to modification in the dosage or composition of the IS protocol. Rapid development of heavy proteinuria, associated with hypertension and decline of renal function, may be symptomatic of pre-eclampsia or acute kidney rejection, with thus totally different therapeutic indications: bed-rest and adequate treatment of hypertension (26) with rapid delivery of the baby; or, on the other hand, high-dose pulse steroid therapy.

Development or aggravation of prepregnancy hypertension is particularly common in patients whose IS protocol includes CSA or FK506. In addition to the maternal risks, prematurity and low birthweight of neonates are also complications resulting from uncontrolled blood pressure in mothers. Treatment of hypertension is similar to that indicated for hypertensive pregnant dialysis patients with the same contra-indications for ACE-inhibitors (*vide supra*).

All IS drugs carry an increased risk for infections, bacterial, viral, and particularly opportunistic complications. Among the latter, CMV maternal infections (although much less frequent beyond 2 years after transplantation) can be transmitted to the fetus with clinical manifestations present at birth (thrombocytopenia, growth or mental retardation, or even death) or later in life (hearing loss, learning disability). Positive testing for IgM-specific CMV antibody cannot differenciate between primary and recurrent infection in the mother and is thus not predictive for infection or damage to the fetus. This also holds true for the presence of CMV virus evidenced by culture or PCR-reaction in the amniotic fluid obtained with amniocentesis. It is, however, recommended to measure anti-CMV IgM and IgC titers in the blood each trimester (1). The efficacy of ganciclovir for prevention of CMV-infectious complications in the fetus rests currently on single-case reports. An *ex vivo* study has shown that ganciclovir crosses the plasma by simple diffusion with per cent fetal levels, compared with maternal levels, ranging between 17.2% and 19.2% at 1 h after perfusion of doses yielding therapeutic maternal levels (64). There are no available data to date on the efficacy and potential side-effects of foscarnet in pregnancy.

Pregnant transplant recipients should be serologically screened for toxoplasmosis each trimester, since transmission of the disease results in neonatal infection in 25–65% of the newborns whose mothers presented a primary infection during pregnancy (1). Prenatal diagnosis can also be made with PCR-analysis of cultured cells obtained via amniocentesis (52). The incidence of congenital infections increases with the months of pregnancy, but the severity of the disease is greater in early pregnancy. Toxoplasmosis may provoke miscarriage or intra-uterine death and deafness, blindness, or mental retardation after birth. Treatment of toxoplasmosis diagnosed after primary infection or in case of rising antibody titers in prepregnancy positive women with sulfadiazine, pyrimethamine, or spiromycine is reported as reducing the transmission of the disease to the fetus in up to 60% of cases (1, 52).

The risk for neonatal herpes simplex infection occurs only if maternal infection develops close to the onset of labor. Women who experience their first genital herpes outbreak during gestation benefit from acyclovir treatment with a decrease of an otherwise possible need for cesarean delivery. By contrast, the beneficial effect of acyclovir as prophylactic treatment in patients with prepregnancy herpes infection is not firmly proven. No short-term adverse fetal or neonatal effects have been recorded in more than 1800 infants exposed to varying amounts and duration of maternal acyclovir suppression. Acyclovir is also well-tolerated with a wide margin of safety in infants, even if premature (65).

Hepatitis B remains a very frequent disease in large parts of the world, where populations are exposed to unscreened blood products and/or have no access to anti-hepatitis B vaccination. Neonates born to hepatitis B-positive mothers are infected at the time of delivery and thus become virus carrier themselves. Emergency treatment is thus mandatory within 48h after delivery. Hepatitis B immune globulin, in association with anti-hepatitis B vaccine, are very effective for prevention of chronic hepatitis B in infants.

Hepatitis C is nowadays much more commonly encountered in the Western World than hepatitis B among the ESRD population. From studies conducted in anti-HCV-positive non-transplant pregnant women, it appears that preterm deliveries are not more frequent than in anti-HCV-negative women, APGAR scores, ombilical pH, and birthweight are similar in neonates from anti-HCV-positive and negative mothers. While all tested babies from anti-HCV-positive mothers were found positive at birth, the percentage fell to 10% at 12–18 months of age, with only one infant remaining HCV-RNA-positive beyond 12 months, yielding a 5% vertical transmission rate among HCV-RNA-positive mothers (66).

Pregnancy in female pancreas–kidney recipients

Apart from single-case reports, pooled information on this subject is available mainly through the International Pancreas Transplant Registry (67) and from the USA-based National Transplantation Pregnancy Registry (68). When 28 pregnancies in kidney-only recipients were compared with 12 pregnancies in pancreas–kidney recipients, the latter presented no difficulty for blood glucose control during pregnancy in contrast to 20% of the kidney-only recipients, but maternal infections were more frequent in pancreas–kidney transplanted women (67% vs. 15%). Newborns from pancreas–kidney-grafted mothers had a lower birthweight but fewer complications than those born to kidney-only recipients (67). Among 19 cases of pregnancy in 17 recipients of pancreas–kidney transplants with 19 live births, metabolic control was reported as good in all cases, but worsening of retinopathy developed in one patient. Mean birthweight of the neonates was 2150 ± 680 g and mean duration of gestation 35 ± 2.2 weeks. Acute rejection caused the loss of one pancreas graft at delivery (66). Successful pregnancy is thus possible and documented in female pancreas–kidney recipients. Prematurity and low birthweight of the infants are of greater concern than an increased risk of maternal complications related to the presence of two solid grafted organs.

References

1. Hou, S. (1999). Pregnancy in chronic renal insufficiency and end-stage renal disease. *American Journal of Kidney Diseases*, **33**, 235–52.
2. Palmer, B.F. (1999). Sexual dysfunction in uremia. *Journal of the American Society of Nephrology*, **10**, 1381–88.

3. Schmidt, R.J. and Holley, J.L. (1998). Fertility and contraception in end stage renal disease. *Advances in Renal Replacement Therapy*, **5**, 38–44.

4. Schaefer, R.M., Kokot, F., Kuerner, B., Zech, M., and Heidland, A. (1989). Normalization of serum prolactin levels in hemodialysis patients on recombinant human erythropoeitin. *International Journal of Artificial Organs*, **12**, 445–49.

5. Steffensen, G. and Aunsholt, N.A. (1993). Does erythropoietin cause hormonal changes in hemodialysis patients? *Nephrology Dialysis Transplantation*, **8**, 1215–18.

6. Maruyama, H., Shimada, H., Obayashi, H., Nakamaru, T., Miakawa, Y., Gojo, S. *et al.* (1998). Requiring higher doses of erythropoeitin suggests pregnancy in dialysis patients. *Nephron*, **79**, 413–19.

7. Hussey, M.J. and Pombar, X., (1998). Obstetric care for renal allograft recipients or for women treated with hemodialysis or peritoneal dialysis during pregnancy. *Advances in Renal Replacement Therapy*, **5**, 3–13.

8. Bagon, J.A., Vernaeve, H., De Muilder, X., Lafontaine, J.J., Martens, J., and Van Roost, G. (1998). Pregnancy and dialysis. *American Journal of Kidney Diseases*, **31**, 756–65.

9. Okundaye, I., Abrinko, P., and Hou, S. (1998). Registry of pregnancy in dialysis patients. *American Journal of Kidney Diseases*, **31**, 766–73.

10. Toma, H., Tanabe, K., Tokumoto, T., Kobayashi, C., and Yagisawa, T. (1999). Pregnancy in women receiving renal dialysis or transplantation in Japan: a nationwide survey. *Nephrology Dialysis Transplantation*, **14**, 1511–16.

11. Souqiyyeh, M.Z., Huraib, S.O., Saleh, A.G., and Aswad, S. (1992). Pregnancy in chronic hemodialysis patients in the Kingdom of Saudi Arabia. *American Journal of Kidney Diseases*, **19**, 235–38.

12. Hou, S.H. (1994). Frequency and outcome of pregnancy in women on dialysis. *American Journal of Kidney Diseases*, **23**, 160–63.

13. Giatras, I., Levy, D.P., Malone, F.D., Carlson, J.A., and Jungers, P. (1998). Pregnancy during dialysis: case report and management guidelines. *Nephrology Dialysis Transplantation*, **13**, 3266–72.

14. Chan, W.S., Okun, N., and Kjellstrand, C.M. (1998). Pregnancy in chronic dialysis: a review and analysis of the literature. *International Journal of Artificial Organs*, **21**, 259–68.

15. Blowley, D.L. and Warad, B.A. (1998). Neonatal outcome in pregnancies associated with renal replacement therapy. *Advances in Renal Replacement Therapy*, **5**, 45–52.

16. Jungers, P. and Chauveau, D. (1997). Pregnancy in renal disease. *Kidney International*, **52**, 871–85.

17. Hou, S. and Firanek, C. (1998). Management of the pregnant dialysis patient. *Advances in Renal Replacement Therapy*, **5**, 24–30.

18. Romao Jr, J.E., Luders, C., Kamale, S., Pascoal, I.J.F., Abensur, H., Sabbaga, E. *et al.* (1998). Pregnancy in women on chronic dialysis. *Nephron*, **78**, 416–22.

19. Okundaye, I. and Hou, S. (1996). Management of pregnancy in women undergoing continuous ambulatory peritoneal dialysis. *Advances in Peritoneal Dialysis*, **12**, 151–55.

20. Castillon, A.A., Lew, S.Q., Smith, A.M., and Bosch, J.P. (1999). Women issues in female patients receiving peritoneal dialysis. *Advances in Renal Replacement Therapy*, **6**, 327–34.

21. Hou, S. (1996). Pregnancy in women treated with peritoneal dialysis: Viewpoint 1996. *Peritoneal Dialysis International*, **5**, 442–43.

22. Reisenberger, K., Egarter, C., Sternberger, B., Eckenberger, P., Eberle, E., and Weissenbacher, E.R. (1996). Placental passage of angiotensin-conventing enzyme inhibitors. *American Journal of Obstetrics and Gynecology*, **174**, 1450–55.

23. Shotan, A., Widerhorn, J., Hurst, A., and Elkayam, U. (1996). Risks of angiotensin-converting enzyme inhibitor during pregnancy: experimental and clinical evidence potential mechanisms and recommendations for use. *American Journal of Medicine*, **96**: 451–56.

24. Unsigned. (1997). Postmarketing surveillance for angiotensin-converting enzyme inhibitor during the first trimester of pregnancy—United States, Canada and Israel, 1987–1995. *MMWR, Morbidity, Mortality. Weekly Report*, **46**, 240–42.

25. Pryde, D.G., Sedman, A.B., Nugent, L.E., and Barr, M. Jr. (1993). Angiotensin-converting enzyme inhibitor fetopathy. *Journal of the American Society of Nephrology*, **3**, 1575–82.

26. Vermillion, S.T., Scardo, J.A., Newman, R.B., and Chauchan, S.P. (1999). A randomized double-blind trial of oral nifedipine and intravenous labetabol in hypertensive emergencies of pregnancy. *American Journal of Obstetrics and Gynecology*, **181**, 858–61.

27. Visser, W. and Wallenburg, H.C. (1995). A comparison between the hemodynamic effects of oral nifedipine and intravenous dihydralazine in patients with severe pre-eclampsia. *Journal of Hypertension*, **13**, 791–95.

28. Knight, M., Duley, L., Henderson-Smart, D.J., and King, J.F. (2000). Antiplatelet agents for preventing and treating pre-eclampsia. *Cochrane Data Base System Review*, **2**, CD 000492.

29. Heyborne, K.D. (2000). Pre-eclampsia prevention, lessons from the low-dose aspirin therapy trials. *American Journal of Obstetrics and Gynecology*, **183**, 523–28.

30. Schneider, H. and Malek, A. (1995). Lack of permeability of the human placenta for erythropoietin. *Journal of Peritoneal Medicine*, **23**, 71–6.

31. Working Party for European. (1999). Working Party for European best practice guidelines for the management of anemia in patients with chronic renal failure. *Nephrology Dialysis Transplantation*, **14**, (Suppl. 5), 1–50.

32. Brookhyser, J. and Wiggins, K. (1998). Medical nutrition therapy in pregnancy and kidney disease. *Advances in Renal Replacement Therapy*, **5**, 53–63.

33. Norton, M.E., Merrill, J., Cooper, B.A., Kuller, J.A., and Clyman, R.I. (1993). Neonatal complications after the administration of indomethacin for pre-term labor. *New England Journal of Medicine*, **329**, 1602–07.

34. Norton, M.E. (1997). Teratogen update, fetal effects of indomethacin administration during pregnancy. *Teratology*, **56**, 282–92.

35. Lu, J.F. and Nightingale, C.H. (2000). Magnesium sulfate in eclampsia and pre-eclampsia, pharmacokinetic principles. *Clinical Pharmacokinetics*, **38**, 305–14.

36. Rizzoni, G., Ehrich, J.H., Broyer, M., Brunner, E.P., Brynger, H., Fassbinder, W. *et al.* (1992). Successful pregnancies in women on renal replacement therapy, report from the EDTA Registry. *Nephrology, Dialysis, Transplantation*, **7**, 279–87.

37. Armenti, V.T., Moritz, M.J., and Davison, J.M. (1998). Medical management of the pregnant transplant patient. *Advances in Renal Replacement Therapy*, **5**, 14–23.

38. Owda, A.K., Abdallah, H., Al-Suliman, M.H., al-Hawas, F., Mousa, D.H., Fedail, H. *et al.* (1998). No evidence of functional deterioration of renal graft after repeated pregnancies. A report on three women with 17 pregnancies. *Nephrology, Dialysis, Transplantation*, **13**, 1281–84.

39. Ehrich, J.H., Loirat, C., Davison, J.M., Rizzoni, G., Wittkop, B., Selwood, N.M. *et al.* (1996). Repeated successful pregnancies after kidney transplantation in 102 women (report by the EDTA Registry). *Nephrology, Dialysis, Transplantation*, **11**, 1314–17.

40. Armenti, V.T., Wilson, G.A., Radomski, J.S., Moritz, M.J., McGrory, C.H., and Coscia, L.A. (1999). Report from the National Transplantation Pregnancy Registry (NTPR), outcomes of pregnancy after transplantation. *Clinical Transplants*, 111–19.

41. Rischen, J., Hoitsma, A.J., de Fijter, J.W., Surachno, S., Tegzess, A.M., Van Hooff, R.J. *et al.* (1999). Pregnancy in renal transplant in the Netherlands (1969–1998). *Journal of the American Society of Nephrology*, **10**, (Abstract), 745 A.

42. Armenti, V.T., McGrory, C.M., Cater, J.R., Radomski, J.S., and Moritz, M.J. (1998). Pregnancy outcomes in female renal transplant patients. *Transplantation Proceedings*, **30**, 1732–34.

43. Davison, J.M. (1985). The effect of pregnancy on kidney function in renal allograft recipients. *Kidney International*, **27**, 74–79.

44. Crowe, A.V., Rustom, R., Gradden, C., Seus, R.A., Bakran, A., Bone, J.M. *et al.* (1999). Pregnancy does not adversely affect renal transplant function. *Quarterly Journal of Medicine*, **92**, 631–35.

45. First, M.R., Combs, C.A., Weiskittel, P., and Miodovnik, M. (1995). Lack of effect of pregnancy on renal allograft survival or function. *Transplantation*, **59**, 472–76.

46. Barrou, B., Sylla, C., Ourahma, S., Benalia, H., Mouquet, C., Luciani, J. *et al.* (1996). Pregnancy after renal transplantation, Impact on graft function. *Transplantation Proceedings*, **28**, 2835.

47. Davison, J.M. (1994). Pregnancy in renal allograft recipients. Problems, prognosis and practicabilities. *Baillieres Clinical Obstetrics and Gynaecology*, **2**, 501–25.

48. Armenti, V.T., Ahlswede, K.M., Ahlswede, B.A., Cater, J.R., Jarrell, B.E., Moritz, M.J. *et al.* (1995). Variables affecting birthweight and graft survival in 197 pregnancies in cyclosporine treated female kidney transplant recipients. *Transplantation*, **59**, 476–79.

49. Sturgiss, S.N. and Davison, J.M. (1995). Effect of pregnancy on the long-term function of renal allografts, an update. *American Journal of Kidney Diseases*, **26**, 54–6.

50. Kozlowska-Bozko, B., Durlik, M., Kuczynka-Sicinska, J., and Lao, M. (1996). Predictor of transplanted kidney deterioration following pregnancy: daily urine protein loss or serum creatinine concentration? *Annals of Transplantation*, **1**, 30–1.

51. Gaughan, W.J., Moritz, M.J., Radomski, J.S., Burke, J.F. Jr., and Armenti, V.T. (1996). National Transplantation Pregnancy Registry, Report on outcomes in cyclosporine-treated female kidney transplant recipients with an interval from transplant to pregnancy greater than five years. *American Journal of Kidney Diseases*, **28**, 266–69.

52. Ghandour, F.Z., Knauss, Th.C., and Hricik, D.E. (1998). Immunosuppressive drugs in pregnancy. *Advances in Renal Replacement Therapy*, **5**, 31–8.

53. Ramsay-Goldman, R. and Schilling, E. (1997). Immunosuppressive drug use during pregnancy. *Rheumatic Diseases Clinics of North America*, **23**, 149–67.

54. Thomas, A.G., Burrows, L., Knight, R., Panico, M., Lapinski, R., and Lockwood, C.J. (1997). The effect of pregnancy on Cyclosporine levels in renal allograft patients. *Obstetrics and Gynecology*, **90**, 916–19.

55. Kozlowska-Boszko, B., Gaciong, Z., Serafinowicz, A., Majchrzak, J., Durlik, M., Rowinski, W. *et al.* (1998). Cyclosporine A blood concentration during pregnancy in renal allograft recipients. *Transplant International*, **11**, (Suppl. 1), S90–3.

56. Little, M.A., Abraham, K.A., Kavanagh, J., Connolly, G., Byrne, P., and Walshe, J.J. (2000). Pregnancy in Irish renal transplant recipients in the Cyclosporine-era. *Irish Journal of Medical Sciences*, **169**, 19–21.

57. Lo Giudice, P., Dubourg, L., Hadj-Aissa, A., Said, M.H., Claris, O., Audra, Ph. *et al.* (2000). Renal function of children exposed to Cyclosporine in utero. *Nephrology, Dialysis, Transplantation*, **15**, 1575–79.

58. Fehrman-Ekholm, I. and Nisell, H. (1998). A successful pregnancy in a kidney recipient with Tacrolimus (Prograf, FK 506) therapy. *Nephrology, Dialysis, Transplantation*, **13**, 2982–83 (letter).

59. Jain, A., Venkataramanan, R., Fung, J.J., Gartner, J.C., Lever, J., Balan, V. *et al.* (1997). Pregnancy after liver transplantation under Tacrolimus. *Transplantation*, **64**, 559–65.

60. Kainz, A., Harabacz, I., Cowlrick, I.S., Gadgil, S.D., and Hagiwara, D. (2000). Review of the course and outcome of 100 pregnancies in 84 women treated with Tacrolimus. *Transplantation*, **70**, 1718–21.

61. Gonin, J.M. (2000). Maintenance immunosuppression, New agents and persistent dilemmas. *Advances in Renal Replacement Therapy*, **7**, 95–116.

62. Morelon, E., Mamzer-Bruneel, M.F., Peraldi, M.N., and Kreis, H. (2001). Sirolimus, a new promising immunosuppressive drug, towards the rationale for its use in renal transplantation. *Nephrology, Dialysis, Transplantation*, **16**, 18–20.

63. Saunders, R.N., Metcalfe, M.S., and Nicholson, M.L. (2001). Rapamycin in transplantation, A review of the evidence. *Kidney International*, **59**, 3–16.

64. Gilstrap, L.C., Bawdon, R.E., Roberts, S.W., and Sobhi, S. (1994). The transfer of the nucleoside analog ganciclovir across the perfused human plasma. *American Journal of Obstetrics and Gynecology*, **170**, 972–73.

65. Scott, L.L. (1999). Prevention of perinatal herpes, Prophylactic antiviral therapy. *Clinical Obstetrics and Gynecology*, **42**, 134–48.

66. Hillemanns, P., Dannecker, C., Kimming, R., and Hasbargen, U. (2000). Obstetric risks and vertical transmission of hepatitis C virus infection in pregnancy. *Acta Obstetrica et Gynecologica Scandinavica*, **79**, 543–47.

67. Barrou, B., Gruessner, A.C., Sutherland, D.E., and Gruessner, R.W. (1998). Pregnancy after pancreas transplantation in the Cyclosporine era, Report from the International Pancreas Transplant Registry. *Transplantation*, **65**, 524–27.

68. Armenti, V.T., McGrory, C.H., Cater, J., Radomski, J.S., and Moritz, M.J. (1997). The National Transplantation Pregnancy Registry, Comparison between pregnancy outcomes in diabetic Cyclosporine-treated female kidney recipients and CYA-treated female pancreas-kidney recipients. *Transplantation Proceedings*, **29**, 669–70.

7

Optimal renal replacement therapy in elderly patients

Claude Jacobs and Françoise Mignon

No universal consensus currently prevails for the definition of elderly people. A 65-year age-limit is widely recognized in many countries for designating people as such on social, professional, or administrative grounds. In many persons, old age cannot be strictly identified with civil age, as an elderly condition is also largely a state of mind. Similar difficulties and complications of dialysis treatments can be encountered in patients aged 40 or 75 years depending on their individual past history, presence of co-morbid diseases, and social environment.

Nowadays, at least in the developed countries of the world, the life–expectancy (at birth) of the populations at large has increased steadily over the past 50 years, being currently estimated at around 80–82 years for females and around 75 years for males. It may thus be quite appropriate to distinguish between seniors persons aged 60–75 years and truly old patients aged 75 years or more. However, for the sake of homogeneity with most of the reports that have been published during the past 25 years on the results of renal replacement therapies (RRT) in elderly patients, we shall comply here with the widely accepted lower age-limit of 65 years for defining the segment of elderly patients.

Demographic profile

Among the 84 435 patients who started some form of RRT in the USA during the year 1998, 49% were aged at least 65 years versus 37. 8% of those accepted for therapy in 1990 (Table 7.1). Expressed per million population (pmp) the incidence rate of all the patients newly treated for ESRD in the USA rose from 195 to 312 between 1990 and 1998, whereas it soared at 1323 and 1385 pmp in 1998 for patients aged 65–74 years and 75+years, respectively (1). The percentage of patients aged ≥ 65 years taken onto RRT in 1998 was 87. 4% of the total ESRD population (all ages combined) taken onto RRT in 1990. Of note, the proportion of patients aged ≥ 85 years, increased by 228%. Actually, the population with terminal renal failure starting RRT in the USA is indeed, for its vast majority, belonging to the elderly people category, based on the fact that in 1997 the mean and median ages of the incident ESRD patients were 61 years and 65 years, respectively.

Table 7.1   Incidence rates of elderly patients starting renal replacement therapy in the USA

	1990		1998		Δ% 1990–98
	(*n*)	(%)	(*n*)	(%)	
Patients of all ages	47 054	100.0	84 435	100.0	+79.4
All patients ≥65 years	17 795	37.8	41 141	48.7	+131.0
Patients 65–74 years	9 864	21.0	21 973	26.0	+122.0
Patients 75–84 years	6 967	14.8	16 015	19.0	+130.0
Patients 85+ years	962	2.0	3 153	3.7	+228.0

Source: USRDS Report (2000).

Table 7.2   Prospects for persons alive (million) aged >75 years

	Years								
	2000 Total population >75 years			2010 Total population >75 years			2020 Total population >75 years		
		(*n*)	(%)		(*n*)	(%)		(*n*)	(%)
Europe	729	43.1	5.9	724	53.1	7.3	712	58.1	8.2
North America	310	18.3	5.9	332	20.4	6.1	364	23.9	6.7
Latin America	510	9.9	1.9	595	14.0	2.3	665	19.6	2.9
Asia	3682	68.2	1.9	4136	100.8	2.4	4535	133.8	2.9

Source: World Population Prospects. 1998 Revision, Vol. II (1999).
      Department of Economic and Social Affairs, United Nations, New York, USA.

On the basis of historical data from 1982 through 1997, the projected growth of US ESRD patients is estimated between the years 2000 to 2010 at a 4.1% yearly rate for incidence, 6.4% for prevalence thus reaching in 2010, 129 000 and 651 000 patients, respectively (2). The demographic and epidemiological trends observed in the ESRD population during the last two decades having no foreseeable reason to change significantly during the next 10 years, it is thus certain that the vast majority of these new patients will be older than 65 years, with an increasing proportion of truly old persons aged 75 years or more. Of note, the populations of very old persons are foreseen to grow in all continents (with the exception of Africa) within the next two decades, the highest increases being anticipated in the European and Asian countries (Table 7.2). Among 46 677 patients who were reported as starting RRT in 1995 in the European countries still participating to the EDTA registry at that time, the overall percentage of patients aged ≥60 years was 52%, ranging from 53% in France up to 61% in Italy, where 25% of the newly treated patients during that year were in the 70–79 years age

Table 7.3 Point prevalence rates of patients aged ≥65 years treated with renal replacement therapies in the USA

	December 1990		December 1998		Δ% 1990–98
	(*n*)	(%)	(*n*)	(%)	
Patients of all ages	172 569	100.0	319 515	100.0	+85.0
All patients ≥65 years	52 743	30.6	110 581	34.6	+110.2
Patients 65–74 years	34 673	20.0	65 190	20.4	+88.0
Patients 75–84 years	15 978	9.2	38 734	12.1	+142.4
Patients 85+years	2 092	1.2	6 667	2.1	+218.7

Source: USRDS Report (2000).

range (3). A survey conducted in France in the greater Paris area during the year 1998, revealed that 54.7% of the incident ESRD patients were older than 60 years; 21.6% were aged 75 years or more (4).

In the USA, the point prevalence on 31 December 1998 for patients aged≥65 years was 34.6% of the total treated ESRD population versus only 30.6% in December 1990 (Table 7.3). In the European countries as of December 1995, 40% of all patients treated for ESRD were older than 60 years, ranging from 37% in France up to 51% in Italy. Of the ESRD population, 14% were in the 70–79 years age range: 19% in Italy, 16% in Spain, and 13% in France (2).

Causes of ESRD in elderly patients

The distribution of underlying renal diseases leading to ESRF in elderly patients has been recently reviewed according to data collected from January 1980 to December 1994 in four of the world's largest dialysis and transplant registries (Europe, USA, Australia, New Zealand (5) (Table 7.4). Arteriopathic renal diseases and infective obstructive nephropathies were reported most frequently among the elderly USA patients, whereas diabetic nephropathy and glomerulonephritis were more frequently diagnosed in patients aged 35–64 years at start of RRT. In the European countries, all these four underlying renal diseases were more frequently reported in middle-aged patients, and no investigated cause of ESRD was found as specifically prominent in elderly patients.

Optimal use of dialysis methods in elderly patients

HD, as well as PD, can be considered equally suitable options for the treatment of ESRF in elderly patients. The nephrological team in charge of elderly patients has, however, to pay even greater attention than for young patients, to many non-strictly medical criteria for counseling (and finally selecting) the modality of RRT. Of key importance for the future success, difficulties, or failure of a given dialysis treatment,

Table 7.4   Distribution according to age of primary renal diseases in patients taken onto RRT (01.1980–12.1994)

	Australia–New Zealand			European Countries			USA		
	15–34 (%)	35–64 (%)	65+ (%)	15–34 (%)	35–64 (%)	65+ (%)	15–34 (%)	35–64 (%)	65+ (%)
Arteriopathic renal diseases	3.5	57.4	39.1	4.7	5.1	44	5.1	36.9	57.9
Glomerulonephritis	26.9	56.4	14.3	30.9	51.5	12.9	23.3	45.1	29.5
Diabetes	12.4	74.9	12.7	9.7	59.1	31.0	8.2	54.6	37.2
Infective obstructive nephropathies	39.5	43.4	9.3	16.0	52.4	28.8	13.6	37.0	46.6
Familial hereditary renal diseases	11.0	73.5	11.1	9.8	71.7	14.9	8.2	66.9	22.9

Adapted from Maisonneuve *et al.* (*2000*) *American Journal of Kidney Diseases*, 35-1, 157-165.

are comprehensive and objective assessments of each individual patient's psychological and cognitive status, quality of familial and social environment, acceptance or refusal of the mere principle of undergoing RRT, or objection to the mode and/or location of the treatment (in-center, satellite unit, or home) (6, 7). It has to be remembered that an elderly person is fragilized in many ways by the mere effect of aging, which pledges strongly for an early initiation of dialysis to prevent the devastating effects of long-term, frequently concealed malnutrition, or of uncontrollable hypertension or fluid overload. Some widely used biological parameters may be misleading, e.g. a low concentration of serum creatinine may in fact reflect a significant reduction of muscular mass, a low serum urea concentration and a normal/high serum bicarbonate may be second to a poor protein intake. Some mode of dialysis should be commenced at short notice if any significant change is recorded for one or several of these criteria, which cannot be adequately corrected by medical or dietary measures.

Hemodialysis (HD) turns out as the elective mode of dialysis therapy for patients who are unable to perform self-care for peritoneal dialysis or who have no support available from spouse, relatives, or other caregivers to assist them for their daily technical requirements. Depending on the patient's clinical and psychological status, and on the additional burden imposed by co-morbidities or disabilities, hemodialysis treatment will be delivered either in hospital-based or in limited-care facilities.

Vascular access is best achieved with a native arteriovenous (AV) fistula. Arteriovenous synthetic grafts, especially if they are placed in proximal segments of the limbs, may provoke arterial-steal syndromes favored by pre-existing atherosclerotic lesions and lead to distal ischemic gangrenous lesions. Efficient vascular access for HD can be obtained for prolonged periods with the use of percutaneously placed jugular-vein catheters, if an internal vascular access is difficult to create or keep patent.

It has been well demonstrated that older age is a significant potential risk factor for the development of clinical signs and symptoms of dialysis related amyloidosis (DRA), besides the time elapsed since start of dialysis and the type of dialysis membrane used (8). The most effective prevention of the consequences of β2-microglobulin accumulation is an early successful renal transplantation, a treatment modality from which the vast majority of elderly ESRD patients unfortunately cannot benefit. The use of high-flux biocompatible membranes, which provide a greater clearing of β2-microglobulin than cellulosic membranes, together with sterile ultra-pure dialysis fluids (9) or of convective blood purification techniques, such as hemodiafiltration, is thus recommended in elderly patients not suitable for renal transplantation (10).

Profound and frequently sudden, unexpected, falls of blood pressure occuring during hemodialysis sessions are particularly dangerous for elderly patients. These incidents result mainly from a fluid removal from the vascular space too rapid to be compensated adequately by an adequate refilling rate from the interstitial space (11, 12). The phenomenon is amplified by the frequent insufficiency of the cardiac output to compensate for the decrease of peripheral vascular resistance. Autonomic dysfunction, mainly present in diabetic patients, and low cardiac reserve due to left ventricular hypertrophy, dilated or hypertrophic cardiomyopathy, or ischemic heart disease, are among the main factors that preclude an adapted response to rapid fluid removal. Hypotensive episodes are furthermore triggered by existing arrhythmias and also by the transient hypoxemia that occurs in the early phases of dialysis sessions performed with acetate dialysate and cellulosic membranes (13).

Because of this vascular instability, frequently present in elderly patients, HD sessions should be performed very smoothly with a slow, volumetrically controlled fluid removal, bicarbonate-buffered dialysate, with a minimal and adjustable sodium concentration not lower than 140 mmol/l, in order to avoid hypotensive episodes, which can precipitate the occurrence of angina, myocardial infarction, or cerebrovascular accidents (14). Re-evaluation of dry weight is mandatory in case of an increasing frequency of hypotensive episodes. Recent studies have well demonstrated the improved tolerance and better control of clinical and biological parameters yielded by daily dialysis techniques, which unfortunately can be proposed only to the very small group of elderly patients who can or wish to perform home HD (15). Addition of glucose to the dialysate (up to 200 mg/dl) may provide better hemodynamic tolerance and some frequently needed caloric supplementation. Per-dialytic supply of amino-acid solutions, or other nutritional compounds/mixtures, can also be helpful for malnourished patients.

Peritoneal dialysis (PD) has proved in recent years its excellent suitability as RRT for elderly patients. Actually, PD should be considered as the first-line mode of treatment for terminally uremic patients with coronary heart disease, arrhythmias, for those who cannot tolerate hemodialysis for any medical reason, or whose place of residence is distant from a dialysis center and who wish to preserve their personal and family life-style (16, 17). As described in detail in Chapter 2, PD techniques are now very diversified, ranging from conventional three to four daily exchanges, to nightly automated PD performed with sophisticated cyclers. Novel dialysis fluid solutions ensure better tolerance, less metabolic adverse effects, and improved control of the patients' fluid and electrolyte balance. On-going advances in connectology and reduced hazards of bacterial contamination, thanks to the diminution of daily manipulations achieved with automated techniques, render PD increasingly more efficient and safer. Dialysis regimens are now prescribed on individual patient criteria, depending mainly on body size, residual renal function, performances of the peritoneal membrane regarding solute removal and ultrafiltration capacity, and also patient's technical ability, and compliance.

Adhesions resulting from previous intra-abdominal operation(s) are the major medical contra-indication to PD; extensive diverticulosis, severe peripheral vascular disease, major obesity, non-surgically curable hernias, very voluminous liver/renal polykystosis, blindness, or other major disability, are all transient or definitive medical contra-indications to PD. Loneliness, chronic depression, overt malnutrition, poor hygienic or lodging conditions, are strong arguments against home-performed PD, which in turn can be practised in nursing homes or other institutions. Lastly, the patient's personal acceptance and adhesion to the treatment, as well as that of the familial environnment, plays a pivotal role for the success or failure of the method. It proves uselessly time- and energy-consuming, and furthermore dangerous, to oblige an unwilling patient to perform a demanding, daily, long-term treatment modality. Technical, medical, or psychological complications will then end up in a more or less rapid drop-out of the method, with patients by then often plunged in worsened clinical conditions (18, 19).

Whatever the dialysis method used, the elderly patient is more exposed than his/her younger counterparts to the shortcomings and complications of long-term RRT. A special emphasis has here to be given to underdialysis, which is quite common due to often several combined factors. An inadequate dialysis prescription may result from misleading interpretations of spuriously satisfactory biological parameters. Insufficient delivery of dialysis dose in hemodialysis patients may result from vascular access dysfunction or early ending of dialysis sessions entailed by clinical or psychological intolerance. Moreover, in the case of acute or chronic shortage of in-center dialysis facilities, elderly patients are often the first in line for whom the number of weekly sessions or the duration of sessions will be reduced. Peritoneal dialysis patients treated at home are also exposed to underdialysis, being usually medically monitored at longer time-intervals than hemodialysis patients. Underdialysis may develop insidiously either through personal or familial non-compliance with the peritoneal dialysis regimen, incorrect evaluation of dialysis efficiency through underestimation of the performances of the peritoneal membrane, or wrong adjustment of the number or volume of daily fluid exchanges in keeping with a progressive loss of residual renal function.

Malnutrition greatly enhances the risk of complications. Infections are very common in all dialysis patients but to a greater extent in the elderly, whose immunological defenses are reduced. Persistent anorexia, with a particular loss of taste for meat or other foods of animal origin, a frequent overt or concealed depressive state aggravated by clinical problems (adverse effects of medications on digestive tract mobility, interdialytic persistent sensations of malaise due to hemodynamic instability), or low financial resources, often aggregate to the development of severe malnutrition. Assessment of nutritional status rests on the determination of anthropometric parameters, body mass index, serum albumin concentration, and dietary protein intake normalized to actual (dry) body weight (20). An active support from a dietician/nutritionist team is of paramount importance for counseling the patients and their familial environnment on the requested qualitative and quantitative nutritional requirements of the patients, bearing in mind that caloric requirements of elderly persons are frequently underestimated. Actually, the nutritional intake for elderly dialysis patients is considered only slightly different from their younger counterparts and should thus include at least 30–35 kcal/kg/day with at least 1.0 g/kg/day of protein, of which >60% should be of high biologic value. A sufficient protein intake is particularly necessary in patients treated with PD in whom protein loss, via the peritoneal exchanges, has to be considered. Vitamin B supplementation (folic acid 1 mg/day, pyridoxine 10 mg/day) may be indicated to compensate for defective dietary supply (21).

Iatrogenic complications arise frequently in the case of inadequate prescription or monitoring of numerous medications, especially hypnotics, analgesics, some classes of antibiotics, or anti-hypertensives. The risk of overdosage is enhanced by the great variability of drug removal capacity by dialysis methods, according mainly to the molecular weight and the protein-binding level of the compounds (22, 23). Neurological, psychiatric, cardiac, and/or digestive complications of iatrogenic origin are thus particularly frequent in elderly dialysis patients, and may present with very misleading symptomatologies.

The successful treatment of anemia with erythropoietin (EPO) in patients with advanced/end-stage renal disease is one of the prominent advances achieved during the past 10 years for improving the clinical condition and the quality of life of dialysis patients. The beneficial impact of correcting renal anemia on the quality of life (QL) of elderly patients has been found very comparable to that achieved in younger patients (less than 50 years) using the Karnofsky performance scale and the sickness impact profile (SIP) tests (24). Actually, the hematocrit values after administration of EPO are positively related to improvement in the SIP global score, suggesting that the higher the hematocrit (or hemoglobin concentration), the better the QL. Tolerance of elderly patients to EPO is very good, with only a small minority of patients either becoming hypertensive or worsening a pre-existing hypertension. The recently circulated European best-practice guidelines for the treatment of renal anemia with EPO, certainly apply to the vast majority of elderly dialysis patients with a mean target hemoglobin of at least 11 g/dl for 85% of the patients, corresponding to a median/mean concentration of 12–12.5 g/dl (25). Setting the upper optimal limit of hemoglobin concentration remains controversial, and no specific study has been done thus far for elderly patients. Close follow-up of iron status is particularly important in the elderly population exposed to nutritional deficiencies. Additional oral/IV iron supply is mandatory to achieve a transferrin saturation of at least 20% and a serum ferritin concentration not lower than 100–150 ng/ml for obtaining optimal results with EPO therapy and minimizing the cost.

The psychological tolerance to the different modalities of ESRD treatment is highly variable among patients of any age-range, according to a great number of individual medical, environmental, behavioral, and spiritual factors. Depression is, however, particularly common in elderly dialysis patients, of whom most of them realize that they have no way out to renal transplantation and that the dialysis machine or the PD bags/cycler will be their mandatory ultimate companion to the end of their life. The technical constraints of dialysis therapies and their consequences on patients' life styles, are often less responsible for the development of a depressive state than the functional impairment(s) resulting from co-morbidities such as peripheral vascular disease having led to amputations, limitation of de-ambulation due to arthrosis, sequalae of cerebral vascular accidents, reduction of cognitive functions, and so on. Such functional impairments, interfering to a variable extent with the patient's autonomy, imposes frequently a heavy dependence on the medical/nursing staff and even more on family members, relatives, institution staff. Poor economic conditions, loneliness, and feelings of exclusion from society, increase in many patients their dissatisfaction with life. The psychological status of each patient and his/her family is thus of crucial importance for selecting as first choice an in-center or home dialysis method. For some socially isolated patients, the contacts with caregivers and fellow patients in the treatment facility may revive a positive social link, whereas other patients will feel more psychologically comfortable in remaining in their personal environment with home dialysis therapy. Close attention should be extended for home-treated patients for detecting early enough the signs or symptoms of a burn-out syndrome, which would develop either in the patient him/herself or in the spouse or other family members. Increasing anorexia, a worsened nutritional status, irritability, insomnia, decrease in drug or dietary compliance, shortening or skipping dialysis sessions, are all features that may actually express a depressive state. In recent years, at least as many patients are reported as dropping out of home PD treatment and are switched to hemodialysis because of the consequences of psychological intolerance or true depression as those who have to switch because of infections or technical complications (19). Elderly functionally dependent patients require a particularly strong and demanding support from all the members of the team providing for their care, including dietitian, social worker, and psychologist (26). The evaluation of cognitive functions is one of the most difficult problems. Dementia affetcs one woman out of two and one man out of three in the general population after the age of 85 years. Little is known about the incidence of dementia in elderly dialysis patients. The multitude of factors that may cause cognitive problems in elderly ESRD patients should be analyzed with great care before a definitive diagnosis of dementia is made. In particular, ischemic abnormalities may cause brain atrophy (evidenced on brain CT scan or MRI imaging), which is more important in ESRD patients than in control subjects. In difficult situations, it is very important to consult the members of the patient's family who may have noticed changes in the behaviour of the patient in the previous months. It may take several weeks of well-conducted dialysis treatment before a confirmed diagnosis of dementia will finally be made.

The diagnosis is based on simple screening tests, such as the Mini Mental Status examination (MMS) (27). In the case of clear abnormalities, the patient should be referred to a specialist's team who will provide a diagnosis, always probabilistic by nature: vascular dementia, Alzheimer's disease, or dementia of other type. Anti-depressive medications or anticholinesterase drugs in cases of Alzheimer's disease, may prove useful for many patients; their prescriptions have, however, to be monitored very closely for avoiding potentially severe adverse side-effects in case of overdosage or conflicting combinations (23). Actually, the optimal reduction of functional impairments is often the most sucessful means against depression, both factors being significantly related in dialysis patients (27). A well-demonstrated example is given by the tremendously positive effect on the feeling of well-being reported by so many patients following the correction of anemia with epoietin. Long-lasting depression has been individualized as a significant factor associated with increased patient mortality, in the same order of magnitude as medical risk factors (28). Death by suicide in elderly dialysis patients is reported as more frequent than in the younger age-groups in several single-center, as well as in large-scale national or international, reports (1).

No unequivocal conclusion can be drawn from the tens of papers published in the literature over the past 15 years on the respective superiority in terms of morbidity/mortality of HD or PD for the ESRD population in general, at least during the first 5 years following the commencement of RRT, and this holds true for the elderly patients as well (29–32). Results in terms of survival vary greatly between single-center experiences and that recorded in large national or international dialysis registries. Multiples biases in patient-selection policies, differences in the degree of expertise for several modes of treatment, or mere availability of dialysis equipment, positive or negative influences of socio–cultural and environmental factors, all contribute to the difficulty of providing a clear-cut answer regarding the most appropriate mode of dialysis treatment for elderly ESRD patients, as well as for a truly objective overall statement on comparative morbidity/mortality data.

Similar statements are valid for the issues pertaining to the quality of life offered to elderly patients by dialysis therapies. This issue is indeed of particular importance for this segment of ESRD patients, since a poor quality of life provided by dialysis methods is an argument more easily taken into account by healthcare providers or healthcare funding bodies for denying or withdrawing dialysis in elderly patients, thus substantiating an age-selection process (33–35).

A recent meta-analysis performed on the prolific literature published on this theme during the past two decades, evidenced significant differences between the various renal replacement therapies on two fundamental quality of life dimensions: psychological well-being and emotional distress. Overall results from 49 published comparative studies, show that CAPD adult patients reported more psychosocial well-being than those on hospital-based hemodialysis, and those on hospital hemodialysis reported more emotional distress than those receiving home hemodialysis. However, the meta-analysis review led to the conclusion that it remains unclear whether the quality of life differences accross alternative renal replacement therapies result from valid differences accross treatment modalities, or from pre-existing differences in case-mix among the populations studied, or a combination of these two alternatives (36). A recent study performed in the UK, involving several hundreds of patients aged 70 years or over at start of renal replacement therapy, evidenced that the mental quality of life of the patients remained, in fact, intact and was similar to that in elderly people in the general population, both in the initial stages after the first 3 months of dialysis and after having been on dialysis for some years (37). Age alone should not be used as a barrier to dialysis. The medically, socially, and humanely unjustified age-based rationing of dialysis treatment is further discussed extensively in Chapter 10.

Thus, much more important than trying to loudly promote the superiority of HD or PD for elderly patients on data that are quickly challenged most of the time, it is more essential to enforce the concept according to which optimal management of ESRD in elderly patients requires a fully integrated HD + PD program available in each treatment facility, since a switch to an alternative mode of RRT may become necessary for many of them according to modifications that may occur over time in their physical or mental status, or in case of changes in their socio-familial environment such as death of a spouse or other usual companion, or if leaving the home for moving into an institution (38).

The age-adjusted 5-year survival probability for patients aged 75 or more years, who started dialysis (all types) in the USA in 1992, was 9.56%, and 19.26% for those aged 65–74 years (1). These figures differed only slightly from that reported in the USA patients who started dialysis 8 years earlier, which were 10.12% and 19.48%, respectively. However, during this timespan, the number of very old patients, aged 80 or more years, has soared from 1031 up to 4466 (+333%). It can thus be postulated that the selection-criteria for taking very old patients on dialysis therapy have been widely expanded during the past decade, with more debilitated patients having thus a shorter survival on dialysis. Conflicting results are reported regarding the outcome of very elderly patients treated with RRT: the 1-year survival rate of 58 patients aged 75 years or over who commenced dialysis in a single facility in the UK between 1991 and 1995 was 53.5% vs. 72.6%, and 90.6% for individuals aged 65–74 years and less than 65 years at start of RRT. The 5-year survival rates in the three groups were 2.4%, 18.8%, and 61.4%, respectively. The very elderly spent 20% of their survival time in the hospital (39). Much more encouraging results are reported in several single-center studies: a 30% 2-year survival was thus achieved in 30 consecutive patients aged 83 ± 3 years, who started dialysis in France in 1995 and 1996 (40). The mean patient-survival time on dialysis in a series of 47 patients aged 80 or more years, who began dialysis in Germany, was 28.8 months (34). Patient survival rates of 73.6%, 59.6%, and 45%, at 1, 2, and 3 years, respectively, were reported in a series of 213 patients treated with PD in eight French centers, whose mean age at start of PD was 79.4±3.6 years and mean time on PD treatment was 21.4±19.8 months (19). Technical survival on PD in these series was 68%, 53%, and 35%, at 1, 2, and 3 years. Cardiac arrest, acute myocardial infarction, and cerebro-vascular accidents are among the leading causes of death in most of the reported series. More specific to this age-group of patients is the high death-rate following withdrawal from dialysis. During the years 1995–97 in the USA, the death rate of dialysis patients, reported as due to withdrawal from dialysis, was about three times higher in patients aged 65+years than in those aged 45–64 years (70.5 vs. 24 per 1000 dialysis-patient years). Failure to thrive is the leading reason reported for withdrawal from dialysis, this terminology accounting often for a combination of deteriorated clinical condition associated in many cases with loss of overall autonomy and absence or poor social/familial support (1).

Renal transplantation in the elderly

Among the very rapidly growing segment of the ESRD population aged more than 65 years accepted for RRT, quite a substantial proportion do not suffer from co-morbid conditions that could strongly and definitely contra-indicate organ transplantation. Selecting the age of 65 years for addressing the issue of renal transplantation in elderly persons, rests on the same rationale as that set forward for maintenance-dialysis patients. However, many transplant teams lower the ceiling for elderly patients down to 60 years, probably in accordance with their own perception of old-age (particulary regarding their physician-colleagues'). On the other hand, renal transplantation is very rarely done for truly old patients aged 75 years or more, the vast majority of elderly renal-transplant recipients belonging thus to the 60–70 year age group. Rationing renal transplantation by age, by restricting or excluding elderly patients from transplantation programs, is still common practice in many countries grounded on poor survival and/or quality of life of transplant recipients, and on priorities set for allocating scarce organ resources to patients with a predictably longer lifespan and better graft survival. This latter reason will, unfortunately, remain valid for many years to come, whereas the denial of renal transplantation for elderly people on purely medical grounds may become less frequently justified due to a better global medical management of patients with renal insufficiency pre- and during maintenance-dialysis treatment, and technical advances at all stages of the transplantation process. An extension of organ transplantation to a larger segment of elderly patients is thus inseparable from an expansion of the pool of organ donors, which fuels lively controversies concerning the limits set for the harvesting of organs from elderly donors and the practice of age-matching between kidney donors and recipients (*vide infra*).

Top experts in the field of organ transplantation kept asking the same question from the beginning to the end of the last decade:

- Cadaveric renal transplantation in elderly recipients: is it worthwhile? asked Sir Roy Calne in 1991 (41).
- Should renal transplantation be offered to older patients? asked Claudio Ponticelli in 2000 (42).
- Current data on the results achieved in recent years for this population of patients allow some contributive answers to these debated issues to be presented.

Demographic overview of renal transplantation in the elderly

Data collected over the years by the USRDS registry clearly demonstrate the steep rise of renal transplantation for treating ESRD in elderly patients: between 1990 and 1998 the percentage of patients aged 65 years and older, alive with a functioning kidney, rose in the USA from 3.4% ($n=5232$) up to 8.4% ($n=8104$). Of the first cadaveric kidney transplants performed in the USA in 1990 ($n=5865$, 23.5 pmp), 4.26% were allocated to patients aged 65+ years. This percentage doubled in 1998 with 8.78% of the 7718 first cadaveric kidney grafts (28.6 pmp) being implanted into elderly patients. In 1997, the mean time-interval between start of ESRD treatment and first cadaveric transplantation was 949 days, 100 days shorter than that reported for recipients aged 40–44 years, whilst it was only 517 days for youngsters aged 15–19 years (1). Whether this shorter waiting time for elderly versus younger patients is linked to using less than optimal or marginal organs for elderly patients for the sake of expanding the donor pool, is a tempting but not easily provable hypothesis. Only 1.1% of living donor kidneys were grafted in the USA in patients aged 65+ years in 1990 ($n=20$), this percentage increased four-fold in 1948: 4.4% ($n=160$).

There were 51 490 and 103 582 patients aged 65 years and over alive on dialysis in the USA at the end of 1990 and 1998, respectively, accounting for 40% and 42% of the whole dialysis population alive on those dates. Assuming that only one-third of the 57 784 dialysis patients aged 60–70 years, alive at the end of 1998, could be deemed reasonable candidates for transplantation, more than 18 200 elderly patients would thus have to be squeezed into the kidney transplant waiting-list, more than twice the number of all the cadaveric kidney harvested in the USA in 1998!

The frequency of kidney transplantation for elderly patients varies greatly among the developed countries where organ transplantation is widely practised. The main factors accounting for those differences are the wide variations of the overall transplantation activity, the size of the dialysis population deemed as potential candidates, and, very importantly, a complex interplay of social, psychological, and economical debated issues, which strongly influence the willingness to expand or restrict the indications of kidney transplantation to less than ideal transplant candidates, on single-facility, regional, or national levels. The annual renal transplant rate in Canada was 32.1 per million in 1996, 5.75% of the living and cadaveric donated kidneys were allocated to patients aged 65 years and over (43). In Australia, where 24 transplant operations pmp were performed in 1999, 2.2% (10/453) concerned patients aged 65 years or more. Of all the 5042 patients alive at the end of that year with a functioning kidney graft, 12.5% belonged to the elderly age-group (44). Norway has had, for decades, a very active transplantation program with 38–46 kidneys transplanted pmp annually: among 801 first cadaveric renal transplants performed between 1989 and 1997, 244 (30.4%) were allocated to patients aged 65 years or more (45). In Catalonia, patients aged 65+ years alive with a functioning renal transplant were practically non-existent in 1984. By the end of 1997 they accounted for 13.8% of all renal transplant recipients alive by the end of that year (46). France had a renal transplantation rate of 30.7 pmp in 1999, but only 2.1% of the 1842 kidneys transplanted during that year benefited to patients aged 65 years or more (47).

Survival issues in elderly patients

To achieve a good (and even more than just good!) patient and graft survival, is a particularly compelling goal to justify the allocation of scarce organ resources to patients who have a natural shorter life-expectancy than younger ones, are most of the time retired from professional activities, have fullfilled their essential familial com-mittments, and may, therefore, not be considered as first-line candidates in the hard competition for receiving a donated organ.

The results of renal transplantation in elderly patients are even more difficult to analyze objectively than those reported for young patients. The selection criteria applied by transplantation teams for placing elderly patients on waiting-lists, the cri-teria for accepting organs from older donors, the immunosuppressive drug regimens prescribed in the early and long-term post-transplantation, are extremely variable among transplantation facilities and over time. These differences account for the con-trasted results presented in large national or international registries with that based on single-center studies, the center effects on graft and patient survival being usually most significant within the first year post-transplantation (48).

In a normal Western world population, the life-expectancy of 65-year-olds is reported as 13–15 years (49). Predictions for ESRD patients treated with any mode of RRT cannot realistically be anything but worse. Survival of elderly renal transplant patients can be compared with that of three main categories of people:

1. A general population of the same age-range living in the same geographical area and societal environment.
2. Transplanted patients belonging to younger age-groups.
3. Dialysis patients placed on a transplant waiting-list and not transplanted during the same observation period for the sole reason of lack of suitable donor.

The markedly increased mortality risk of renal transplant recipients versus a general population is documented in a recent Dutch study: in a cohort of 916 cadaveric kidney recipients followed-up between 1966 through 1996, the standardized mortal-ity ratio versus the general Dutch population was 14 times greater during the first year post-transplantation and remained four times greater in the following year (50). A more focused view on elderly renal transplant patients is provided by a single-center study at the University of Wisconsin: 57% of 146 kidney transplant recipients aged >60 years (122 cadaveric, 24 living donors) followed between 1966 through 1995 reached their median observed/expected lifespan, based on the Wisconsin state-specific life-tables (51). This percentage was significantly lower than that found for patients aged less than 21 years (67%), but did not differ significantly from that of patients of intermediate age-categories, 49% and 47% in the 21–40 years and 41–60 years of age, respectively. Kidney-recipient age was not signaled out as a statistically significant risk factor reducing the median observed/expected lifespan, according to a Cox proportional hazard model applied to the whole cohort of transplanted patients.

The data reported to the UNOS Scientific Transplant Registry in the USA during the period 1991–97 yield that the half-life of cadaveric renal transplant recipients aged >60 years was 9.7 years, whereas it was longer than 30 years in patients aged up to 30 years at time of transplant, 29.4 years in those aged 31–45 years, and 16.5 years in those aged 46–60 years (52). The data shown in Table 7.5 illustrate the changes that have occured in two age-groups of the USA renal transplant population over 10-year time-intervals: the 5-year survival of cadaveric renal transplant recipients has increased 15.4% between 1983 and 1993, vs. only 11.2% in young adults; the absolute difference between the two groups remaining, however. 32.8%. In Norway, the 5-year patient-survival rate in 244 first cadaver kidney recipients aged >65 years transplanted from 1989 to 1997 was close to 50% vs 82% in 577 patients aged less than 55 years (45). Among 559 patients who received a cadaveric renal transplant in Catalonia in the years 1984–94, the 5-year patient-survival rates were 87% and 66% in those aged 60–65 years and 65–70 years, respectively (53).

In the results reviewed by Cameron in six single-center studies published between 1989 and 1995, the 5-year patient-survival rates of cadaveric renal transplant recipients aged over 60 years, and receiving cyclosporine, ranged between 59% and 80%. Four studies published between 1995 and 1999 involving patients treated with tacrolimus instead of cyclosporine yielded a 5-year patient-survival rate in recipients aged >60 years ranging between 54% and 86%. Among 106 patients older than 70 years of age who were transplanted in Norway from 1983 through 1993, the patient-survival rates were 80% and 74% at 1 and 5 years for those who received a living donor kidney, and 80% and 54% for cadaveric kidney recipients. This outcome was found as good as in patients 55–70 years old for at least 5 years after transplantation (54).

Data reported from the vast majority of single- and multi-center studies thus concur in demonstrating that elderly patient survival post-transplantation in recipients aged 60–65 years at transplantation, is significantly lower than that recorded in patients aged less than 55–60 years (55–59). However, the results of the group from Rotterdam well highlight the pitfalls that have to be avoided in the interpretation of crude survival data based on survival tables built up with data collected over a prolonged period of time. In their single-center homogenous series of 509 cadaveric renal transplantations performed between 1983 and 1997, with cyclosporine as primary immunosuppressor, the raw comparisons of patient (and graft) survival according to age distribution of the recipients, by means of a Kaplan–Meier analysis, is very misleading in the absence of a proper adjustment for the transplantation year. The improvements achieved overall in kidney transplantation over the years, exceed by far the influence of age: using a Cox proportional hazards analysis, the authors established that the relative risk of a 20-year-old patient, who underwent renal transplantation between 1983 and 1990, was equal to that of a 70-year-old patient, who underwent transplantation between 1991 and 1993 (60).

Table 7.5 1-, 2-, and 5-year patient-survival probabilities in first cadaveric kidney recipients according to age at transplantation (last follow-up: December 1998)

Age-groups (Years)	1 Year		2 Years		5 years	
	(1987) (%)	(1997) (%)	(1986) (%)	(1996) (%)	(1983) (%)	(1993) (%)
25–34 years	96.4	98.2	90.8	95.5	77.7	88.9
65+ years	84.8	86.3	78.0	82.4	40.7	56.1

Source: USRDS Report (2000).

A retrospective nationwide longitudinal study has been conducted in the USA aimed at comparing the mortality of patients receiving long-term dialysis with that of the subgroup of dialysis patients placed on a transplant waiting-list and that of the patients having received a first cadaveric renal transplant between 1991 and 1997. In all dialysis patients aged 60 years and over ($n=46022$), the death rate per 100 patient-years was 23.2; it was 10.0 in those placed on the waiting-list and not transplanted ($n=1053$), and only 7.4 in the 622 patients who received a renal transplant. With an enrolment date set at the time of initial placement on the waiting-list, transplanted patients aged 60–74 years had a projected increase in their lifespan of 4 years and a decrease in the long-term risk of death of 61%, compared to that of those who were stuck on the waiting-list (61). These favorable results of renal transplantation in elderly patients are, however, somewhat fragilized by the fact that the causes of death of all the three categories of patients have not been analyzed, leaving unclear whether a lesser co-morbidity (particularly concerning cardiovascular complications) was not present in the transplanted patients, which could have strongly influenced their lower mortality rate post-transplantation.

Other recent studies from Canada (62), Catalonia (53), and Australia (63), concur in reporting substantial survival advantages in elderly transplanted patients, compared with dialysis patients maintained on a transplant waiting-list. In 284 patients aged 60 years and over having received a renal transplant in Canada between 1987 and 1993, the death rate was 54 per 1000 patients-years of post-transplant follow-up vs. 294 per 1000 patients-years in 6116 patients stuck on a waiting-list. In the Catalan experience, a 10% increase in survival was observed vs. patients maintained on dialysis but only in the subgroup aged 60–64 years and only in the long-term (87% vs. 77% at 5 years). No difference, however, was observed in patients aged 65–70 years. Univariate and multivariate analyzes revealed that patients maintained on the waiting-list and not transplanted, had a two-fold greater risk of death compared to that of transplanted patients. The survival rates of 67 patients aged over 60 years, having received a cadaveric renal transplant in a single Australian center between January 1993 and December 1997, were 98%, 95%, and 90% at 1, 3, and 5 years post-transplant, respectively, vs. 92%, 62%, and 27% at the same time intervals in 107 carefully matched patients remaining on the center's waiting-list (63).

These encouraging results of recent studies contrast sharply with the quite dismal ones reported in series published more than 15 years ago, with which any comparison can be deemed useless and misleading, so important have been the changes that have occured within this timespan in all the aspects of renal transplantation.

Renal-graft survival in elderly patients

A substantial increase in the short- and long-term graft survival is evidenced in a nationwide study that includes 93 394 renal transplantations performed in the USA between 1988 and 1996. The projected half-life of cadaveric renal grafts increased from 7–9 years in 1988, up to 13.8 years in 1995 (+ 42%), and from 11.0 years to 19.5 years after censoring of data for patients who had died with a functioning transplant

(+77%) (64). Data from the USRDS report for the year 2000, show improvements for renal-graft survival over 10-year time-intervals in elderly patients that reached +12.4% and 15.6% at 1 and 3 years post-transplantation, respectively (Table 7.6). The lesser gain in survival at 5 years (+7.8%) has to be accounted for, at least in part, by the absence of data censoring for patients who have died more than 3 years post-transplantation with a functioning renal transplant.

Single-center reports on renal-graft survival in elderly patients vary considerably between transplant facilities, due to the already mentioned great variability in recipient-selection criteria, and also a rapidly growing heterogeneity in organ donor selection policies, with an expanding tendency to allocate marginal kidneys to elderly recipients and an increasing diversification of immunosuppressive protocols. Very importantly, a proper interpretation of the results of renal-graft survival in the older segment of the population requires a clean distinction between those that take into account all graft losses and those in which the graft loss is caused by the death of the patient with a functioning renal transplant (censored graft survival). This distinction is supported by the results of a study reported by the UNOS Scientific Renal Transplant Registry and the USRDS: among 7040 adult transplanted patients, the relative risk of dying with graft function was seven times higher in patients aged >65 years and over, than in patients aged 18–29 years (65). Total and death-censored cadaveric renal-graft survival was thus 81% and 90% at 2 years, respectively, in a French series of 58 patients whose mean age was 64±3 years at transplantation (56). Among 69 patients older than 60 years (mean 64.4 years ±4.1) transplanted in a New York center between 1985 and 1997, cumulative renal-graft survival was 68.4% and 42.6% at 1 and 5 years post-transplant, respectively, compared with 77.6% and 55.2% for a control-group of 724 patients 18–59 years of age. After censoring for patients who died with a functioning graft, the difference in graft survival between the two subgroups was no longer significant (58). A similar profile is observed in the series at Guy's Hospital in London, where, after adjustement for death of the patients with a functioning kidney, the survival of the graft itself remains almost constant at all age-ranges, being 70% at 5 years in 117 patients aged 61–75 years vs. 73% and 76% in patients aged 51–60 years (n=106) and 41–50 years (n=114), respectively (49). In a series of 49 cadaveric renal transplants performed in patients aged >60 years at

Table 7.6 1-, 2-, and 5-year graft-survival probabilities in first cadaveric renal transplant recipients according to age at transplantation

Age-groups (years)	1 Year		2 Years		5 years	
	(1987) (%)	(1997) (%)	(1985) (%)	(1995) (%)	(1983) (%)	(1993) (%)
20–44 years	74.5	90.0	60.4	72.4	40.1	61.1
45–64 years	75.2	87.8	60.4	70.5	34.8	57.2
65+years	67.7	80.1	48.2	63.8	35.6	43.4

Source: USRDS Report(2000).

Geneva University Hospital between 1983 and 1993, 1-, 5-, and 10-year graft survival was, after censoring for patient death with a functioning graft, 96%, 85%, and 81%, respectively. Renal function, as assessed by serum creatinine, was not different between patients aged less or more than 60 years, at 1 and 5 years post-transplantation (59).

Among 126 patients aged >70 years, 106 received a cadaveric donor renal transplant in Norway from 1983 to 1993 (mean age: 73.1 years). Graft survival was 78% and 52% at 1 and 5 years post-transplant, respectively, percentages that were not statistically different from those recorded in the group of 340 patients aged 55–70 years (54).

Impact of donor age

The negative impact of donor age on graft survival is documented in several studies (57, 66). In a series of 83 patients who received a cadaveric renal transplant in the same center between 1992 and 1998, the course of renal function was analyzed over a continuum over time after transplantation (67). A univariate mixed-effects regression analysis, taking into account exclusively non-immunologic parameters, disclosed that donor age significantly influenced the time course of the recipients' creatinine clearance. When rejection episodes were included in the list of variables, an analysis done mith multiple explanatory variables yielded that donor age had the greatest impact on recipients' creatinine clearance at all time points up to 3 years post-transplantation, exceeding that of rejection, gender, and donor creatinine clearance. Recipients of kidneys from older donors had a lower creatinine clearance when compared with recipients of kidneys from ideal adult donors aged 20–55 years.

In donors aged more than 55 years, a reduction of creatinine clearance ($<80\,ml/mn$) and/or a previous history of hypertension of more than 10 years duration, are very significant risk factors for decreased graft-survival in cadaveric renal recipients (68).

A similar conclusion on the negative impact of donor age on graft function can be drawn from the study conducted in Pittsburgh on 230 patients aged 60 years and older, who received a cadaveric renal transplant between 1990 and December 1996: the 1- and 5-year overall graft-survival rate was 84% and 64%, respectively. It was 73% and 52% in kidneys from donors over the age of 60 years, and 87% and 66% when donors were less than 60 years old (69). The inferior outcome observed with organs from older donors allocated to older recipients, thus raises ethical concerns about the concept of a targeted allocation of age-matched kidney to elderly patients.

Although this strategy is advocated by several authors (65, 66), its sole possible justification rests actually in the dearth of donated organs for all the patients who could benefit from renal transplantation. Such is particularly the case for transplants performed with a single kidney from very old donors (aged up to 74 years), in whom a pre-transplant biopsy shows only a limited extent of glomerulosclerosis ($<15\%$ of the glomeruli) (70), or the simultaneous transplantation of two marginal kidneys (Dual Kidney Transplants) with a total sclerosis of glomeruli up to 40% (71).

Besides donor age, the recipient age by itself has an independant effect on the development of chronic renal allograft failure. A Cox proportional hazards model, designed for a large analysis involving 2907 patients having survived 5 years post first cadaveric transplantation performed in the UK between 1983 and 1993, highlighted that in all age-ranges from 35 years onwards, including 1024 patients aged >60 years, older recipient age was associated with a worse graft outcome (72).

Apart from donor and recipient age, a recipient's past history of hypertension, diabetes, non-skin malignancy, cerebro or peripheral vascular disease, current tobacco use, cold ischemia times, acute cellular rejection within 6 months post-transplantation, high peak panel reactive antibodies, and (inconsistently) degree of HL-A matching, are the most commonly identified risk factors evidenced by means of the Cox-proportional hazard models, designed in many studies for identifying predictors of graft and patient survival (65, 66, 72, 73).

Whereas in younger patients (<50 years), graft rejection is the predominant cause of graft loss, death with a functioning graft is the leading cause of graft loss in most of the published series. For example, in a recent Swiss report, graft loss due to patient death was 29% among 48 patients aged >60 years, as compared to 6% in the <60 years age group. In contrast, kidney transplants were lost to acute or chronic rejection in 22% of patients in the <60 years group (*n*=239), compared to 10% for those in the >60 years group (59). A similar profile of renal-graft outcome is described in other single-center series (55, 56). The great predominance of patient death as cause of graft failure in elderly patients, is also confirmed in large nationwide surveys, such as in Norway, where patient death accounted for 83% of graft loss in patients aged >65 years, compared to 41% in younger ones (45). In the USA during the period 1994–98, 65% of the transplants that failed after the first year of transplantation, in patients aged >60 years, were due to patient death, compared with 18% among 19–45 olds (52).

Mortality and morbidity in elderly transplanted patients

Cardio-vascular disease is reported in most studies as the leading cause of death in this population with acute myocardial infarction heading the list (56, 58, 69, 74). Differences in the frequency and distribution of causes of cardio-vascular and cerebro-vascular deaths exist between single-center reports, which reflect the great variability of the selection criteria applied to the transplant candidates, based on more or less comprehensive pre-transplant evaluation of their cardiac, and vascular status (*vide infra*).

Infections (mainly septicemias and pulmonary infections) most commonly rank second as causes of death, especially within the first year post-transplantation (55, 75), but may equal—or even exceed—cardiac causes in some studies (56, 76). An analysis of the causes of death recorded in patients having undergone a primary renal transplantation compared with that of patients maintained on a waiting-list in the USA, shows that death related to infections soars exponentially in transplanted patients with increasing age, while it increases only linearly for those on the waiting-list. This increased risk of dying of an infectious cause in older transplant-recipients, to a much greater degree than in patients on a waiting-list, is attributed to their greater vulnerability to immunosuppression (76). Whilst-non lethal skin cancers are the most frequent malignancies that develop in elderly transplant-patients, solid-tumor related deaths and lymphomas account for 12–16% of all deaths in several single-center series

(49, 54). Table 7.7 shows the profile of death rates (per 1000 patient-years at risk) among patients who have died in the USA with a functioning kidney during the years 1996–98. The overall death rate is more than 100% greater in patients aged 65 + years, compared with those aged 45–64 years. Death rates due to all cardiac causes combined amount to 14.4 per 1000 patient-years at risk in the elderly group vs. 8.5 per 1000 patient-year and 3.1 per 1000 patient-years in patient aged up to 44 years. Death rates from malignancies are close to three-fold in elderly vs. middle-aged patients. Such a profile is, however, at variance with data from a large European series in which the percentage of deaths among elderly transplant-recipients was indeed much greater than in younger patients, but with no significant differences in the distribution of the causes of deaths between the age-groups (60).

Impact of immunodeficiency on the post-transplantation clinical course and outcome in elderly patients

Modifications of the immune system related to aging are widely considered as playing an important role on the increasing incidence of infections and malignancies in the elderly general population. Extensive studies of the immune system have been performed in recent years on very old persons, particularly in centenarians, giving issue to the concept of immunosenescence, which is being considered more as a remodeling-reshaping of the immune system, rather than a true deterioration (77–79).

The concept of immunosenescence, its strict identification with immunodeficiency, and its clinical significance, are matters of current debates among geriatricians and immunologists, who can only agree on the statement according to which a direct causal relationship between changes in immunity and the occurrence of specific diseases in humans remains poorly understood, and even yet unproven (80–81).

Table 7.7 Death rates (per 1000 patient-years at risk) in patients dying with a functioning transplant in the USA (1996–98)

	Age groups (years)		
	20–44	45–64	65+
All causes	17.0	45.3	94.5
Acute myocardial infarction	1.1	3.2	5.0
Other cardiac causes	0.7	1.9	3.5
Cardiac arrest	1.3	3.4	5.9
Septicemia	1.1	2.8	5.1
Pulmonary infection	0.4	1.0	2.0
Cerebro vascular accident	0.6	1.6	2.7
Malignancy	0.7	2.7	6.6

Source: Annual USRDS Report (2000).

The mechanisms underlying age-related changes in immunity are deemed multi-factorial, involving both genetic and environmental factors (77, 82).

Whilst their true clinical relevance thus remain controversial, the changes of humoral and cellular immunity related to aging have been extensively investigated in animal models and humans, and recently reviewed (77–79). Deterioration of humoral immunity comprises mainly a decrease of the number of peripheral B lymphocytes, various modifications among IgG and IgA subclasses, and of the ability of B cells to generate antibody responses to specific antigenic challenges. Disorders of humoral immunity are held responsible for the reduced resistance of elderly people to bacterial infections and a poor response to vaccination. Actually, age-related immunodeficiency is primarily associated with a decrease in the total number of T lymphocytes, alterations of T-cell phenotype, and modifications of T-cell responses. There is a decrease in the proportion of naïve T cells, with a concomitant increase of T cells with an activated/memory phenotype, resulting in the reduction of the ability of the host to respond to not previously encountered antigens. The functions of macrophages and granulocytes are also impaired, along with complex dysregulations in the cytokine-network production system (IL-1, IL-4, IL-6, tumor necrosis factor), with, in particular, an over-production of IL-8 (83). These defects in T cell-mediated immune responses are deemed to play an important role for the enhanced risk of cancer, viral infections, and infections due to intra-cellular bacterial pathogens, such as *Mycobacterium tuberculosis*.

The mandatory use of immunosuppressive drugs (ID) for ensuring tolerance of a grafted organ superimposed on the age-related immunodeficient state, greatly worsens the risk of infectious complications in elderly transplant-recipients. Data collected in a large survey, involving close to 74 000 primary transplant-recipients followed up between 1988 and 1997, clearly show the increased immunosuppressive vulnerability of elderly patients: the relative risk for death due to infection within the first 24 months of post-transplant follow-up is more than six times greater in patients above age 65 than in those aged 18–29 years, and even higher (8.7-fold) for deaths due to opportunistic infections. By contrast, the incidence of acute rejection episodes during the first 6 months post-transplant decreased from 28% in the youngest group down to 19.7% in the elderly patients (76). In the large series of patients followed-up at Guy's Hospital in London, the number of biopsy-proven rejection episodes documented during the first year post-transplantation falls from 1.62 episodes per patient aged 18–30 years down to 0.97 episode in recipients aged 61–75 years (49).

The objectives of immunosuppressive protocols designed for transplant patients in general, and elderly ones in particular, are thus to ensure an optimal long-term good tolerance and function of the grafted organ, together with minimizing the risk for patient morbidity/mortality. The choice between immunosuppressive regimens has become much larger in recent years, ranging from monotherapy with calcineurin inhibitors to quadruple drug immunosuppression. One very important goal is attempting to reduce, as much as possible, the administration of corticosteroids, which favor the occurrence of infectious complications but also the development of diabetes, osteoporosis, cataracts, and so on. The availability of cyclosporine (and now Neoral®), in association with low doses of steroids and azathioprine, has markedly improved the outcome of renal transplantation, compared with the historic combination of steroids + azathioprine. Moreover, excellent graft and patient survival have been achieved with cyclosporine monotherapy (84, 85). Recently, a 76% 5-year patient-survival rate, along with a 64% graft-survival rate, have been reported in a series of 230 patients aged 60 years and over treated with a tacrolimus-based immuno-suppressive regimen (74), with also excellent 5-year patient and graft survival in 25 patients aged 60+years, who underwent renal retransplantation (86). Drug combinations consisted of: tacrolimus+steroids; or tacrolimus+steroids+mycophenolate mofetil; or tacrolimus+steroids+azathioprine. The results achieved with the recent drugs still require further evaluations, as shown in a study that disclosed a significantly greater risk factor for the occurrence of infectious complications (particularly cytomegalovirus and fungal) in a cohort of 46 patients aged >60 years submitted to a protocol associating steroids+cyclosporine+mycophenolate mofetil, compared with a matched control group receiving cyclosporine+steroids+azathioprine. Whereas the number of infections requiring patient hospitalization was markedly greater in the mycophenolate mofetil group, the 1-year patient- and graft-survival rates turned out not to be significantly different between the two groups (87).

An increasing panel of anti-lymphocytic antibodies has become available in recent years, either for immunosuppressive induction therapy or for treating corticosteroid-resistant rejection episodes (muronomab, polyclonal anti-lymphocyte globulins), or for prophylactic use against early post-transplant acute rejection episodes (basiliximab, duclizumab). Data on the use of this class of drugs in elderly transplant recipients are scanty, their beneficial effects remaining to be challenged in a frail population with the gravity and frequency of their acute side-effects (muronomab, anti-lymphocyte globulins), and with their yet undetermined long-term effects on the incidence of infections and malignancies (85).

In choosing among the plethora of immunosuppressive protocols designed for transplanted patients, the main concern to be kept in mind when treating elderly recipients is the risk for over-immunosuppression. The key recommendations are thus to attempt at tapering, as early as possible, the high dosages of corticosteroids, and to exert great caution in the prescription and surveillance of calcineurin inhibitors, in order to avoid their acute and chronic nephrotoxic adverse effects.

How can the outcome of elderly transplant-patients be optimized?

The facts and figures collected over the past 10 years, well demonstrate that older age *per se* is far from necessarily representing a formal contra-indication to renal transplantation. Main reasonable exclusion criteria remain active (not eradicable) infection, significant cardiac abnormability, severe chronic obstructive respiratory insuffisiency, previous non-skin malignancy with a disease-free period of less than at least 5 years, and overt psychiatric disorders. Steady progress remains, however, necessary for reducing morbidity/mortality in these patients and for improving their quality of life. Moreover, increasingly better results need to be permanently demonstrated for defending the allocation of scarce organ-resources to elderly patients when, in our time of age-discrimination, there is a predominant trend for privileging the young against the old. Careful selection of transplant candidates, smart post-transplant management of immunosuppression, and excellent global medical and social care, are the mandatory conditions for a successful transplantation program in this fragilized population.

A comprehensive evaluation of cardiovascular risk factors is of critical importance for elderly transplant candidates, bearing in mind that deaths of cardiovascular cause account for more than 50% of all deaths in most of the published reports, and that this high percentage remains unchanged over the years despite the advances made in the overall management of organ transplantation: hypertension, left ventricular hypertrophy, diabetes mellitus, obesity, cigarette smoking, dyslipidemia, family history of premature cardiovascular diseases/death, are among the most commonly recognized risk factors for post-transplant severe complications and death. Some of these risk factors are accessible to efficient preventive measures, consisting in modifications in life-style or adequate control with medical treatment (88). Cigarette smoking, for example, has been associated with a significant increase of cardiovascular deaths post-transplantation (89), which leads some transplant groups to exclude from the waiting-list patients who are unable, or unwilling, to quit smoking. Basic cardiac screening should include echocardiography and dipyridamole-thallium stress testing. Abnormal results (particularly of thallium testing) make coronary angiography necessary. This (invasive) investigation is very often practised routinely, irrespective of symptoms and age, for diabetic patients and by some groups for all elderly transplant candidates in whom thallium-testing has yielded incomplete results. If indicated, coronary revascularization, either with bypass grafting or angioplasty with/without stenting, should then be performed pre-transplantation (88). Doppler investigation of cerebral and iliac arteries should also be standard procedures, aiming at detecting and treating appropriately stenotic lesion(s) by endarterectomy or bypass grafting. Among other abnormalities that need to be more specifically investigated in elderly patients are: lower urinary tract obstruction, due to prostatic hypertrophy in men and extensive colonic diverticular disease, which has to be evaluated with barium enema or colonoscopy. Preventive treatment (either medical or surgical, according to each case) should then minimize the risk of acute diverticulitis and colonic perforation, often a life-threatening complication in elderly immunosuppressed patients. Similarly, cholelithiasis has to be diagnosed, prior to transplantation, with gallbladder ultrasound. If present, cholecystectomy is indicated to prevent post-transplant acute cholecystitis. Prevention of possibly very severe/lethal cytomegalovirus (CMV) infections requires that a prophylactic antiviral treatment with ganciclovir be given to sero-negative patients who receive a CMV-positive transplant.

Conclusions

A clearly positive answer can definitely be given to the two questions quoted at the beginning of this section: *yes,* renal transplantation should indeed be offered to elderly patients. The body of accumulated evidence demonstrates that it is *indeed worthwhile,* provided that patient selection is properly carried out, according to currently well-established criteria, and that excellent global medical management is ensured for efficient prevention and early appropriate treatment of post-transplant incident complications.

References

1. US Renal Data System (1990–99). *USRDS Annual Data Reports*. National Institutes of Health, National Institute of Diabetes and Digestive and Kidney Diseases. Bethesda. Maryland, USA.
2. Xue, J.L. and Collins, A.J. (2000). Projecting the number of patients with end-stage renal disease in the United States to the year 2010. *Peritoneal Dialysis International*, **20**, (Suppl. 1), S109.
3. Berthoux, F., Gellert, R., Jones, E., Mendel, S., Valderrabano, F., Briggs, J.D. *et al.* (1998). Epidemiology and demography of treated end-stage renal failure in the elderly, from the European Renal Association (ERA-EDTA) Registry. *Nephrology Dialysis Transplantation*, **13**, (Suppl. 7), 65–8.
4. Jungers, P., Massy, Z., Man, N.K., Labrunie, M., Taupin, P., Guin, E. *et al.* (2000). Incidence of end-stage renal disease in Ile-de-France, a prospective epidemiological survey. *Presse Medicale*, **11**, 589–92.
5. Maisonneuve, P., Agodoa, L., Gellert, R., Stewart, J.H., Buccianti, G., Loewenfels, A.B. *et al.* (2000). Distribution of primary renal diseases leading to end-stage renal failure in the United States, Europe, and Australia/New-Zealand, results from an International Comparative Study. *American Journal of Kidney Diseases*, **35**, 157–65.
6. Latos, D.L. (1996). Chronic dialysis in patients over age 65. *Journal of the American Society of Nephrology*, **7**, 637–46.
7. Ismail, N., Hakim, R., Oreopoulos, D.G., and Patrikarea, A. (1993). Renal replacement therapies in the elderly, Part. 1. Hemodialysis and chronic peritoneal dialysis. *American Journal of Kidney Diseases*, **22**, 759–82.
8. Van Ypersele De Strihou, C., Jadoul, M., Malghem, J., Maldague, B., and Jamart, J. (1991). Effects of dialysis membranes and patients'age on signs of dialysis-related amyloidosis. The working party on dialysis amyloidosis. *Kidney International*, **39**, 1012–19.
9. Schiffl, H., Fisher, R., Lang, S.M., and Mangel, E. (2000). Clinical manifestations of AB-amyloïdosis, effects of biocompatibility and flux. *Nephrology Dialysis Transplantation*, **15**, 840–5.
10. Lornoy, W., Becaus, I., Billiow, J.M., Sierens, L., Van Malderen, P., and D'Haenens, P. (2000). On-line hemodiafiltration. Remarkable removal of beta 2-microglobulin. Long term clinical observations. *Nephrology Dialysis Transplantation*, **15**, (Suppl. 1), 49–54.
11. Daugirdas, J. (1991). Dialysis hypotension, a hemodynamic analysis. *Kidney International*, **39**, 233–46.
12. Maggiore, Q., Pizzarelli, F., Dattolo, P., Maggiore, U., and Cerrai, T. (2000). Cardiovascular stability during hemodialysis, hemofiltration and hemodiafiltration. *Nephrology Dialysis Transplantation*, **15**, (Suppl. 1), 68–73.
13. De Broe, M.E. (1994). Hemodialysis induced hypoxemia. *Nephrology Dialysis Transplantation*, **9**, (Suppl. 2), 173–5.
14. Coli, L., La Manna, G., Dalmastri, V., De Passacis, A., Pace, G., Santese, G., *et al.* (1998). Evidence of profiled hemodialysis efficacy in the treatment of intra-dialytic hypotension. *International Journal of Artificial Organs*, **21**, 389–402.

15. Pierratos, A., (1999). Nocturnal home hemodialysis, an update on a 5-year experience. *Nephrology Dialysis Transplantation*, **14**, 2835–40.

16. Brown, E.A. (1999). Peritoneal dialysis versus hemodialysis in the elderly. *Peritoneal Dialysis International*, **19**, 311–12.

17. Winchester, J.F. (1999). Peritoneal dialysis in older individuals. *Geriatric Nephrology and Urology*, **9**, 147–52.

18. Malberti, F., Conte, F., Limido, A., Marcelli, D., Spotti, D., Lonati, F. *et al.* (1997). Ten years experience of renal replacement treatment in the elderly. *Geriatric Nephrology and Urology*, **7**, 1–10.

19. Issad, B., Benevent, D., Allouache, M., Durand, P.Y., Aguilera, D., Milongo, R., *et al.* (1995). 213 elderly uremic patients over 75 years of age treated with long-term peritoneal dialysis, a French multicenter study. *Peritoneal Dialysis International*, **16**, (Suppl. 1), S414–18.

20. K/DOQI (2000). Clinical practice guidelines for nutrition in chronic renal failure, evaluation of protein- energy nutritional status. *American Journal of Kidney Diseases*, **35**, (Suppl. 2), S17–S36.

21. K/DOQI (2000). Management of protein and energy intake in maintenance hemodialysis and peritoneal dialysis patients. *American Journal of Kidney Diseases*, **35**, (Suppl. 2), S40–6.

22. Bohler, J., Donauer, J., and Keller, F. (1999). Pharmacokinetic principles during continuous renal replacement therapy. *Kidney International*, **72**, (Suppl.), S24–8.

23. Aronoff, G.R., Berns, J.S., Brier, M.E., Golper, Th.A., Morrison, G., Singer, I. *et al.* (1999). *Drug prescribing in renal failure, Dosing Guidelines for Adults*, Vol. 1, (4th edn). American College of Physicians, Philadelphia.

24. Moreno, F., Aracil, J., Perez, R., and Valderrabano, F. (1996). Controlled study on the improvement of quality of life in elderly hemodialysis patients after correcting end-stage renal disease related anemia with erythropoietin. *American Journal of Kidney Diseases*, 27, S48–56.

25. Working Party for European Best Practice Guidelines for the Management of Anemia in Patients with Chronic Renal Failure (1999). European best practice guidelines for the management of anemia in patients with chronic renal failure. *Nephrology Dialysis Transplantation*, **14**, (Suppl. 5), S1–50.

26. Sankarasubbaiyan, S. and Holley, J.L. (2000). An analysis of the increased demands placed on dialysis health care team members by functionally dependent hemodialysis patients. *American Journal of Kidney Diseases*, **35**, 1061–7.

27. Fosltein, M.F., Folstein, S.E., and Mc Hugh, P.R. (1975). Mini mental status examination. A pratical method for grading the cognitive state of patients for the clinician. *Journal of Psychiatric Research*, **12**, 189–98.

28. Kutner, N.G., Brogan, D., Hall, W.D., Haber, M., and Daniels, D.S. (2000). Functional impairment, depression and life satisfaction among older dialysis patients and age-matched controls, a prospective study. *Archives of Physical Medical Rehabilitation*, **81**, 453–9

29. Kimmel, P.L., Peterson, R.A., Weihs, K.L., Simmens, S.J., Alleynes, S., Cruz, I. *et al.* (2000). Multiple measurements of depression predict mortality in a longitudinal study of chronic hemodialysis outpatients. *Kidney International*, **57**, 2093–8.

30. Bloembergen, W.A., Port, F.K., Mauger, E.A., and Wolfe, R.A. (1995). A comparison of mortality between patients treated with hemodialysis and peritoneal dialysis. *Journal of the American Society of Nephrology*, **6**, 177–83.

31. Fenton, S.S., Schaubel, D.E., Desmeules, M., Morrison, H.I., Mao, I., Copleston, P. *et al.* (1997). Hemodialysis versus peritoneal dialysis, a comparison of adjusted mortality rates. *American Journal of Kidney Diseases*, **30**, 334–42.

32. Murphy, S.W., Foley, R.N., Barrett, B.J., Kent, G.M., Morgan, J., Barre, P. *et al.* (2000). Comparative hospitalization of hemodialysis and peritoneal dialysis patients in Canada. *Kidney International*, **57**, 2557–63.

33. Biesen, W., Van Holder, R., Debacker, G., and Lameire, N. (2000). Comparison of survival on CAPD and hemodialysis, statistical pitfalls. *Nephrology Dialysis Transplantation*, **15**, 307–11.

34. Schaefer, K. and Röhrich, B. (1999). The dilemna of renal replacement therapy in patients over 80 years of age. *Nephrology, Dialysis, Transplantation*, **14**, 35–6.

35. Mallick, N. and El Marasi, A., (1999). Dialysis in the elderly, to treat or not to treat. *Nephrology, Dialysis, Transplantation*, **14**, 37–9.

36. Cameron, J.I., Whiteside, C., Katz, J., and Devins, G.M. (2000) Differences in quality of life across renal replacement therapies, a meta-analytic comparison. *American Journal of Kidney Diseases*, **35**, 629–37.

37. Lamping, D.L., Constantinovici, N., Roderick, P., Norman, C., Henderson, L., Harris, L. *et al.* (2000). Dialysis outcome, quality of life, and costs in the North Thames dialysis study of elderly people on dialysis, a prospective cohort study. *The Lancet*, **356**, 1543–50.

38. Van Biesen, W., Van Holder, R., Dhont, A.M., Veys, N., and Lameire, N. (2000). An evaluation of an integrative care approach for the treatment of ESRD patients. *Journal of the American Society of Nephrology*, **11**, 116–25.

39. Munshi, S.K., Visayakumar, N., Taub., N.A., Bhullar, H., Nelson Lo, T.C., and Warwick, G. (2000). Outcome of renal replacement therapy in the very elderly. *Nephrology, Dialysis, Transplantation*, **16**, 128–33.

40. Sturm, J.M., Maurizi-Balsan, J., Foret, M., and Cordonnier, D. (1998). Dialysis in octogenarians, search for mortality risk factors. Consecutive series of 30 patients. *Presse Medicale*, **16**, 748–52.

41. Morris, G.E., Jamieson, N.V., Small, J., Evans, D.B., and Calne, R. (1991). Cadaveric transplantation in elderly patients, is it worthwhile? *Nephrology, Dialysis, Transplantation*, **6**, 887–92.

42. Ponticelli, C. (2000). Should renal transplantation be offered to older patients? *Nephrology, Dialysis, Transplantation*, **15**, 315–17.

43. Parsons, D.A., Tracy, S.E., Handa, K.A., and Greig, P.D. (1998). An update of the Canadian organ replacement register (1998). *Clinical Transplants*, 97–106.

44. Russ, G. (2000). In *Anzdata Registry Report* (ed. A.P.S. Disney), pp.67–90. Adelaide, South Australia.

45. Bentdal, O.H., Leivestad, T., Fauchald, P., Albrechtsen, D., Pfeffer, P., Lien, B. *et al.* (1998). The National kidney transplant program in Norway still results in unchanged waiting lists. *Clinical Transplants*, 221–8.

46. Vela, E. and Cleries, M. (1999). Renal transplantation in Catalonia from 1984 to 1997. *Transplantation Proceedings*, **31**, 2354–7.

47. Etablissement Français des Greffes. (2000). *Rapport d'Activité 1999.*

48. Ismail. N., Hakim. R.H., and Helderman. J.H. (1994). Renal replacement therapies in the elderly, II. Renal transplantation. *American Journal of Kidney Diseases*, **23**, 1–15.

49. Cameron, J.S. (2000). Renal transplantation in the elderly. *International Urology and Nephrology*, **32**, 193–201.

50. Arend, S.M., Mallat, M.J., Westendorp, R.J., Van der Woude, F.J., and Van E.S., L.A. (1997). Patient survival after renal transplanttaion, more than 25 years follow-up. *Nephrology, Dialysis, Transplantation*, **12**, 1672–9.

51. Becker, B.N., Becker, Y.T., Pintar, T.J., Collins, B.H., Pirsch, J.D., Friedman, A. *et al.* (2000). Using renal transplantation to evaluate a simple approach for predicting the impact

of end-stage renal disease therapies on patient survival, observed/expected life span. *American Journal of Kidney Diseases*, **35**, 653–9.

52. Cecka, J.M. (1998). The UNOS Scientific Renal Transplant Registry. *Clinical Transplants*, 1–16.

53. Bonal, J., Cleries, M., Vela, E., and The Renal Registry Committee (1997). Transplantation versus hemodialysis in elderly patients. *Nephrology, Dialysis, Transplantation*, **12**, 261–4.

54. Albrechtsen, D., Leivestad, T., Bendtal, O., Berg, K.J., Brekke, I., Fauchald, B. *et al.* (1995). Kidney transplantation in patients older than 70 years of age. *Transplantation Proceedings*, **27**, 986–8.

55. Nyberg, G., Nilson, B., Norden, G., and Karlberg, I. (1995). Outcome of renal transplantation in patients over the age of 60, a case-control study. *Nephrology, Dialysis, Transplantation*, **10**, 91–4.

56. Mourad, G., Cristol, J.P., Vela, C., Hauet, T., Iborra, F., and Chong, G. (1995). Cadaveric renal transplantation in patients 60 years of age and older, experience with 58 patients in a single center. *Nephrology, Dialysis, Transplantation*, **10**, (Suppl.6), 105–7.

57. Lufft. V., Kliem. V., Tusch. G., Dannenberg, B., and Brunkhorst, R. (2000). Renal transplantation in older adults, is graft survival affected by age, a case control study. *Transplantation*, **69**, 790–4.

58. Basu, A., Greenstein, S.M., Clemetson, S., Mallis, M., Kim, D., Schechner, B. *et al.* (2000). Renal transplantation in patients above 60 years of age in the modern era. A single center experience with a review of the literature. *International Journal of Urology and Nephrology*, **32**, 171–6.

59. Saudan, P., Bernay, Th., Leski, M., Morel, Ph., Bolle, J.F., and Martin, P.Y. (2001). Renal transplantation in the elderly, a long-term, single-center experience. *Nephrology, Dialysis, Transplantation*, **16**, 824–28.

60. Roodnat, J.I., Zietze, R., Mucder, P.C., Rischen-Vos, J., Van Gelder, J., Ijzermans, J.N. *et al.* (1999). The vanishing importance of age in renal transplantation. *Transplantation*, **67**, 576–80.

61. Wolff, R.A., Ashby, V.B., Milford, E.L., Ojo, A.O., Ettenger, R.E., Agodoa, L.Y. *et al.* (1999). Comparison of mortality in patients on dialysis, patients on dialysis awaiting transplantation and recipients of a first cadaveric transplant. *New England Journal of Medicine*, **341**, 1725–30.

62. Schaubel, D., Desmeules, Mao, Y., Jeffery, J., and Fenton, S. (1995). Survival experience among elderly end-stage renal disease patients. A controlled comparison of transplantation and dialysis. *Transplantation*, **60**, 1389–94.

63. Johnson, D.W., Herzig, K., Purdie, D., Brown, A.M., Rigby, R.J., Nicol, D.L. *et al.* (2000). A comparison of the effects of dialysis and renal transplantation on the survival of older uremic patients. *Transplantation*, **69**, 794–9.

64. Hariharan, S., McBride, M.A., Bennett, L.E., and Cohen, E.P. (1997). Risk factors for renal allograft survival from older cadaver donors. *Transplantation*, **64**, 1748–54.

65. Ojo, A.O., Hanson, J.A., Leichtman, A.B., Agodoa, L.Y., and Port, F.K. (2000). Long-term survival in renal transplant recipients with graft function. *Kidney International*, **57**, 307–13.

66. Waiser, J., Schreiber, M., Budde, K., Fritsche, L., Böhler, T., Hauser, H., and Neumayer, H.H. (2000). Age-matching in renal transplantation. *Nephrology, Dialysis, Transplantation*, **15**, 696–700.

67. Kouli, F., Morrell, H., Ratner, L.E., and Kraus, E.S. (2001). Impact of donor/recipient traits independent of rejection on long-term renal function. *American Journal of kidney Diseases*, **37**, 356–65.

68. Carter, J.T., Lee, C.M., Weinstein, R.J., Dafoe, D.C., and Alfrey, E.J. (2000). Evaluation of the older cadaveric kidney donor, the impact of donor hypertension and creatinine clearance on graft performance and survival. *Transplantation*, **70**, 765–71.

69. Basar, H., Soran, A., Shapiro, R., Viva, C., Scantlebury, V.P., Jordan, M.L. *et al.* (1999). Renal transplantation in recipients over the age of 60, the impact of donor-age. *Transplantation*, **67**, 1191–3.

70. Andres, A., Morales, J.M., Herrero, J.C., Praga, M., Morales, E., Hernandez, E., Ortuno, T. *et al.* (2000). Double versus single renal allografts from aged donors. *Transplantation*, **69**, 2060–6.

71. Lu, A.D., Carter, J.T., Weinstein, R.J., Stratta, R.J., Tyalor, R.J., Bowers, V.D. *et al.* (2000). Outcome in recipients of dual kidney transplants. *Transplantation*, **69**, 281–5.

72. Morris, P.J., Johnson, R.J., Fuggle, S.V., Belger, M.A., and Briggs, J.D. (1999). Analysis of factors that effect outcome of primary cadaveric renal transplantation in the UK. HLA task force of the kidney advisory group of the United Kingdom Transplant Support Service Authority. (UKTSSA). *Lancet*, **354**, 1147–52.

73. Doyle, S.E., Matas, A.J., Gillingham, K., and Rosenberg, M.E. (2000). Predicting clinical outcome in the elderly transplant recipient. *Kidney International*, **57**, 2144–50.

74. Sora, A., Shapiro, R., Basar, H., Vivas, C., Scantlebury, V.P., Jordan, M.L. *et al.* (1999). Outcome of kidney transplantation under tacrolimus-based immunosuppression in elderly patients. *Journal of Transplant Coordination*, **2**, 101–3.

75. Jassal, S.V., Opelz, G., and Cole, E. (1997). Transplantation in the elderly, a review. *Geriatric Urology and Nephrology*, **7**, 157–65.

76. Meier-Kriesche, H.U., Ojo, A.O., Hanson, J.A., and Kaplan, N.B. (2001). Exponentially increased risk of infectious death in older renal transplant patients. *Kidney International*, **59**, 1539–43.

77. Franceschi, C., Monti, D., Barbieri, D., Salvioli, S., Grassili, E., Capri, M. *et al.* (1996). Successful immunosenescence and the remodelling of immune responses with ageing. *Nephrology, Dialysis, Transplantation*, **11**, (Suppl. 9), 18–25.

78. Ginaldi, L., De Martinis, M., D'Ostillio, A., Marini, L., Loreto, M.F., Corsi, M.P. *et al.* (1999). The immune system in the elderly, I specific humoral immunity. *Immunological Research*, **20**, 101–8.

79. Ginaldi, L., De Martinis, M., D'Osillio, A., Marini, L., Lorejo, M.F., Martorelli, V. *et al.* (1999). The immune system in the elderly, II specific cellular immunity. *Immunological Research*, **20**, 109–15.

80. Voets, A.J., Turner, L.R., and Lighart, G.J. (1997). Immunosenescence revisited. Does it have any clinical significance? *Drugs Aging*, **11**, 1–6.

81. Castle, S.C. (2000). Clinical relevance of age-related immune dysfunction. *Clinical Infectious Diseases*, **31**, 578–85.

82. Burns, E.A. and Goodwin, J.S. (1997). Immunodeficiency of aging. *Drugs Aging*, **11**, 394–7.

83. Khanna, K.V. and Markham, R.B. (1999). A perspective on cellular immunity in the elderly. *Clinical Infectious Diseases*, **4**, 710–13.

84. Cantarovich, D., Baatard, E., Baranger, T., Tirouvanziam, A., Lesant, J.N., Hourmant, M. *et al.* (1999). Cadaveric renal transplantation after 60 years of age. A single center experience. *Transplant. International*, **7**, 33–8.

85. Morales, J.M., Campistol, J.M., Andres, A., and Herrero, J.C. (2000). Immunosuppression in older renal transplant patients. *Drugs aging*, **16**, 279–87.

86. Soran, A., Basar, H., Vevas, C., Scantlebury, V.P., Jordan, M.L., Gritsch, H.A. *et al.* (2000). Renal retransplantation in elderly patients under tacrolimus-based immunosuppression. *Transplantation Proceedings*, **32**, 663–4.

87. Meier-Kriesche, H.U., Friedman, G., Jacobs, M., Mulgaonkar, S., Vaghela, M., and Kaplan, B. (1999). Infectious complications in geriatric transplant patients, comparison of two immunosuppressive protocols. *Transplantation*, **68**, 1496–502.

88. Stewart, G., Jardine, A.G., and Briggs, J.D. (2000). Ischemic heart disease following renal transplantation. *Nephrology, Dialysis, Transplantation*, **15**, 269–77.

89. Kasiske, B.L. and Klinger, D. (2000). Cigarette smoking in renal transplant recipients. *Journal of the American Society of Nephrology*, **11**, 753–9.

8

Renal replacement therapy for diabetic patients with end–stage renal disease (ESRD)

Claude Jacobs

The course of events that have developed over the past 20 years in the domain of ESRD in diabetic patients, well illustrates the current popular saying, according to which 'one should never make predictions, especially for the future'. Indeed, the paper authored by W.J. Kolff *et al.* in 1972, based on the outcome of nine insulin-receiving diabetic patients treated with maintenance hemodialysis (HD) for a maximum duration of 20 months, stated that 'Dialysis for such patients should be considered as a palliative measure with little likelihood of long-term survival or improvement in quality of life' (1). A quarter-century later, diabetic patients account for 15–40% of all the new patients taken yearly on renal replacement therapy (RRT) in most of the economically developed countries, and their survival rates on dialysis or transplantation come steadily closer to that of non-diabetic patients of comparable age-range.

Diabetics, however, still constitute a specific segment within the population of patients undergoing RRT, due to greater difficulties encountered for their technical and overall medical management, the high rate of diabetes-induced target-organ damage, poorer quality of life, and worse overall outcome, compared with non-diabetic patients. Except for the happy few successful recipients of combined renal and pancreas transplantation (TX), the persistance of the diabetic state will combine its deleterious effects with that of sustained uremia in dialysis patients or the adverse effects of immunosuppressive drugs in renal transplant patients, to cast a gloom on the outcome of this group of patients.

Over the past 20 years, the management of ESRD diabetic patients with various modes of RRT has given issue to a prolific literature, unique in its abundance compared to any other category of patients with terminal uremia. During this period, considerable changes have occured in the demography of diabetic patients, major advances have been made in dialysis techniques, and in the domain of renal or combined renal and pancreas TX.

This chapter will thus focus more specifically on the current status of RRT in diabetic patients, referring mainly to the more recent reports from the literature. Actually, changes have been so fast in many areas that the results of many studies, completed no later than 10 years ago, may not reflect anymore the current spectrum and may even be misleading if taken as a basis for the practice of RRT for diabetic patients.

Demographics and definitions

Diabetic nephropathy (DN) has become, by the end of the twentieth century, the leading cause of ESRD in the developed countries. Actually, the rapid and relentless growth of the number of diabetic patients requiring RRT has been qualified as a medical catastrophe of world-wide dimensions (2). Table 8.1 displays the percentages of diabetic patients, among all the patients taken onto RRT in various countries across the world, in the late 1990s, ranging from 17.5% in the French-speaking part of Belgium, up to 36% in Japan, and 40% in New-Zealand. Table 8.2 shows the changes that have occurred over a 10-year time interval in the USA regarding the yearly incidence rates for the three most common causes of ESRD: the rise in the percentage (per million population, pmp) of incident diabetic patients was 110% higher in 1998 than in 1989, almost double of that of the whole population of patients taken on RRT.

The prevalence of diabetic patients alive on all types of RRT in the USA increased by 136% between December 1989 and December 1998 (154 vs. 364 pmp), whilst it rose only by 96% for the total RRT population and by 31% for patients with glomerulonephritis (Table 8.3) (3). Diabetic patients accounted for 35% of all patients alive on dialysis in the USA in December 1998 vs. only 25% of those thus treated in December 1989. In contrast, the percentage of diabetic patients alive with a functioning kidney graft at these dates remained at the same level: 17.5% vs. 15.5%. However, the absolute numbers of patients have changed considerably during this 10-year time-interval (Table 8.4). The prevalence of diabetic patients was even greater in Japan,

Table 8.1   Diabetic patients as percentages of all patients taken onto renal replacement therapy (RRT) in various countries in the late-1990s

Country/region	Year	Diabetics type I %	Diabetics type II %	All diabetics %
Austria	1998	7	24	31
Germany	1999	6	18	24
Spain	1997	NA	NA	19
Sweden	1999	13	12	25.0
Finland	1999	18.2	5.7	23.9
French-Speaking Belgium	1999	3.5	14.0	17.5
France (Ile de France)	1998	NA	NA	20.6
Japan	1999	NA	NA	36
Australia	1999	4.2	20.4	24.6
New Zealand	1999	5.8	34.2	40
USA	1998	NA	NA	40.3

NA: not available.

Table 8.2   Yearly incidence rates of patients with diabetic nephropathy, glomerulonephritis, and hypertension-related renal disease, starting renal replacement therapy in the USA

	1989			1998			Δ pmp%
	(*n*)	(%)	(pmp)	(*n*)	(%)	(pmp)	1989–98
All patients starting RRT	44 569	100.0	188	86 438	100.0	310	+64.9
Diabetic nephropathy	14 313	32.1	60	34 874	40.3	126	+110.0
Glomerulonephritis	7 325	27.8	31	9 493	10.1	34	+9.7
Hypertensive renal disease	12 373	16.4	53	18 273	21.1	66	+24.5

Source: USRDS Annual Report (2000).

Table 8.3   Point prevalence of all patients on RRT, patients with diabetic nephropathy, glomerulonephritis and hypertension-related renal disease treated in the USA with renal replacement therapy (RRT)

	December 1989			December 1998			Δ pmp%
	(*n*)	(%)	(pmp)	(*n*)	(%)	(pmp)	1989–98
All patients on RRT	150 332	100.0	609	323 159	100.0	1195	+96.2
Diabetic nephropathy	36 241	24.1	154	101 550	31.4	364	+136.4
Glomerulonephritis	37 327	24.8	156	57 004	17.6	205	+31.4
Hypertensive renal disease	35 712	23.7	156	64 629	20.0	233	+49.3

Source: USRDS Annual Report (2000).

Table 8.4   Patients alive on renal replacement therapy in the USA

	December 1989		December 1998		Δ%
	(*n*)	(%)	(*n*)	(%)	1989–98
Total dialysis patients	117 100	100.0	245 910	100.0	+ 109
Diabetics on dialysis	29 718	25.4	85 350	34.7	+ 187
Total patients with functioning graft	45 795	100.0	100 543	100.0	+ 119
Diabetics with functioning graft	7 083	15.5	17 592	17.5	+ 148

Source: USRDS Annual Report (2000).

around 380 pmp by the end of 1999 (personal communication), much lower figures being recorded in the European countries: 134 pmp in Germany 1999, 98 pmp in Catalonia in 1999, and 79 pmp in Denmark in 1997 (2, 4).

In most of the countries, the vast majority of adult diabetic patients on RRT are classified as type 2, non-insulin dependent diabetes mellitus (NIDDM). The rising tide of new diabetic patients having started RRT in recent years is indeed composed of type 2 diabetics, whereas no significant increase of juvenile-type 1 insulin-dependent patients has been observed (2). The incidence/prevalence of patients with NIDDM nephropathy type 2 is not geographically equally distributed, and also varies among social and ethnic groups: in the USA, the frequency is highest among African-American elderly women, African-American males, Hispanic and Native Americans (3). There are also wide differences between the European countries, with a significantly lower incidence observed in the South European countries (Spain, Italy) in contrast with Germany or Belgium, with the greatest proportion of juvenile type 1 diabetics being recorded in the Nordic/Scandinavian countries (2).

Several explanations are commonly set forward for the apparently unlimited growth of patients with NIDDM-associated nephropathy, mainly: the increasing prevalence of NIDDM among the aging population of the Western World; the important decrease in early cardiac and cerebrovascular mortality, thanks to the beneficial effects of anti-hypertensive therapy and efficient therapeutic procedures for coronary heart disease; and, last but not least, the more widespread availability of RRT. This key factor is well demonstrated by the rapid changes in the demographic profiles of ESRD patients that followed the political and economical shifts that occurred in the East European countries since the early 1990s. The true frequency of NIDDM-associated ESRD may even be under-estimated, since many patients maintained on insulin are erroneously classified as insulin-dependent, whereas they may be only insulin-requiring or even non-insulin-requiring patients. Clinical criteria may require confirmation by results of measurements of C-peptide plasma concentration, to rule out the persistance of residual insulin secretion. Following the injection of 1 mg of glucagon, a concordance of C-peptide response with clinical criteria for the classification of diabetic status has been established in 89% of 346 prospectively investigated patients (5). An accurate classification of the diabetic state is particularly important for selecting the patients for pancreas transplantation (see below and Chapter 4).

Diagnostic problems may be all the more complicated by the fact that non-diabetic renal disease may either occur or be surimposed on, in patients with type 2 diabetes. The clinical diagnosis of diabetic nephropathy rests on a long history of diabetes, evidence of multi-target organ damage, and proteinuria preceding the development of renal insufficiency. While this profile is well-established for IDDM patients, it can be very different in patients with NIDDM. The majority of patients with diabetic renal disease also have diabetic retinopathy, but the reverse is not true—the incidence of diabetic retinopathy being much greater than that of diabetic nephropathy. Moreover, biopsy studies have shown that 25–50% of proteinuric patients with NIDDM have glomerular lesions unrelated with, or additional to, diabetic nephropathy, while such a finding is much less prevalent in IDDM patients (6). In NIDDM-proteinuric patients, the absence of retinopathy, autonomic neuropathy, or a short time-course (less than 5 years) since the onset of diabetes, may cast a doubt on the diabetic origin of the renal symptomatology and thus lead to a confirmation by renal biopsy, which will then frequently reveal a non-specific glomerular lesion, such as membranous or IgA glomerulopathy. Due to its totally silent development, the discovery of NIDDM may become effective only several years after the onset of the diabetic state, which fragilizes greatly the time-course criterion in many patients.

Many epidemiological studies conducted during the past 20 years in the USA and in Europe have clearly shown that the natural history of diabetic nephropathy and its evolution towards ESRD are very comparable in IDDM and NIDDM patients (7). The cumulative incidence of ESRD was thus 40% at 10 years and 61% at 15 years following the onset of proteinuria in the extensively studied population of Pima Indians, similar to the 50% incidence of ESRD after 10 years of proteinuria in IDDM patients followed up at the Joslin Clinic in Boston (8). The lower incidence of ESRD observed in white NIDDM patients, in whom persistent proteinuria developed after the diagnosis of NIDDM (11% at 10 years and 17% at 15 years), is attributed to a lower risk of death from coronary heart disease or CVA in the relatively young NIDDM Pima Indians and IDDM whites, compared with that of the older NIDDM white patients, who may thus have died before reaching the terminal stage of uremia.

When approaching the advanced end-stage of renal insufficiency, the majority of surviving IDDM and NIDDM patients, having experienced a similar duration of diabetes, have actually been exposed to well-individualized risk factors, such as long-term hyperglycemia, hypertension, micro- and macro-angiopathy, proteinuria (often in the nephrotic range), dyslipidemia, malnutrition, and so on. The younger age-range of the majority of IDDM patients should have a favorable impact on their outcome, which is all too often offset by the combined devastating effects of chronic uremia associated with the multiple end-organ damages caused by long-lasting diabetes. Still, many young IDDM patients reach the stage of ESRD in a clinical status, which may not really be better that of NIDDM patients, particularly those living in poor socio-economic or psycho-social conditions, who have little or no access to (or do not follow) adequate medical care. The medical management of diabetic patients with ESRD is thus quite comparable, regardless of the type of diabetes, the only important difference lying in the possibility of performing renal or combined pancreas and renal transplantation, according to the variable age-barrier and the nature and degree of gravity of co-morbidities.(see below).

The therapeutic options that are currently available (at least in the most medically advanced countries) for diabetic ESRD patients, have far more important consequences for their future life-course than for non-diabetic patients. Indeed, with dialysis treatment, the diabetic patient remains diabetic and uremic, with the persistant adverse effects of both diseases. His/her key benefit is survival, generally shorter than in non-diabetic patients and with often a poorer quality of life. A successful renal transplant relieves the patient from uremia, but the detrimental effects of diabetes on target-organs persist, to which are then added the risk factors associated with the immunosuppressive regimens. Finally, only a very few who will benefit from a successful combined pancreas and renal transplantation procedure, may expect a very substantial improvement of their health status, long-term survival, and quality of life.

Dialysis therapy in diabetic patients with ESRD

There is certainly no other category of uremic patients for whom as many papers and presentations have been produced, since RRT became an established method of treatment of ESRD. After more than a quarter-century of world-wide experience, diabetics do remain a special group of patients, because the management of any mode of RRT is more complex for them, severe complications are more frequent, and their outcome, in terms of survival and quality of life, remains poorer than for age-, and gender-matched non-diabetic patients of similar socio-economic status.

The list of the main co-morbidities that are present, to a variable degree of severity, in most diabetic ESRD patients, quite easily explains why diabetics are clearly separated from all other patients in the reports dealing with the results of any mode of RRT. In a recent series of 84 consecutive type 2 diabetic patients, aged 67 ± 10 years, taken on dialysis in a single French center between 1995 and 1998, 67% had diabetic retinopathy documented at fundoscopy; the same percentage had presented at least one episode of acute left-ventricular dysfunction; 64% were hypertensive, despite anti-hypertensive treatment, and heavily overhydrated; 36% had angina; 26% had suffered a previous myocardial infarction; 37% were unable to walk independently; and 16% had already undergone at least one limb-amputation operation (9). Such a dismal profile is common in many other reports of the literature, positive changes over time are far too modest and slow, due to sub-optimal medical follow-up and too late referral of many diabetic patients to nephrological facilities. The terrible threat of blindness for diabetic patients has greatly diminished in recent years, if the patients have an early enough, and sustained, access to laser treatment and/or vitreous surgery, as appropriate. Among other prominent complications related to diabetes, autonomic neuropathy causes, at the same time, impairment of motricity and, sometimes, severe pain not easily alleviated by drugs; orthostatic hypotension renders de-ambulation hazardous; gastroparesis precludes adequate food intake, and thus worsens an already deteriorated nutritional status. Chronic diarrhea, or alternation of obstination and diarrhea, often co-exist with gastroparesis. In some patients, diabetic cystopathy, due to detrusor malfunction, entails voiding problems and bladder enlargement with chronic urine retention, which favors urinary tract infections that may interfere with a future kidney or pancreas–kidney TX.

Actually, most of the persistent excess mortality recorded for ESRD diabetic patients is due to macro-angiopathic cardiac, cerebrovascular, or peripheral vascular causes. Diabetes mellitus is known as an independent risk factor for coronary heart disease in non-uremic patients. There is a sound evidence for a specific cardiomyopathy characterized by a ventricular thickness beyond that expected from blood pressure levels. Whether this specific feature is preventable by good glycemic control remains undetermined (10).

Which dialysis therapy for diabetic patients?

The long-lasting controversies on the respective advantages and drawbacks of HD vs. PD techniques, which delight or worry advocates or opponents of either method, are at their highest when addressing diabetic patients. They concern not only survival criteria (see below) but also their respective efficiency for the better control of the clinical and metabolic disturbances induced by the association of uremia with the diabetic state, the frequency and gravity of treatment-induced morbidities, psychological tolerance, and quality of life. The final choice for a dialysis modality is thus the result of a complex interplay, including the patient's clinical condition and preferences, sociofamilial environment, availability of dialysis techniques, and the nephrologist's own personal convictions or biases.

Table 8.5 shows the trend in the distribution of diabetic ESRD treatment modalities in the USA during the period 1990–98. A steadily increasing percentage of diabetic patients are treated with in-center HD (up to 73.6% in 1998), while out-of-center HD has halved in 1998 its already very marginal role as recorded in 1990. The use of PD has declined substantially in recent years. This disfavor for PD looks surprising at first glance, given the attractive technical advances made for managing PD in recent years, towards better safety and adaptability (11). Actually, the trends observed for diabetic patients do not differ from that of the whole population on RRT in the USA during the same time-interval, with a similar increase in percentages of center HD-treated patients, slump of home HD, decline of PD, with, as sole difference, a greater percentage of patients alive with a functioning TX (Table 8.6).

Older age of diabetic patients, with more extended acceptance criteria (regardless of severe co-morbidities) are first-line explanations for this trend in the use of RRT modalities. In contrast, the European scene is somewhat different, PD being used in the years 1995–97 in up to 32.5% of diabetic patients in Lombardy, 25% in Denmark, 14% in France, but in only 6.5% in Norway, and 5.5% in Catalonia (2).

Table 8.5 Distribution of modes of treatment in diabetic patients alive with renal replacement therapy in the USA

	December 1990		December 1994		December 1998	
	(n)	*(%)*	*(n)*	*(%)*	*(n)*	*(%)*
All diabetic patients	42909	100.0	72122	100.0	102942	100.0
Centre HD	28246	62.8	47832	66.3	75725	73.6
Out-of-centre HD	642	1.5	911	1.3	846	0.8
CAPD/CCPD	4991	11.6	8016	11.1	7590	7.4
Renal transplant	8149	19.0	12753	17.7	17502	17.0

Source: USRDS Annual Report (2000).

Table 8.6 Distribution of modes of treatment in the whole population patients alive with renal replacement therapy in the USA

	December 1990		December 1994		December 1998	
	(*n*)	(%)	(*n*)	(%)	(*n*)	(%)
All patients	180986	100.0	271914	100.0	346453	100.0
Centre HD	103063	56.9	149061	54.8	208133	60.0
Out-of-centre HD	3651	2.0	3990	1.5	3546	1.02
CAPD/CCPD/APD	18318	10.1	27041	9.9	25273	7.3
Renal transplant	52312	28.9	77463	28.5	100543	29.0

Source: USRDS Annual Report (2000).

Medical and technical management of hemodialysis

A steadily increasing part of the bulk of diabetic type 2 patients with ESRD share the co-morbidities and handicaps of elderly persons, and thus belong to a population of frail patients who require similar procedures and precautions for HD therapy (see Chapter 7). Several points deserve, however, to be particularly emphasized.

The construction and maintenance of a vascular access delivering a blood-flow rate ensuring satisfactory performances of the HD/filtration system, is of crucial importance. Special difficulties are frequent in diabetic patients, due to extensive peripheral arterial calcifications and/or exhausted superficial veins, resulting from repeated venous samplings and previous vessel-aggressive infusions. The use of native vessels should be priviledged at all times, with, as first choice, a radiocephalic arteriovenous (AV) fistula created at the wrist. A calcified, narrowed, distal artery may, however, deliver an insufficient blood-flow rate, thus leading to the use of more proximal vessels at the upper-third of the forearm or the elbow region (12). The placement of the vascular access has to be performed well in advance of the anticipated date of HD, since several months may be necessary before a sufficient development of the vascular access is effective. Careful pre-operative work-up is mandatory, which includes, in addition to the clinical evaluation of the arterial and venous status of the upper limbs: plain X-ray of both arms, to detect arterial calcifications; ultrasonic evaluation of the arterial and venous systems of both arms; and dual/Doppler investigation, which yields the best informative status of the vessels (13). Concurrent old-age and diabetes mellitus markedly increase the risk of an AV fistula primary failure. Nevertheless, experienced surgical teams achieve similar results in diabetic and non-diabetic patients for patency and lifespan of internal vascular accesses, if the first operation is well planned, the elective site well chosen, and the strategies for revisions, stenoses, thromboses, infections, aneuvrysms, etc., well-defined, either with surgical or interventional percutaneous techniques (13, 14). Most unfortunately, due to too frequent late referral of patients to nephrological facilities, a well-scheduled program for vascular access placement cannot be respected, resulting in the use of prosthetic vascular grafts, which are expensive and have a shorter trouble-free function than native vascular accesses. Emergency situations have to be handled, with jugular vein cannulation having to be maintained for some time—several weeks or months—until a permanent access becomes usable. Careful attention has to be paid for preventing, detecting, and caring for distal ischemia of the access limb, which may be caused by obstructive arterial disease, vascular steal syndrome, or ischemic monomelic neuropathy (15). A risk of gangrene of the hand may result from severe peripheral ischemia in patients with proximal internal AV fistulas or prosthetic grafts diverting too high a blood-flow from the distal portion of the limb, rendering surgical correction by banding or ligation of the access mandatory (16).

Sudden and sharp falls of blood pressure (BP) during HD sessions are frequent and may generate immediate acute cardiac, cerebral, or visual complications. Intradialytic vascular instability results from several factors, among which the key role is played by a too rapid fall in plasma osmolality, due to excessive extracellular volume depletion not adequately compensated by the refilling rate from the intravascular space. Associated risk factors for cardiovascular instability are: reduced ejection fraction, due to coronary heart disease; diastolic dysfunction, related to diabetic cardiomyopathy, autonomic neuropathy precluding the normal increase of heart rate, and peripheral resistance in case of impending drops in BP; anemia, which also decreases peripheral vascular resistance; and hypoalbuminemia, resulting from nephrotic syndrome or malnutrition. Hypotensive episodes are furthermore triggered by cardiac arrythmias or the transient hypoxemia, which develops in the early phases of dialysis sessions performed with acetate dialysate and cellulosic membranes. Hypotensive episodes often occur despite obvious fluid overload and interdialytic HTA, requiring anti-hypertensive medications. They sometime lead to a therapeutic deadlock with repeated early termination of dialysis leaving the patient with sustained fluid overload, underdialyzed, and exhausted. The association of intradialytic hemodynamic instability with gastroparesis symptoms and swings in blood glucose levels, has a strongly negative impact on the psychological and nutritional status of the patients, entailing loss of appetite and reduction of caloric intake.

HD sessions should thus be performed with a slow, volumetrically controlled, fluid removal, bicarbonate-buffered dialysate, with a minimal and adjustable sodium concentration of 140 mmol/l. The use of dialyzers with high-permeability, biocompatible membranes, allows a greater clearing of middle-molecular weight neurotoxic compounds, β2-microglobulin, and also of advanced-glycation-end-products (AGES), such as pentosidine, AGE peptides, and AGE β2-microglobulin, which are considered as having a contributive role for the development of diabetic microvascular complications (17).

Furthermore, it has been shown that the decline of residual renal function (RRF) is slower in patients receiving HD with dialysers fitting a biocompatible membrane (High-Flux Polysulfone) than in those for whom dialysis is performed with filters equipped with a bioincompatible (cellophane) membrane (18). Maintenance of RRF has a very positive impact on the patients' quality of life, it contributes favorably to the overall clearance of small and middle molecular weight compounds and for keeping an adequate fluid and electrolyte balance.

Recent studies have shown a substantial reduction of intradialytic hypotensive episodes obtained by using either sodium modeling in a step-wise protocol with a dialysate sodium concentration starting at 152 mmol/l at onset of the HD session and declining to 140 mmol/l in the last 30 min of dialysis, or with using a high sodium dialysate (144 mmol/l) throughout the dialysis session, or by cooling the dialysate to 35 °C (19). The main drawback of the two former procedures is to produce an increased interdialytic thirst, resulting in excessive increment of body weight and worsening of volume-dependent hypertension; and of the latter procedure, to cause shivering and cramps in some patients. In contrast, a dialysis protocol made of 1 h of isolated ultrafiltration followed by 3 h of isovolumic dialysis, was found much less effective for preventing hypotensive episodes. Recently developed depurative methods, such as acetate-free biofiltration, have been shown as very effective for reducing intra- and interdialytic symptoms in diabetic patients compared with conventional bicarbonate buffered HD (20). Additional preventive measures include adequate correction of anemia with administration of Rhu-EPO and iron salts for raising the Hb level up to at least 12 g/dl, refraining from taking anti-hypertensive drugs during the hours preceding dialysis, as well as from food intake immediately before or during dialysis. α-Agonist medications, such as midodrine, have been credited with beneficial results (21).

A well-functioning vascular access, and stable hemodynamic conditions during the HD sessions, are mandatory prerequisites for the delivery of an adequate/optimal dialysis dose, which is of key importance for maintaining the best possible clinical status and preventing the development of complications related to underdialysis, such as fluid overload, malnutrition, aggravation of neuropathy, and so on. The beneficial effect on survival of increased dialysis doses has been well-documented in several studies (22, 23). The recently updated NKF/DOQI guidelines do thus recommend a delivery HD dose amounting to a Kt/V of 1.3, corresponding to a urea reduction rate (URR) of 70% (24). Maintaining these HD criteria in the long term is of utmost importance to improve survival in this fragile group of patients.

Malnutrition is very common in diabetic patients at the onset of dialysis treatment, due to the combined effects of uremia, metabolic disturbances related to diabetes, and of the clinical and psychological impact of disabling co-morbidities, as described above. Low albumin, pre-albumin, and creatinine concentrations, at onset and during further courses of dialysis treatment, are among the strongest predictors of morbidity and mortality in diabetic ESRD patients (25). A daily intake of a diet providing at least 35 kcal/kg and 1.2 g/kg of protein is thus absolutely essential. Oral or per-dialytic parenteral caloric/protein supplementation may be required if spontaneous food intake is quantitatively or qualitatively insufficient, particularly in case of gastroparetic symptoms. Carbohydrates should account for 50–60% of the daily caloric supply. The dialysate should be enriched with 1.5–2 g/l of glucose compensating for the 30–40 g of glucose lost during the dialysis session, and also to limit too wide pre- and post-dialysis swings of blood glucose levels. Lipid and lipoprotein abnormalities are well-documented risk factors for coronary and other vascular diseases, and as such contribute to the high mortality risk of ESRD patients (26). Reduction of high-cholesterol-containing food components, preference given to the use of polyunsaturated fat, and the use of lipid-lowering medications (statins), are generally recommended measures.

Maintaining a good glycemic control by careful, individually tailored, insulin dosage and timing of administration (usually two subcutaneous injections daily, with adjustments made according to the dialysis sessions schedule), is of great importance for reducing the progression of micro-angiopathic complications, especially retinopathy. A good blood-glucose control has been documented as a significant predictor for better survival in a recent prospective study conducted in 150 diabetic ESRD patients (27). The risk of hypoglycemia, however, over-rides a too tight blood-glucose control, a preprandial level of between 6 and 12 mmol/l is an acceptable compromise (28). Hypoglycemia-inducing medications, such as beta blockers, should be used with great care, and only if absolutely necessary. Glycosylated hemoglobin has been validated as a reliable index of integrated glycemia levels in uremic diabetics when measured with techniques that do not use electrical charges to separate the different hemoglobin fractions (photometry, radioimmunoassay), and thus do not provoke interferences with carbamylated hemoglobin (29). A glycosylated Hb1Ac value at 7–8% is thus considered as a reasonable compromise, in that, for this level, the incidence of clinically symptomatic hypoglycemic episodes is low (30).

Infections rank second in the causes of death in diabetic (as well as in non-diabetic) patients (31). Mortality caused by sepsis is higher among diabetic patients across all dialysis populations and is approximately 50-fold higher in diabetics on ESRD, compared with diabetic patients in the general population in the USA (31). Older age of the diabetic type 2 population, uremia-related impairment of host defense mechanisms, and malnutrition, are common causes of the increased susceptibility to infections in dialysis patients (32), to which is added the specific fragility due to the diabetic state. Temporary vascular accesses (jugular vein catheters), prosthetic arteriovenous grafts, and dialyzer re-use, are dialysis-related independent risk factors that have been singled out as elective entry sites for the development of septicemia (32). Life-threatening dissaminated infections may also take their starting point from initially very small cutaneous lesions located in ischemic distal segments of the limbs, toes, or fingers in patients with vascular access-induced stealing syndrome. Regular follow-up of diabetic patients by a podiatrist is mandatory, adequate foot care being aimed at preventing or caring for even the smallest local abnormality, which, if neglected, can lead to catastrophic consequences.

An adequate global management of diabetic dialysis patients thus requires the close co-operation of a large panel of specialists with the medical/nursing staff of the dialysis facility, mainly cardiologist, vascular surgeon, diabetologist, ophtalmologist, neurologist, nutritionist, and dietitian, podiatrist, etc., all of whom should be easily available and able to co-operate mutually, thereby avoiding conflicting therapeutic prescriptions. An on-going support from an efficient and dedicated social worker is also always necessary, given the often very severe psychosocial problems that are present in heavily disabled patients and their overburdened families (33). The complexity of such a global management explains why a majority of diabetic ESRD patients remain treated as in-center HD patients, whereas those whose clinical status is less severe and/or more stable, may receive adequate dialysis treatment with out-of-center PD.

Medical and technical management of peritoneal dialysis

From the onset of the introduction of CAPD into clinical practice, 25 years ago, this mode of RRT has been considered as particularly suitable for both IDDM and NIDDM patients, being devoid of the twice–thrice weekly repeated acute clinical and metabolic imbalances induced by intermittent HD methods, and replaced by a depurative technique coming closer to that achieved by the native kidney in terms of permanence of function. However, over the years, lively controversies have persisted about the clear superiority of PD techniques over HD as the preferential RRT for diabetic patients, not only concerning survival criteria, but also in terms of their respective efficacy for controlling the clinical and metabolic disturbances of ESRD and diabetes, on the frequency and severity of technique-induced morbidities, psychological tolerance, and quality of life. The debate remains all the more timely as important technical advances have been introduced in recent years in the domain of PD, regarding novel dialysis fluid compositions, connectology, assessment of dialysis adequacy, prevention and treatment of abdominal complications, which all have rendered the use of PD safer and acceptable to more extended fractions of the ESRD population. It is thus somewhat disappointing that, as among the whole ESRD population of the USA, the use of PD has steadily declined percentagewise during the recent 10-year interval, even if the absolute number of diabetic patients treated with PD was 52% greater by the end of 1998, compared to December 1990 (Table 8.5).

The main benefits drawn from the use of PD over HD in diabetic patients are summarized in Table 8.7. On the other hand, one should not conceal several drawbacks of PD, such as an increased risk for peritoneal and catheter exit-site infections, the

Table 8.7   Reasons for priviledging peritoneal dialysis vs. hemodialysis for diabetic patients with ESRD

- No vascular access.
- No systemic anticoagulation.
- Better hemodynamic stability.
- Better control of blood-glucose equilibrium.
- Better preservation of residual renal function.
- Only out-of-centre dialysis method devoid of acute potentially life-threatening complications.
- Lower cost than in-centre hemodialysis.

negative impact of the continuous loss of protein through the dialysate on an already, often very deteriorated, nutritional status, along with the clinical and metabolic consequences of the continuous absorption of glucose from the dialysate. In addition, there is the progressive loss over time of the fluid- and solute-removal capacities of the peritoneal membrane, leading to an insidiously developing state of underdialysis, which makes a transfer to an alternative mode of RRT mandatory. Many of these advantages and shortcomings are common for all the patients who undergo PD treatments (see Chapters 2 and 7). We shall concentrate, in this section, on issues that concern more specifically diabetic patients on PD therapy.

Glucose-containing PD solutions used in conventional dialysis regimens lead to a daily peritoneal absorption of 150–300 g of glucose, which results in sometimes important weight gain and increased insulin-requirements for blood-glucose control. Furthermore, a high peritoneal glucose absorption enhances the hypertriglycemia and other atherogenic lipid abnormalities usually present in patients at the inception of RRT. Glucose-degradation products are generated through heat sterilization of the solutions and concur with the non–enzymatic glycation process of glucose for the formation of AGES, which accumulate in the peritoneal vascular walls. Accumulation of AGES has been found to be positively related to duration of PD treatment, number of peritonitis episodes, and dialysis-fluid glucose concentration. Peritoneal biopsies have disclosed that the AGES level in the peritoneal tissue is significantly higher in diabetics than in non-diabetic PD patients (34). Glucose-induced damages to the peritoneum play an important role for the development of progressive loss of ultra-filtration capacity and of peritoneal sclerosis, which renders the peritoneal membrane inefficient for providing adequate dialysis. Due to their hypertonicity, acidity, and unphysiologic buffer (lactate), glucose-containing PD fluids also express toxicity towards peritoneal mesothelial cells, whose role is to preserve the integrity of the membrane. The hypertonicity of the dialysate also interferes negatively with the peritoneal defense mechanisms by inhibition of phagocytosis and bactericidal activity (35, 36).

Novel PD solutions, with alternative osmotic agents, have been developed in recent years, which are of particular interest for diabetic patients (37, 38). The glucose polymer icodextrin is a very efficient colloid osmotic agent, which advantageously replaces hypertonic glucose solutions in providing slow and sustained ultrafiltration volumes throughout long-dwell periods (39). The use of glycerol-containing solutions is hampered by accumulation of glycerol in the blood and exacerbation of hypertriglycemia. Other formulae, some still under clinical investigation, comprise a combination of glycerol and amino acids, which permit a reduction of caloric uptake and insulin requirements, or a mixture of polyglucose and amino acids. Amino acid–containing solutions contribute to the reduction of peritoneal net loss of proteins and amino acids, and are deemed helpful for improving the nutritional status of malnourished patients. Finally, bicarbonate or bicarbonate/lactate-buffered mixed solutions are also promising advances aimed at minimizing the toxicity and bioincompatibility properties of PD solutions.

PD allows the more physiologic intraperitoneal (i.p.) administration of insulin, given the similarities between the absorption kinetics of i.p. insulin and the normal insulin secretion of insulin by the pancreatic islet cells. The method is, however, unapplicable to the increasing fraction of patients treated with automated dialysis methods (see Chapter 2) who can receive insulin only subcutaneously. Intraperitoneal insulin, preferably administered in an empty peritoneal cavity before meals, is absorbed by diffusion across the visceral peritoneum into the portal-venous circulation and also through the capsule of the liver (40). Intraperitoneal administration of insulin is credited with improved control of blood-glucose levels and less hypoglycemic episodes, compared with subcutaneous insulin (41), but its effects on lipid abnormalities remain debated (38). Whether i.p. administration of insulin increases by itself the incidence of peritonitis is difficult to establish unequivocally, given the conflicting results reported in single- or multi-center studies. However, a large Italian multi-center study, conducted in the late 1980s, did not show a significantly different incidence of peritonitis episodes between patients receiving, or not receiving, i.p. insulin (0.67 and 0.77 episode per patient year, respectively) (42).

The continuous, slow, fluid and sodium removal achieved with PD is much better tolerated than the rapid, fluid and electrolyte shifts induced by extra-corporeal ultrafiltration methods. A better and more stable control of blood pressure can thus be obtained in many PD-treated patients in whom anti-hypertensive drugs can often be discontinued. However, increased thirst linked to hyperglycemia. in the case of poor glycemic control, reduction of urinary output, loss of peritoneal ultrafiltration capacity, and inaccurate assessment of dry weight, concur in some patients to the development of an insidiously developing chronic volume overload with elevation of blood pressure. In other patients, orthostatic hypotension, due to autonomic dysfunction and/or heart failure, can be enhanced by excessive PD-induced volume depletion and greatly worsen the symptoms of peripheral vascular disease in the lower limbs. Hypotensive episodes can also trigger falls, cardiac ischemic accidents, or strokes. Clinical symptoms of hypotension have thus to be actively treated, depending on their severity, either with non-pharmacologic interventions or with fludrocortisone, midodrine, sentaline, together with reduction or discontinuation of non-indispensable medications that favor the incidence of orthostatic hypotension (43). Although adequate control of blood pressure is generally more easily obtained than in HD-treated patients, close surveillance and frequent reassessments of dry weight and residual urinary output are mandatory in PD patients, who show a reduction in the control of blood pressure.

The damages induced by diabetic micro-angiopathic lesions on target organs (eyes, peripheral nerves), at best stabilize, and do not worsen, in adequately treated PD patients, with results depending on the severity of the lesions at start of RRT, the quality of blood-pressure and glycemic control, of opthalmologic care, overall nutritional status, and dialysis adequacy (11).

Delivery of an adequate dialysis dose is of key importance for the quality of results in terms of morbidity and mortality (44). The practical guidelines for the delivery of an adequate dose of peritoneal dialysis have been recently updated in NKF/DOQI recommendations (45). The recommended weekly dose of dialysis varies to some extent according to the mode of PD used: CAPD, NIPD, or CCPD (see Chapter 2). PD associated with residual renal function (RRF) should result in delivering to the patient a total Kt/V urea in the 2–2.2 range, and a total creatinine clearance of

60–70 l/week/1.73 m² area. These targets are deemed not to be different in diabetic vs. non-diabetic patients. It has to be remembered that severe malnutrition, common in diabetic patients, may lead to erroneous estimations of total body water (V) and body surface area.

Preservation of residual renal function (RRF) is therefore essential for delivery of an adequate dialysis dose to diabetic patients treated with PD. Whatever the PD modality used, the target indexes of dialysis adequacy will not be met in patients with too low or complete loss of RRF. A slower rate of deterioration of RRF in PD- compared with HD-treated patients, is well-documented: rapid changes in extracellular fluid volume during aggressive ultra-filtration in HD, result in a fall of BP and ischemia in the remaining functioning nephrons, combined with the detrimental effects of the bio-incompatibility of the components of the extra-corporeal dialysis systems (mainly the bio-incompatible membranes), exert a nephrotoxic effect and cause further deterioration of RRF (40). In contrast, the better hemodynamic stability (associated sometimes with a certain degree of extracellular-fluid expansion) and the reduced bio-incompatibility of the PD systems, contribute to maintaining RRF for a longer period of time in PD patients. Nevertheless, deterioration of RRF develops ineluctably over time, with 40% of patients becoming anuric at a mean of 20 months after initiation of dialysis. Diabetes as a cause of ESRD has been found significantly associated with the rate of decline of RRF in a group of 90 diabetic patients among a population of 242 PD patients recently reviewed in a Canadian study (46). Administration of furosemide (250–500 mg/day) had a beneficial effect on the urinary output, but no effect on preservation of GFR (47). There have been controversies concerning a possible negative impact of automated dialysis techniques on preservation of RRF compared with CAPD/CCPD modalities (48). Results of recent studies tend to indicate that actually the rate of decline of RRF is equal in CAPD and APD patients (49–51).

The most frequent technique-related complications that occur during PD treatment are peritonitis and exit-site infections. Apart from their immediate potential hazards, such as bacterial dissemination, repeated peritoneal infections contribute to an accelerated loss of the depurative abilities of the peritoneal membrane, which will lead to patient drop-out and transfer to HD. An increased incidence of peritonitis episodes remains reported in some large series of diabetic patients compared with non-diabetics (52), but great difference in case-mix, connectology, and PD techniques, prevent any generalizations from these findings. The use of automated PD techniques has been shown to reduce the risk of peritoneal infections (53). Worsening of peripheral vascular disease with ischemic gangrene may lead to extended amputations, small ischemic lesions are often the starting point for sepsis. Persistent malnutrition, associated with disabling co-morbidities and depression (burn-out syndrome), result in the development of cachexia, which pays a high toll to morbidity. It is thus of paramount importance to decide early enough a transfer to HD for patients who run into repeated technical complications or who become non-compliant or intolerant to the constraints of PD therapy. The poor quality of life that is reported, particularly for many elderly type 2 diabetic patients, is actually due to the association of various co-morbidities that had developed prior to the initiation of RRT, and are not improvable by dialysis techniques, with the iatrogenic complications of PD or HD. On-going technical advances, accumulated physician and nursing staff experience at selecting for each patient his/her best adapted mode of RRT, early diagnosis and expert care of complications, highly beneficial effects of recently available new medications, such as Rhu-EPO for treating renal anemia, all contribute to improving the rehabilitation and overall quality of life in this fragile group of ESRD patients.

Outcome of diabetic patients on dialysis therapy

In most single-center, national, or international studies published over the past 15 years, the survival rates of diabetic patients treated with ESRD are reported to be 20–25% lower than that obtained in age-adjusted non-diabetic patients (3, 29, 54–56). However, the interpretations of such comparisons must be treated with great caution, particularly because the frequent and severe co-morbidities present in diabetics at the start of RRT are manipulated differently with the statistical tools used in studies addressing populations analyzed in facilities or surveys of variable sizes and origin (55, 57).

Recent data from the annual USRDS report, shown in Table 8.8, yield encouraging results in terms of survival recorded over the past 15 years in diabetic, as well as in other, ESRD patients treated with dialysis methods: the 1-, 2-, and 5-year survival probabilities of diabetic patients (all types and ages combined) have increased by 11.8%, 16.1%, and 6.5%, respectively, while remaining lower, by more than half, at 5 years compared with that recorded in age-, gender-, and race-adjusted non-diabetic subjects. These results are all the more remarkable as the age of incident dialysis patients has markedly increased during this time-interval, and the selection criteria for acceptance on RRT have become more flexible. The death rates and causes of death in patients aged 45–64 years, treated with HD and PD in the USA in the years 1996–98, are shown in Table 8.9: overall, the differences in death-rates for the five most frequently considered causes of death, are much greater among the PD-treated patients than in those receiving HD (286.1/1000 patient-years at risk for PD vs. 193.8 for HD patients). Death rates due to septicemia are greater than that due to myocardial infarction, in both groups of patients. Among homogenous (younger and older) age-groups of

Table 8.8   1-, 2-, and 5-year patient-survival probabilities for dialysis patients (censored at transplant) according to primary renal disease (1987–98)

	1 year			2 years			5 years	
Start of dialysis ⟶	1987	1992	1997	1987	1992	1996	1987	1993
Diabetes (%)	68.5	74.9	80.3	46.5	54.9	62.6	14.8	21.3
Hypertension (%)	72.2	76.1	80.3	53.5	59.1	65.5	21.7	26.0
Glomerulonephritis (%)	77.7	86.0	90.9	68.9	73.7	82.1	35.1	47.5
Total probabilities (%)	72.8	78.4	83.2	54.0	61.8	68.5	22.8	29.5

Source: USRDS Annual Report (2000).

Table 8.9 Death rates by primary cause of death per 1000 patient-years at risk in patients aged 45–64 years treated with dialysis methods in the USA (1996–98)

	Diabetic HD	Non-diabetic HD	Diabetic PD	Non-diabetic PD
Acute myocardial infarction	21.9	12.0	35.6	13.8
Atherosclerotic heart disease	6.0	2.9	10.9	3.6
Cardiac arrest	45.4	27.5	60.5	27.9
Cerebro vascular accident	13.0	7.3	18.2	8.3
Septicemia	23.9	15.2	49.4	25.6
All patients at risk aged 45–64 years	193.8 ($n=104\,408$)	138.0 ($n=113\,272$)	286.1 ($n=16\,159$)	151.5 ($n=19\,567$)

Source: USRDS Annual Report (2000).

Table 8.10 Death rates per 1000 patients years at risk of patients treated with dialysis methods in the USA in 1998 according to age and primary renal disease

Age-range (years)	Diabetes	Hypertension	Other	All patients
30–34	137.9	40.8	54.8	68.2
45–49	170.2	87.3	91.7	115.0
65–69	299.3	252.2	249.9	275.8
75–79	422.0	377.9	360.3	388.9

Source: USRDS Annual Report (2000).

patients, the death rates for diabetic patients are notably higher than that recorded for patients with other underlying renal diseases (Table 8.10). In a recent single-center report, diabetics had a six-fold higher cardio-vascular mortality and three-fold higher infectious mortality than non-diabetic patients, this excess of mortality rates being generated mostly by diabetic type 2 patients (56).

Survival analyses performed in Europe and in North America, regarding diabetic patients on RRT, thus yield conflicting results. An abysmal prognosis is, for example, described in a series of 84 diabetic patients taken on dialysis in a single French center in the years 1995–98, with a 32% mortality observed during an average follow-up period of only 211 days (9). On the other hand, survival rates ranging between 21% and 45% at 5 years, are reported in many single- or multi-center studies (3, 11, 57–59). Comparisons of survival rates or other criteria, such as annual hospitalization days, published in different studies are most of the time inappropriate, since the results are heavily influenced by selection biases, and stratifications of the investigated populations according to type of diabetes, age, co-morbidities, dose of dialysis, nutritional status, and so on. Confusion must also be avoided between technique survival and overall patient survival: young type 1 diabetic patients may have their dialysis technique survival shortened if treated in facilities that have an active transplantation program, whereas the technique survival is negatively influenced in older type 2 PD patients having a high transfer rate to HD.

PD-treated diabetic type 1 and 2 patients enrolled in the CANUSA study thus had a 2-year survival probability of 83.3% and 65.5%, respectively, whereas the combined patient and technique survival probabilities were only 61.7% and 46.8%, respectively (60). Regarding the issue of a significantly better outcome provided by one of the dialysis methods over the others, the conclusions of an in-depth nationwide analysis, carried out on data collected through the USRDS, are in accordance with that reported in European and Asian series (58, 59) in that there is little or no difference in overall mortality between PD and HD, at least in male diabetic patients. The risk of death was found to be higher in patients aged less than 50 years treated with HD, whereas PD carried a greater risk in those aged over 50 years (57). The debate about which is the best treatment may remain open for a long time to come, since a prospective, carefully randomized study, designed for addressing this issue, is very unlikely to be carried out within the foreseeable future.

Renal transplantation (Renal TX) in diabetic patients

Over the past 20 years, the practice of renal TX has changed for diabetic patients to a much greater extent than for any other group of patients with ESRD. The availability of new immunosuppressive agents, together with major advances acquired for organ-preservation procedures, and for surgical and intensive-care techniques, have paved the way for moving from the mere replacement of renal function to that of kidney *and* pancreas function. Thus, between October 1988 and June 1997, among 13 467 uremic diabetics type 1 who had been placed on a Renal TX waiting-list in the USA, 70.3% have been transplanted, of whom 49.4% underwent a simultaneous kidney and pancreas transplantation (SPK), 43.4% received a cadaver kidney alone (CAD), 7% a living donor kidney (LKD), and 29.3% were never transplanted (61). Technical management and benefits of renal and SPK transplantation in diabetic patients have been reviewed in Chapters 3 and 4, to which we refer the reader. We shall focus in this section on the evolution of trends observed in this domain during the last two decades, concerning demographics and the (provisional) lessons that can be drawn from the currently reported results for providing guidance for the future.

The changing scene of organ TX for diabetic patients

A few landmark papers illustrate best the extraordinary impulse provided by some pioneering teams who challenged the perilous undertaking of developing organ TX programs for, at first glance, a very unattractive group of ESRD patients.

In 1989, the group headed by John Najarian at the University of Minnesota reported on 265 uremic type 1 diabetic patients who had received a kidney TX between 1966 and 1978. The actual 10-year-patient- and graft-survival rates overall were 40% and 32%, respectively. Of the 100 patients who survived into a second decade, at 15 years post-TX, 51% were alive and 41% had functioning grafts (62). Three years later the same group reported on their 15 years experience, gained in 1275 renal transplants performed in diabetic patients. Their patient and survival rates, obtained in patients treated with cyclosporine (CSA), are displayed in Table 8.11 and well demonstrate that, as far back as 10 years ago, the results achieved by a highly experienced team were little different from large populations of diabetic and non-diabetic kidney recipients (63).

The demographic profile of renal TX in the USA over a recent 10-year interval, is shown in Table 8.12. The percentage of diabetic patients among the cadaveric kidney recipients increased by 8.2% in 1998, compared with 1988, reaching almost 25% of all patients transplanted that year with a cadaveric kidney. The absolute number was 62% greater in 1998 than in 1988. Diabetics, in 1998, accounted for 18.5% of all living donor transplants performed that year; their absolute number rose by 129% compared to 10 years earlier.

This steadily increasing kidney-alone (KA) transplant activity for diabetic patients, has actually become a well-established (routine) mode of treatment, at least in several North American and European transplantation centers, where kidney TX for this

Table 8.11   Kidney transplantation in diabetic patients—the University of Minnesota experience in the cyclosporine era

	Patient survival				Graft survival			
	Cadaveric graft		Living donor graft		Cadaveric graft		Living donor graft[*]	
	1 year (%)	5 years (%)	1 year (%)	5 years (%)	1 year (%)	5 years (%)	1 year (%)	5 years (%)
Diabetic recipients	91	75	93	84	85	64	90	80
Non-diabetic recipients	93	83	98	89	82	61	93	69

[*] All deaths=graft loss
Adapted from: Basadonna *et al.* (1992) *Kidney International*, **42**, (Suppl. 38), S193–6.

Table 8.12   Demographic profile of renal transplantation in the USA (1988–98)

	1988	1998
1. All cadaver TX recipients:	8193	8925
Diabetic patients:	1362 (16.6%)	2215 (24.8%)
2. All living donor TX recipients:	2050	4026
Diabetic patients:	326 (15.9%)	747 (18.5%)
Total 1+2 pmp		
All TX recipients	42	48
Diabetic patients	6.9	10.9

Source: USRDS Report (2000).

subgroup of ESRD patients has been a major theme of clinical research. However, during the last decade, the main interest of the medical community has actually shifted to the widespread expansion of combined kidney and pancreas TX and to the comparative results obtained with this mode of therapy and kidney alone. This change is well illustrated by the fact that less than three papers on KA TX were published in the proceedings of the September 2000 *International Congress of the Transplant Society*, in contrast to more than 30 on combined kidney and pancreas TX.

The magnitude of the changes that have occured within a 10-year time-interval is well demonstrated by quoting three landmark papers: in September 1988 an article from the group at the University of Minnesota bore the following title: 'Renal transplantation is confirmed therapy while pancreas transplantation should be performed only in an investigated setting' (64). In september 1998, the group at the University of Wisconsin reported their experience with 500 SPK transplants (65), and in April 2001, the Minnesota Group draws the lessons learned from more than 1000 pancreas transplantation at a single institution (66). The International Pancreas Transplantation Registry reports, in July 2000, on more than 14 000 pancreas TX performed worldwide since 1987. Of the pancreas TX, 73% were performed in the USA, and 23% in the Western and Nordic European countries (67). Among 3895 pancreas TX performed in the USA between 1996 and 2000, 83.6% were SPK transplants, 11.7% were PAK (pancreatic after kidney) transplants, and 4.7% solitary pancreas TX.

The increased efficacy against rejection, and the advances made for preventing and minimizing the toxicity of new immunosuppressive protocols, are of crucial importance for enlarging the indications of combined K and PTX. The triple association of CSA, AZA, and PRED, which became the most widely used regimen from 1986–87 till the mid-1990s, acted as a real booster for pancreas transplantation. More recently, tacrolimus and mycophenolate mofetil have proven substantially beneficial for reducing rejection rates (65, 68), as well as the use of humanized monoclonal antibodies (daclizumabe–basiliximabe) for immunosuppressive induction therapy (see Chapter 3). Advances in immunosuppressive therapy are inseparable from those gained in surgical and intensive care techniques, for improving the outcome of pancreas TX; the most debated (and yet unsettled) problem lying in the choice of the safest pancreatic duct drainage (bladder or enteric) required for total pancreatic grafts (see Chapter 4).

Current results of renal TX in diabetics

Whatever the success of combined K and PTX, a substantial percentage of diabetic transplant candidates still receive a kidney-only TX. The patient-survival probabilities recorded in the USA for cadaveric kidney diabetic recipients during a 10-year time-interval (all ages and types of diabetes combined), are displayed in Table 8.13. They show that, over the decade, a gain of about 10% in patient survival has been obtained at 2 and 5 years after TX. The diabetic patient survival at 5 years, however, remains lower by 20%, compared to that achieved in patients with primary glomerulonephritis. The same profile in survival rates applies to diabetic living donor kidney recipients: their survivals rate at 2 years is only 5% less than that of patients with primary glomerulonephritis, but comes close to 20% less at 5 years, during the most recent period (Table 8.14).

Many single-center, multi-center, and nationwide studies have addressed, in recent years, the issue comparing the patient-survival and renal-graft function in patients having undergone SPK or KA transplantation.

In a series of patients transplanted at the Department of Surgery of Stanford University between 1992 and 1996, no significant differences were recorded between SPK and KA patients at 1, 2 and 3 years post-TX, regarding serum creatinine, number of rejection episodes, incidence of kidney graft loss, and patient death; the 3-year actuarial patient- and graft-survival rates were similar (69). Among 14 patients having undergone SPK, compared with 15 patients who had received a KA TX and who were followed-up for 10 years at the Karolinska Institute in Stockholm, no difference was noted in patient mortality at 4 years after TX, whereas at 10 years, the mortality rate of KA patients amounted to 80% vs. 20% for the SPK patients (70). This striking difference is attributed by the authors to the beneficial effects of long-term normoglycemia obtained with SPK, on the diabetic late complications. The same contention is set forward by an Italian group, based on the results obtained in 107 SPK and 34 KA transplants, in whom the 7-year patient-survival rates were 75% and 63%,

Table 8.13   1-, 2-, and 5-year patient-survival probabilities for cadaveric kidney transplant recipients according to primary renal disease (1987–98)

	1 year			2 years			5 years	
Year of transplant ⟶	1987	1992	1997	1987	1992	1996	1987	1993
Diabetes (%)	87.4	91.0	93.8	79.1	85.2	88.9	59.3	69.5
Hypertension (%)	91.2	92.6	94.2	87.5	88.5	92.4	69.3	77.3
Glomerulonephritis (%)	94.4	96.6	97.0	91.0	95.2	94.3	82.2	88.5
Total patient probabilities (%)	92.2	94.6	95.8	88.1	91.6	93.2	75.8	82.2

Source: USRDS Annual Report (2000).

Table 8.14   1-, 2-, and 5-year survival probabilities for living donor kidney transplant recipients according to primary renal disease (1987–98)

	1 year			2 years			5 years	
Year of transplant ⟶	1987	1992	1997	1987	1992	1996	1987	1993
Diabetes (%)	92.2	95.0	95.4	83.4	92.1	93.8	70.1	75.4
Glomerulonephritis (%)	96.2	97.7	98.9	95.1	96.9	97.9	90.4	93.0
Total patient probabilities (%)	96.5	96.7	98.2	91.5	95.4	96.1	83.5	87.4

Source: USRDS Annual Report (2000).

respectively (71). The group at the University of Wisconsin reported on the comparative outcome of 379 SPK, 43 HL-A identical, 87 haplotype-identical living related donor (LRD), and 296 cadaveric renal transplants performed in diabetic patients: no significant difference was evidenced in patient or renal-graft survival between patients receiving SPK or LRD transplants, whereas both graft- and patient-survival rates were significantly lower for cadaveric kidney recipients than for the two other groups of patients (72). This profile of survival rates was found constent at each time up to 14 years post-TX (73). However, these results have to take into account that the cadaveric kidney recipients were about 10 years older at the time of TX, than the patients belonging to the SPK and LRD groups.

The results of most of single-center, as well as of large nationwide, studies, thus currently concur in yielding very similar long-term survival rates in diabetic type 1 SPK and LD kidney recipients; the survival of cadaveric kidney recipients being around 20% lower. Among 13 467 uremic type 1 diabetics who underwent SPK (4718), LD kidney TX (671), and cadaveric kidney TX (4127) in the USA between 1988 and 1997, the 10-year patient survival was 67%, 65%, and 46% for SPK, LD, and CAD kidney recipients, respectively. All three forms of kidney TX were associated with a significant increase in life-expectancy when compared with type 1 diabetics who remained on a transplant waiting-list and were never transplanted ($n = 3951$) (74).

Overall, the main conclusions that can be drawn, in early 2001, from the studies published during the past 5 years, are that in diabetics type 1, long-term survival (up to 8 years) is similar for SPK and LD kidney recipients and superior to that achieved for cadaveric kidney recipients, even after adjusting for recipient and donor characteristics. Mortality risk and incidence of complications are greater for SPK recipients during the first year post-TX, whereas that of LD kidney recipients become greater in the long-term. For all patient age-ranges from 20 up to 74 years at time of placement of patients on a transplant waiting-list, transplantation reduces the long-term mortality risk: actually, diabetics get the greatest benefit from being transplanted, as documented in a nationwide USA study, which evidenced a gain of more than 11 years in survival of diabetic patients, compared with an increase of 7 years among those with glomerulonephritis and 8 years among those with other causes of ESRD (75). These brilliant results should not conceal the fact that lesions of diabetic nephropathy recur in transplanted kidneys and may lead to failure of the graft, as shown in a series of 14 diabetic type 1 patients, of whom six were living donor and eight cadaveric kidney recipients. On average, 97 months after TX, all these patients were proteinuric with impairment of renal function, their patient- and graft-survival rates were 59% and 34%, respectively, and graft failure was due to recurrent diabetic nephropathy in seven (50%) of the patients (76).

Uremic diabetic patients and transplantation: a dual society

An overwhelming proportion of patients with diabetes mellitus are type 2 NIDDM patients. Important decreases of early deaths from cardiovascular, infectious, or metabolic causes have been obtained in recent years in this population, resulting in a rapidly growing number of long-term survivors, who may develop renal failure after 20 years duration of diabetes. Most of the studies report on organ transplantation performed in juvenile type 1 diabetics, and few data analyzing results specifically in type 2 diabetics are available. A rather restrictive attitude towards renal TX for type 2 diabetic patients is expressed by a Swedish group on the basis of an experience based on 27 type 2 patients (mean age 53 years). After a follow-up period of 51 ± 27 months, 33% of these patients had died vs. only 17% in matched controls (77). In contrast, the outcome of 90 type 2 diabetic patients, who received a kidney transplant at the University of Minnesota, was compared with that of renal TX performed for type 1 diabetic patients, and with that of non-diabetic patients aged over 50 years. Overall, the patient and survival rates of the type 2 diabetic transplanted patients was 61% and 53%, respectively. They were, however, significantly lower than that achieved in the two other groups of investigated patients (78). The Belgian group at Saint-Luc Hospital in Brussels reports an 81% survival rate at 5 years after TX in type 2 diabetic patients without severe cardiovascular disease at time of TX (79). As for combined P and K TX, the Swedish authors clearly state that this procedure is not indicated for type 2 diabetics (77), while the Belgium group similarly contends that combined P and K TX should be considered for type 1 patients under 50 years of age with no, or only moderate, cardiovascular complications (70). In contrast, the proportion of pancreas TX performed in the USA for recipients older than 45 years has increased from 13% in 1996, up to 25% in 2000, with 1-year graft-survival rates of SPK transplants being 88% and 93% in patients aged more or less than 45 years, respectively. About 4.3% of the pancreas TX performed in the USA between 1996 and 2000 were reportedly done for diabetic type 2 patients, with pancreas graft-survival rates at 1-year post-TX being identical for type 1 and type 2 diabetics, 84% and 83%, respectively, and patient-survival rates 95% and 92%, respectively (67).

The great variations in the results of KA or SPK TX among several published series of patients are closely linked to the more or less cogent selection-criteria applied by the transplant teams for placing their patients on a transplant waiting-list: a previous history of stroke, myocardial infarction, severe peripheral vascular disease, and multiple symptoms of autonomic neuropathy, are all predictors of post-TX severe morbidity and impaired survival, and thus plead against offering TX to these patients, an option that may even be ethically questionable taking into account the shortage of organs constrasting with the steadily growing number of patients-in-waiting for TX. Clearly, diabetic ESRD patients have two different life-expectancies, depending on whether or not they are considered positively as transplant candidates, since, as detailed above, the survival rates of diabetic TX patients (regardless of the type of TX) are consistently better than for those who were deemed fit enough to be placed on a waiting-list and were not transplanted. However, it should not be hastily concluded that Dialysis is Hell and Transplantation is Paradise for diabetic patients, any more than for any ESRD patients. Post-renal TX, coronary events, heart failure, strokes, infectious complications, amputations, lack of reversibility, or even worsening of visual and neurological damages, interfere to a large extent with the return to a truly enjoyable quality of life status. However, in successful SPK TX patients who achieve long-term euglycemia and normalization of other metabolic profiles, recurrence of diabetic lesions in the transplanted kidney is less pronounced and retarded compared to KA recipients, and signs and symptoms of diabetic neuropathy may improve (80).

Situation of kidney and combined pancreas–kidney transplantation in the strategy of treatment of diabetic ESRD patients

Based on the considerable experience gained in this domain over the past 25 years, recently published guidelines summarize the current state of the art on this issue at the turn of the century (81).

1. Kidney TX should be considered as the first therapeutic choice for all suitable diabetic ESRD patients.
2. Patients should be considered for an early (if possible pre-emptive) kidney or SPK TX, when their glomerular filtration rate decreases to 20 ml/min.
3. If SPK is not considered, for whatever reason, the availibility of an LRD should be thoroughly investigated, given the superior results of LRD grafts compared to CAD.

The final decision for TX will depend on the results of an intensive evaluation of comorbid conditions, in particular cardiovascular risk factors. Coronary artery disease, pelvic and peripheral vascular disease have to be thoroughly investigated; with pharmacologic stress echocardiography completed, in most cases, by coronary arteriography. Coronary bypass or angioplasty, with or without stenting, should be performed, as appropriate, before placing the patient on a waiting-list—the same attitude being advised for correcting significant carotid artery stenoses. Evaluation of gastric and bladder emptying are also mandatory.

SPK TX should thus, at the present time, be offered preferably (but not exclusively) as first therapeutic option to type 1 diabetics aged less than 45 years. The indications for older, type 2 diabetics remain much more limited but should not be excluded on principle. Early SPK TX, e.g. for a residual creatinine clearance of 20–25 ml/min requires a delicate medical balancing-exercise in evaluating the beneficial effects of metabolic normalization on the stabilization, or even improvement, of end-organ damages due to the diabetic state, together with the retardation of the development of diabetic lesions in the transplanted kidney, versus the risks of heavy immunosuppression imposed on patients who are not in immediate life-threatening conditions.

The challenge for the future will consist actually in the ability to reduce considerably the needs for renal replacement therapies for diabetic patients, thanks to an improved overall medical patient care instituted from the very onset of diabetes and pursued thereafter during the entire course of life. Another exciting perspective is provided by the promising results recently reported in a small series of patients who benefited from pancreatic islet-cell transplantation, performed via a percutaneous transhepatic portal embolization and whose function was maintained with a glucocorticoid-free immunosuppressive protocol (82). If confirmed on a larger scale, a new way of treatment will thus be opened up—at least for the most endangered fraction of diabetic patients, for whom it is essential to prevent or retard the evolution of renal diabetic lesions to end-stage organ failure. Such a dream should not be considered as utopian, but actively encouraged!

References

1. Ghavamian, M., Gutch, Ch.F., Kopp, K.F., and Kolff, J.W. (1972). The sad truth about hemodialysis in diabetic nephropathy. *Journal of the American Medical Association*, **222**, 1386–9.
2. Ritz, E., Rychlik, I., Locatelli, F., and Halimi, S. (1999). End-stage renal failure in type 2 diabetes: a medical catastrophe of worldwide dimensions. *American Journal of Kidney Diseases*, **34**, 795–808.
3. *US Renal Data System: USRDS Annual Data Reports* (1989–2000). National Institute of Health, National Institute of Diabetes and Digestive and Kidney Diseases, Bethesda MD.
4. Rychlik, I., Miltenberger-Miltenyi, G., and Ritz, E. (1998). The drama of the continuous increase in end-stage renal failure in patients with type 2 diabetes mellitus. *Nephrology, Dialysis, Transplantation*, **13**, (Suppl. 8), 6–10.
5. Service, F.J., Dick, P.J., Rizza, P.A., O. Brien, P.C., Zimmermann, B.R., and Melton III, R.J. (1997). The classification of diabetes by clinical and C-peptide criteria. A prospective population-based study. *Diabetes Care*, **20**, 198–201.
6. Ismail, N., Becker, B., Strzelczyk, P., and Ritz, E. (1999). Renal disease and hypertension in non–insulin-dependent diabetes mellitus. *Kidney International*, **55**, 1–28.
7. Hasslacher, C., Ritz, E., Wahl, P., and Michael, C. (1989). Similar risk of nephropathy in patients with type I or type II diabetes mellitus. *Nephrology, Dialysis, Transplantation*, **4**, 859–63.
8. Nelson, R.G., Knowler, W.C., McCance, D.R., Sievers, M.L., Petit, D.J., Charles, M.A. *et al.* (1993). Determinants of end-stage renal disease in Pima Indians with type 2 (non-insulin-dependent) diabetes mellitus and proteinuria. *Diabetologia*, **36**, 1087–93.
9. Chantrel, F., Enache, I., Bouiller, M., Kolb, I., Kunz, K., Petitjean, Ph. *et al.* (1999). Abysmal prognosis of patients with type 2 diabetes entering dialysis. *Nephrology, Dialysis, Transplantation*, **14**, 129–36.
10. Foley, R.N. and Parfrey, P.S. (1998). Cardiac disease in the diabetic dialysis patient. *Nephrology, Dialysis, Transplantation*, **13**, 112–3.
11. Pasadakis, P.S. and Oreopoulos, D.G. (1998). Continuous ambulatory peritoneal dialysis in 224 diabetics with end-stage renal disease: evidence of improved survival over the past 10 years. In *Diabetic Renal-Retinal Syndrome* (ed. E.A. Friedman and F.A. L'Espérance Jr.), pp.89–115. Kluwer Ac. Publishers, Dordrecht.
12. Konner, K. (2000). Primary vascular access in diabetic patients: an audit. *Nephrology, Dialysis, Transplantation*, **15**, 1317–25.
13. National Kidney Foundation K/DOQI (2000). Clinical Practice guidelines for vascular access: update. *American Journal of Kidney Diseases*, **37**, (Suppl. 1), S137–81.
14. Lin, S.C., Huang, Ch., Chen, H.S., HSU, W.A., Yen, C.J., and Yen, T.S. (1998). Effects of age and diabetes on blood flow rate and primary outcome of newly created arteriovenous fistulas. *American Journal of Nephrology*, **18**, 96–100.
15. Miles, A.M. (1999). Vascular steal syndrome and ischemic monomelic neuropathy: two variants of upper limb ischemia after hemodialysis vascular surgery. *Nephrology, Dialysis, Transplantation*, **14**, 297–300.

16. Miles, A.M. (2000). Upper limb ischemia after vascular access surgery: differential diagnosis and management. *Seminars in Dialysis*, **13**, 312–5.

17. Stein, G., Franke, S., Mahiout, A., Schneider, S., Sperschneider, H., Borst, S. *et al.* (2001). Influence of dialysis modalities on serum AGE levels in end-stage renal disease patients. *Nephrology, Dialysis, Transplantation*, **16**, 999–1008.

18. Lang, S.M., Bergner, A., Töpfer, M., and Schiffl, H. (2001). Preservation of residual renal function in dialysis patients. Effects of dialysis technique related factors. *Peritoneal Dialysis International*, **21**, 52–7.

19. Dheenan, S. and Henrich, W.L. (2001). Preventing dialysis hypotension: a comparison of usual protective maneuvers. *Kidney International*, **59**, 1175–81.

20. Verzetti, G., Navino, C., Bolzani, R., Galli, G., and Panzetta, G. (1998). Acatate-free biofiltration versus bicarbonate hemodialysis in the treatment of patients with diabetic nephropathy: a cross-over multicentric study. *Nephrology, Dialysis, Transplantation*, **13**, 955–61.

21. Fynn, J.J., Mitchell, M.C., Caruso, F.S., and Mc Elligott, M.A. (1996). Midodrine treatment for patients with hemodialysis hypotension. *Clinical Nephrology*, **45**, 261–7.

22. Collins, A.L., Liao, A., Umen, A., Hanson, G., and Keshavia, H.P. (1991). Diabetic hemodialysis patients treated with a high Kt/V have a lower risk of death than standard Kt/V. *Journal of the American Society of Nephrology*, **2**, 318.

23. Held, Ph.J., Port, F.K., Wolfe, R.A., Stannard, D.C., Carroll, C.E., Daugidas, J.T. *et al.* (1996). The dose of hemodialysis and patient mortality. *Kidney International*, **50**, 550–6.

24. National Kidney Foundation K/DOQI (2001). Clinical practice guidelines for hemodialysis adequacy: update 2000. *American Journal of Kidney Diseases*, **37**, (Suppl. 1), S27–33.

25. Avram, M.M., Sreedhara, R., Fein, P., OO, K.K., Chattopadhyay, J., and Mittman, N., (2001). Survival on hemodialysis and peritoneal dialysis over 12 years with emphasis on nutritional parameters. *American Journal of Kidney Diseases*, **37**, (Suppl. 2), S77–80.

26. Avram, M.M. (1998). Dialysis in diabetic patients: there decades of experience, from 1964 to 1997. In *Diabetic Renal-Retinal Syndrome* (ed. E.A. Friedman and F.A. L'Esperance Jr.), pp. 67–78. Kluwer Ac. Publishers, Dordrecht.

27. Morioka, T., Emoto, M., Tabata, T., Shoti, T., Tamara, H., Kishimoto, H., Ishimura, E. *et al.* (2001). Glycemic control is a predictor of survival for diabetic patients on hemodialysis. *Diabetes Care*, **24**, 909–13.

28. Miles, A.M.V. and Friedman, E.A. (1997). Managing co-morbid disorders in the uremic diabetic patient. *Seminars in Dialysis*, **10**, 225–30.

29. Tzalamoukas, A.H. (1998). The use of glycosylated hemoglobin in dialysis patients. *Seminars in Dialysis*, **11**, 141–3.

30. Woredekal, Y. and Barth, R.H. (1997). Tiptoeing through a minefield: hemodialysis in the diabetic. *Seminars in Dialysis*, **10**, 219–24.

31. Sarnak, M.J. and Jaber, B.L. (2000). Mortality caused by sepsis in patients with end-stage disease compared with the general population. *Kidney International*, **58**, 1758–64.

32. Powe, N.R., Jaar, B., Furth, S.L., Hermann. J., and Briggs, W. (1999). Septicemia in dialysis patients, incidence, risk factors and prognosis. *Kidney International*, **55**, 1081–90.

33. Jaar, B.G., Herman, J.A., Furth, S.L., Briggs, W., and Powe, N.R. (2000). Septicemia in diabetic hemodialysis patients: comparison of incidence, risk factors and mortality with non-diabetic hemodialysis patients. *American Journal of Kidney Diseases*, **35**, 282–92.

34. Kimmel, P.L. (2000). Psychosocial factors in adult end-stage renal disease patients treated with hemodialysis: correlates and outcome. *American Journal of Kidney Diseases*, **35**, 4, (Suppl. 1), S132–40.

35. Park, M.S., Lee, H.A., Chu, W.S., Yang, D.H., and Hwang, S.D. (2000). Peritoneal accumulation of AGE and peritoneal membrane permeability. *Peritoneal Dialysis International*, **20**, 452–60.

36. Lameire, N., Van Biesen, W., and Vanholder, R. (1998). Consequences of using glucose in peritoneal dialysis fluid. *Seminars in Dialysis*, **11**, 271–5.

37. Cenderoglo, M., Sundaram, S., Jaber, B.L., and Pereira, B.J.G. (1998). Effect of glucose concentration, osmolality and sterilization process of peritoneal dialysis fluids on cytokine production by peripheral blood mononuclear cells and polymorphonuclear cell functions *in vitro*. *American Journal of Kidney Diseases*, **31**, 273–82.

38. Feriani, M., Dell'Aquila, R., and La Greca, G. (1998). The treatment of diabetic end-stage renal disease with peritoneal dialysis. *Nephrology, Dialysis, Transplantation*, **13**, (Suppl. 8), 53–6.

39. Struijk, D.G. and Douma, C.E. (1998). Future research in peritoneal dialysis fluids. *Seminars in Dialysis*, **11**, 207–12.

40. Posthuma, N., Ter Wee, P.M., Donker, A.J.M., Doe, P.L., Peers, E., and Verbrugh, H.A. (2000). Assessment of the effectiveness, safety and biocompatibility of Icodextrin in automated peritoneal dialysis. *Peritoneal Dialysis International*, **20**, (Suppl. 2), S106–13.

41. Khanna, R. (1993). Dialysis considerations for diabetic patients. *Kidney International*, **43**, (Suppl. 40), S58–64.

42. Nevalainen, P.I., Lahtela, J.T., Mustonen, J., and Pasternak, A. (1996). Subcutaneous and intraperitoneal insulin therapy in diabetic patients on CAPD. *Peritoneal Dialysis International*, **16**, (Suppl. 1), S288–91.

43. Viglino, G., Cancarini, G.C., Catizone, L., Cocchi, R., De Vecchi, A., Salomone, M. *et al.* (1994). Ten years experience of CAPD in diabetics. Comparison of results with non-diabetics. Italian cooperative peritoneal dialysis study group. *Nephrology, Dialysis, Transplantation*, **9**, 1443–8.

44. Agrawal, A., Saran, R., and Khanna, R. (1999). Management of orthostatic hypertension from autonomic dysfunction in diabetics on peritoneal dialysis. *Peritoneal Dialysis International*, **19**, 415–7.

45. Canada-USA (Canusa) Peritoneal Dialysis Study Group (1996). Adequacy of dialysis and nutrition in continuous peritoneal dialysis: Association with clinical outcomes. *Journal of the American Society of Nephrology*, **7**, 198–207.

46. National Kidney Foundation. KIDOQI (2001). Clinical practice guidelines for peritoneal dialysis adequacy. Peritoneal dialysis dose: update 2000. *American Journal of Kidney Diseases*, **37**, S84–91.

47. Singhal, M.K., Bhaskaran, S., Vidgen, E., Bargman, J.M., Vas, St.I., and Oreopoulos, D.G. (2000). Rate of decline of residual renal function in patients on continuous peritoneal dialysis and factors affecting it. *Peritoneal Dialysis International*, **20**, 429–38.

48. Medcalf, J.F., Harris, K.P.G., and Walls, J. (2001). Role of diuretics in the preservation of residual renal function in patients on continuous ambulatory peritoneal dialysis. *Kidney International*, **59**, 1128–33.

49. Hufnagel, G., Michel, C., Queffelou, G., Skhiri, H., Damieri, H., and Mignon, F. (1999). The influence of automated peritoneal dialysis on the decrease of residual renal function. *Nephrology, Dialysis, Transplantation*, **14**, 1224–8.

50. De Fijter, C.W., Ter Wee, P.M., and Donker, A.J. (2000). The influence of automated peritoneal dialysis on the decrease in residual renal function. *Nephrology, Dialysis, Transplantation*, **15**, 1094–6.

51. Gallar, P., Ortega, O., Carreno, A., and Vigil, A. (2000). Rate of decline in residual renal function is equal in CAPD and automated peritoneal dialysis patients. *Peritoneal Dialysis International*, **20**, 803–5.

52. Allouache, M., Mallet, A., Bissery, A., Deray, G., and Jacobs, C. (2000). Comparative study between diabetic and non-diabetic patients treated with CAPD/APD: 20 years' experience. *Peritoneal Dialysis International*, **20**, (Abstract), 103.

53. Huang, J.W., Hung, K.Y., Yen, C.J., Wu, K.D., and Tsai, T.J. (2001). Comparison of infectious complications in peritoneal dialysis patients using either a twin-bag system or automated peritoneal dialysis. *Nephrology, Dialysis, Transplantation*, **16**, 604–7.

54. Marcelli, D., Spotti, D., Conte, F., Tagliaferro, A., Limido, A., Lonati, F. *et al.* (1996). Survival of diabetic patients on peritoneal dialysis and hemodialysis. *Peritoneal Dialysis International*, **16**, (Suppl. 1), S283–7.

55. Collins, A.J., Hao, W., Yia, H., Ebben, J.P., Everson, S.E. Constantini, E.G. *et al.* (1999). Mortality risks of peritoneal dialysis and hemodialysis. *American Journal of Kidney Diseases*, **34**, 1065–74.

56. Charra, B., Vovan, C., Marcelli, D., Ruffet, M., Jean, G., Hurot, J.M. *et al.* (2001). Diabetes mellitus in Tassin, France: remarkable transformation in incidence and outcome of ESRD in diabetes. *Advances in Renal Replacement Therapy*, **8**, 42–56.

57. Vonesh, E.F. and Moran, J. (1999). Mortality in end-stage renal disease: a reassessment of differences between patients treated with hemodialysis and peritoneal dialysis. *Journal of the American Society of Nephrology*, **10**, 354–65.

58. Marcelli, D., Spotti, D., Conte, F., Limido, A., Lonati, F., Malberti, F. *et al.* (1995). Prognosis of diabetic patients on dialysis: analysis of the Lombardy Registry Data. *Nephrology, Dialysis, Transplantation*, **10**, 1895–900.

59. Lee, H.B., Song, K.I., Kim, J.H., Cha, M.K., and Park, M.S. (1996). Dialysis in patients with diabetic nephropathy: CAPD versus hemodialysis. *Peritoneal Dialysis International*, **16**, (Suppl. 1), S69–74.

60. Churchill, D.N., Thorpe, K.E., and Teehan, B.P. (CANUSA Peritoneal Dialysis Study group) (1997). Treatment of diabetics with end-stage renal disease: lessons from the Canada–USA (CANUSA) study of peritoneal dialysis. *Seminars in Dialysis*, **10**, 215–8.

61. Ojo, A.O., Meier-Kriesche, J.A., Arndorfer, J.A., Leichtman, A.B., Magee, J.C., Cibrik, D.M. *et al.* (2001). Long-term benefit of kidney-pancreas transplants in type 1 diabetics. *Transplantation Proceedings*, **33**, 1670–72.

62. Najarian, J.S., Kaufman, D.B., Fryd, D.S., McHugh, L., Mauer, S.M., Ramsay, R.C. *et al.* (1989). Long-term survival following kidney transplantation in 100 type 1 diabetic patients. *Transplantation*, **47**, 106–13.

63. Basadonna, G., Matas, A.J., and Najarian, J.S. (1992). Kidney transplantation in diabetic patients: the University of Minnesota experience. *Kidney International*, **42**, (Suppl. 38), S193–6.

64. Najarian, J.S., Canafax, D.M., and Sutherland, D.E. (1988). Renal transplantation is confirmed therapy while pancreas transplantation should be performed only in an investigational setting. *Journal of Diabetic Complications*, **2**, 158–61.

65. Sollinger, H.W., Odorico, J.S., Knechtle, S.J., D'Alessandro, A.M., Kalayoglu, M., and Pirsch, J.D. (1998). Experience with 500 simultaneous pancreas kidney transplants. *Annals of Surgery*, **228**, 284–96.

66. Sutherland, D.E., Gruessner, R.W., Dunn, D.L., Matas, A.J., Humar, A., Kandaswamy, R. *et al.* (2001). Lessons learned from more than 1000 pancreas transplants at a single institution. *Annals of Surgery*, **233**, 463–501.

67. Gruessner, A.C. and Sutherland, D.E. (2001). Report for the International Pancreas Transplant Registry-2000. *Transplantation Proceedings*, **33**, 1643–6.
68. Merion, R.M., Henry, M.L., Melzer, J.S., Sollinger, H.W., Sutherland, D.E., and Taylor, R.J. (2000). Randomized, prospective trial of mycophenolate mofetil versus azathioprine for prevention of acute renal allograft rejection after simultaneous kidney-pancreas transplantation. *Transplantation*, **70**, 105–11.
69. Lee, L.M., Scandling, J.D., Krieger, N.R., Dafoe, D.C., and Alfrey, E.J. (1997). Outcome in diabetic patients after simultaneous pancreas-kidney versus kidney alone transplantation. *Transplantation*, **64**, 1268–94.
70. Tyden, G., Bolinder, J., Solders, G., Brattstrom, C., Tibell, A., and Groth, C.G. (1999). Improved survival in patients with insulin-dependent diabetes mellitus and end-stage diabetic nephropathy 10 years after combined pancreas and kidney transplantation. *Transplantation*, **67**, 645–8.
71. La Rocca, E., Fiorina, P., Astori, E., Rossetti, C., Lucignani, G., Fazio, F. *et al.* (2000). Patient survival and cardiovascular events after kidney-pancreas transplantation: comparison with kidney transplantation alone in uremic IDDM patients. *Cell Transplantation*, **9**, 929–32.
72. Rayhill, S.C., D'Alessandro, A.M., Odorico, J.S., Knechtle, S.J., Pirsch, J.D., Heisey, D.M. *et al.* (2000). Simultaneous pancreas-kidney transplantation and living donor renal transplantation in patients with diabetes: is there a difference in survival? *Annals of Surgery*, **231**, 417–23.
73. Becker, B.N., Brazy, P.C., Becker, Y.T., Odorico, J.S., Pintar, Th.J., Collins, B.H. *et al.* (2000). Simultaneous pacreas-kidney transplantation reduces excess mortality in type 1 diabetic patients with end-stage renal disease. *Kidney International*, **57**, 2129–35.
74. Ojo, A.O., Meier-Kriesche, H.U., Hanson, J.A., Leichtman, A., Magee, J.C., Cibrik, D. *et al.* (2001). The impact of simultaneous pancreas-kidney transplantation on long term patient survival. *Transplantation*, **71**, 82–90.
75. Wolfe, R.A., Ashby, V.B., Milford, E.L., Ojo, A.O., Ettenger, R.E., Agodoa, L.Y. *et al.* (1999). Comparison of mortality in all patients on dialysis, patients awaiting transplantation, and recipients of a first cadaveric transplant. *New England Journal of Medicine*, **341**, 1725–30.
76. Hariharan, S., Smith, R.D., Viero, R., and First, M.R. (1996). Diabetic nephropathy after renal transplantation. Clinical and pathological features. *Transplantation*, **62**, 632–5.
77. Nyberg, G., Hartso, M., Mjornstedt, L., and Norden, G. (1996). Type 2 diabetic patients with nephropathy in a Scandinavian-kidney transplant population. *Scandinavian Journal of Urology and Nephropathy*, **30**, 317–22.
78. Kronson, J.W., Gillingham, K.J., Sutherland, D.E., and Matas, A.J. (2000). Renal transplantation for type II diabetic patients compared with type I diabetic patients and patients over 50 years old: a single-center experience. *Clinical Transplant*, **14**, 226–34.
79. Pirson, Y., Vandeleene, B., and Squifflet, J.P. (2000). Kidney and kidney-pancreas transplantation in diabetic recipients. *Diabetes and Metabolism,* **26**, (Suppl. 4), S86–9.
80. Navarro, X., Sutherland, D.E., and Kennedy, W.R. (1997). Long-term effects of pancreatic transplantation on diabetic neuropathy. *Annals of Neurology*, **42**, 727–36.
81. The EPBG Expert Group on Renal Transplantation (2000). European best practice guidelines for renal transplantation: diabetes mellitus—simultaneous transplantation of kidney and pancreas. *Nephrology, Dialysis, Transplantation*, **15**, (Suppl. 7), 21–2, 35–6.
82. Shapiro, A.M.J., Lakey, J.R.T., Ryan, E.A., Korbutt, G.S., Toth, E., Warnock, G.L. *et al.* (2000). Islet transplantation in seven patients with type 1 diabetes mellitus using a glucocorticoid free immunosuppressive regimen. *New England Journal of Medicine*, **343**, 230–8.

9

Treatment of patients with hereditary and congenital disorders

Yves Pirson, Pierre Cochat, and Eric Goffin

Introduction

A variety of inherited kidney disorders lead to end-stage renal failure (ESRF), at an age ranging from the newborn (such as in the nephrotic syndrome of the Finnish type) to the elderly (such as in type 2 autosomal-dominant polycystic kidney disease). In each instance, the best therapeutic option, maximizing rehabilitation and life-style, is renal transplantation. In most of these disorders, the 5-year graft survival does not differ from transplanted controls, and recurrence of the primary disease in the grafted kidney does not occur (Table 9.1). Unfortunately, it should be emphasized that in most of them the kidney is only one of the affected organs, so that extra-renal involvement continues to progress after renal transplantation. In some diseases, such as the Alport syndrome, this involvement remains clinically silent. In others, such as cystinosis, it jeopardizes patient outcome. The aim of future strategies should be to cure the disease together with renal transplantation—preferably before irreversible renal failure. A first successful example of such strategies is the treatment of primary hyperoxaluria by a combined liver–kidney transplantation. Hemo- or peritoneal dialysis will then be reserved for patients awaiting renal transplantation or in whom this treatment is contra-indicated or has failed.

Congenital malformations of the urinary tract also lead to renal replacement therapy. Among them the most challenging for renal transplantation remains the neurogenic bladder, given the need to provide an adequate capacity reservoir that is both continent and able to empty freely and completely.

Inherited kidney disorders

Cystic diseases

Autosomal-dominant polycystic kidney disease

With a prevalence ranging from 1 in 400 to 1 in 1000, autosomal-dominant polycystic kidney disease (ADPKD) is the most frequent inherited kidney disease. The PKD1 gene, located on chromosome 16, is responsible for 85% of the cases and the PKD2

Table 9.1 Outcome of renal transplantation in patients with the most frequent hereditary nephropathies

Disease	5-year graft survival vs. controls	Recurrence of the disease in the graft	Impact of extra-renal involvement	Special considerations
ADPKD	Equal	No	±	
ARPDK	?	No	+(liver)	
Alport	Equal	No	±	Graft anti-GBM disease in 3%
Tuberous sclerosis	Equal	No	±	Binephrectomy warranted
Von Hippel–Lindau	Equal	No	±	Binephrectomy warranted
Cystinosis	Equal	No	++(growth, eye, CNS)	Cysteamine treatment
PH type 1	?	No	±	Early transplantation better
Fabry	Equal	No	+(c-v)	
Sickle cell	Lower	Yes	+(sickling)	

ADPKD: autosomal-dominant polycystic kidney disease.
ARPKD: autosomal-recessive polycystic kidney disease.
PH1: Primary hyperoxaluria type 1; only combined liver-kidney transplantation is considered.
CNS: central nervous system; c-v : cardio-vascular.

gene, located on chromosome 4, for most of the remaining cases. The disease is characterized by the development of multiple renal cysts that are variably associated with extra-renal (mainly hepatic and cardiovascular) abnormalities (1). Renal involvement leads to end-stage renal failure (ESRF) in 40–75% of patients by age 70 (1). We, and others, have examined the outcome of ADPKD patients during renal replacement therapy (RRT), paying special attention to the course of renal and extra-renal complications, in order to select the optimal strategy (1–3).

Survival

Although large prospective studies comparing the results of dialysis and renal transplantation (RT) in ADPKD patients are lacking, it appears from available reports that similar survival is obtained with both modalities (1). ADPKD itself has no negative impact on overall survival in RRT: as compared to age-matched patients with other primary renal diseases, 5-year survival of ADPKD patients is equivalent, or slightly better, on hemodialysis (HD) (2, 4) and equivalent after RT (2).

Renal complications

Kidney size tends to increase with time on long-term HD—probably due to superimposed development of acquired cystic disease—whereas it gradually decreases after successful RT (5). Every renal manifestation of ADPKD may be encountered during RRT. After starting HD, the 5-year actuarial risk for acute pain, gross hematuria, and infection is 57%, 51%, and 12%, respectively (4). Both gross hematuria and infection occur more frequently among patients with such a history before RRT, than among those without. Gross hematuria is best managed by rest. Renal infection can be controlled by appropriate antibiotics, such as fluoroquinolones, in most dialyzed patients; rarely, either recurrent bleeding or severe infection require nephrectomy (1). Excluding preparation for RT, nephrectomy is required in only 4% of ADPKD patients on HD (4). With a policy of selective removal of problematic kidneys before RT (see below), complications due to polycystic kidneys are infrequent after RT, leading to post-RT nephrectomy in only 7% of patients in our experience (2).

ADPKD does not seem to be associated with an increased risk for development of renal malignancies (6). No case of renal cancer was observed in our HD and RT patients, confirming that this complication is at most very rare, even after years of immunosuppression (2). In a review of renal cancer in ADPKD, Keith *et al.* (6) recorded only four patients who were on RRT.

Extra-renal complications

Liver cysts are rarely symptomatic. Acute pain or infection occur in less than 5% of patients on RRT (2, 4). In the occasional patient with either incapacitating or complicated massive polycystic liver or symptomatic Caroli disease, liver transplantation is increasingly considered, especially when RT is concurrently planned (7). Polycystic liver disease may occasionally be complicated by hepatic venous outflow obstruction, due to compression of the inferior vena cava and hepatic veins by hepatic cysts, and sometimes precipitated by nephrectomy (8). This complication requires appropriate management, including surgical decompression (8).

There is a slightly increased risk of stroke among ADPKD patients on RRT, possibly accounted for, at least partially, by ADPKD-associated intra-cranial aneurysm (2). Major valvular heart disease occurs in less than 1% of patients on RRT and the prevalence of coronary events is not increased (2). Rare patients with polycythemia should be treated with ACE-inhibitors.

The incidence of colonic perforation is not increased on HD, while it has been found either increased—occurring in up to 5% of patients—(9) or not (2) after RT. The previously reported association between ADPKD and diverticular disease remains questionable (1).

Selection of RRT modality

As RT provides a better quality of life, it should be considered in any ADPKD patients with a life-expectancy of more than 5 years in the absence of contra-indication to surgery or immunosuppression.

Pre-transplant work-up should include abdominal CT, echocardiography, myocardial stress scintigraphy and, in patients with signs or symptoms of arteriosclerosis, aorto-iliac angiography. Screening for intra-cranial aneurysm is restricted to 18–45-year-old patients with a family history of ADPKD-associated intra-cranial aneurysm; based on current decision analyses (taking into account aneurysm prevalence, annual risk of rupture, life-expectancy, and risk of prophylactic treatment), this attitude might have to be revised with further information on the natural history of intra-cranial aneurysm and the results of endovascular treatment (1). We do not screen our transplant candidates for diverticular disease, since post-RT colonic perforation is not predicted by the presence of pre-transplant diverticula (1); pre-RT elective colon resection should only be considered in patients with symptomatic, severe diverticular disease.

Since the vast majority of kidneys from ADPKD patients left *in situ* do not lead to major complications after RT, pre-transplant nephrectomy, once routinely per-formed, is now restricted to patients with a history of cyst infection, recurrent major bleeding or complicated lithiasis (1).

Living-related donor RT may be considered, provided the existence of ADPKD has been formally excluded on clinical or genetic (to be advised in donors less than 30 years old) grounds (1).

Patients either awaiting RT or not eligible for RT may opt for HD or peritoneal dialysis (PD). Short-term survival and complication rates on PD were found to be similar in ADPKD and age-matched controls (10). PD is, however, less desirable for patients with very large kidneys, since the larger the kidney volume the lesser the available effective peritoneal surface area. Furthermore, tolerance of PD may be affected by excessive abdominal distension. HD should also be preferred in patients with colonic diverticular disease or abdominal hernia.

Autosomal-recessive polycystic kidney disease

With a prevalence of 1 in 40 000, autosomal-recessive polycystic kidney disease (ARPKD) is a rare disease, whose gene maps to chromosome 6. The condition is char-acterized by the development of renal cysts originating from collecting tubules and ducts that are invariably associated with hepatic abnormalities consisting of biliary dysgenesis and periportal fibrosis (11).

Renal involvement leads to ESRF by the age of 15 in 33% of patients surviving the first month of life (12). PD, the preferred option in infants, may be successful even in the face of large kidneys (11). RT is the treatment of choice.

Long-term outcome of ARPKD patients on RRT is dominated by the progression of hepatic complications. Of a total of 15 patients surviving 3–21 (mean: 8) years after starting RRT at a mean age of 17 (2–43) years, 40% had bleeding from esophageal varices, requiring portocaval anastomosis in most of them, and 13% had recurrent cholangitis complicating Caroli disease (12, 13; personal experience). In patients with severe portal hypertension and/or Caroli disease at the time RT is contemplated, combined liver–kidney transplantation should be considered. In patients with mild, asymptomatic liver involvement, close monitoring for complications of portal hyper-tension is warranted: treatment of bleeding esophageal varices includes sclerotherapy, portocaval shunting, and ultimately liver transplantation (11–13).

After isolated RT, hypersplenism-induced leukopenia may require tapering or withdrawal of azathioprine/mycophenolate treatment. Fever and increase in liver enzymes should raise the suspicion of cholangitis.

In summary, patients with ARPKD and ESRF should be offered RT as the first choice therapy. With prolongation of survival, hepatic complications increasingly dominate the clinical picture, requiring, in a few cases, combined or metachronous liver transplantation.

Other cystic kidney diseases

Other rare inherited cystic kidney diseases include (autosomal-recessive) nephronophthisis, (autosomal-dominant) medullary cystic kidney disease, glomerulocystic kidney disease, and orofaciodigital syndrome. They do not raise special problems, as regards RRT, except for the occasional patient with nephronophthisis associated with liver fibrosis, in whom a combined liver–kidney transplantation may be considered.

Glomerular diseases

Alport syndrome

Alport syndrome (AS) is characterized by a progressive glomerulonephritis erratically associated with various extra-renal features, mainly deafness and ocular defects (14). Estimated prevalence is $1:5000$ to $10\,000$. A disease of type IV collagen (the major component of glomerular basement membranes, GBM), AS includes two main genetic varieties: one X-linked (XL) and the other one autosomal-recessive (AR). The probability of developing ESRF by the age of 40 is 90% in both hemizygotes and AR homozygotes, and 12% in XL heterozygotes (14). Though the outcome of AS patients following RT is generally excellent (15), two specific issues have to be addressed: the risk of anti-GBM disease in the graft and the donation of a kidney from a related heterozygote.

Occurring in about 3% of AS patients, crescentic anti-GBM nephritis appears within the first months following RT and most often leads to graft destruction. It is presumably caused by exposure to type IV collagen antigens from the donor, for which the recipient has not established immune tolerance (16). The clinical and genetic profiles of patients developing this complication have been reviewed (14, 16). Roughly, 90% are hemizygotes with severe XL disease, including deafness, and 10% are AR homozygotes. Nearly all patients have a mutation resulting in a truncated type IV collagen chain. Still, the majority of patients with such a mutation do not develop anti-GBM nephritis, indicating that factors other than the type of mutation might determine the immune response. In practice, there is currently no reason to deny any AS patient a first RT. By contrast, attempting a second transplant after the loss of the first one from anti-GBM nephritis should be discouraged, since recurrence is almost constant (16).

Allowing a related heterozygote to serve as kidney donor should rely on the clinical expression of the disease in this individual. Those without any clinical sign of AS, including microscopic hematuria (5% of XL and 50% of AR heterozygotes), should be accepted as a donor since they will never develop renal failure. Since those with isolated microscopic hematuria have a very low risk of developing late renal failure, they should only be accepted if strongly motivated and well-informed about this risk. Those with any additional clinical manifestation of AS should be rejected (14, 16).

In summary, any AS patient with ESRF should be offered RT. The few patients losing the graft from anti–GBM nephritis should be discouraged from attempting further RT. Related AS carriers wishing to donate a kidney must be carefully evaluated and advised.

Hereditary nephrotic syndromes

Nephrotic syndrome (NS) is said to be congenital when present at birth, and infantile when it appears within the first year of life. Different varieties of hereditary NS may be distinguished according to clinical, histological, and, very recently, genetic criteria. The molecular basis of three of them has been identified, involving proteins that are critical to the function of the podocyte.

Congenital nephrotic syndrome of the Finnish type (CNF)   CNF is the most common form of congenital NS, with an incidence of 1:10000 live births in Finland (founder effect), and a much lower incidence in other countries. CNF is an autosomal-recessive disease whose gene NPHS1 maps to chromosome 19q13.1 and encodes a transmembrane protein, called nephrin, localized to the slit diaphragm of podocytes (17). Prenatal diagnosis is therefore available from DNA analysis. CNF is responsible for massive proteinuria in utero and NS from birth. Antenatal proteinuria results in both placental enlargement and low birth weight (placenta >25% of birth weight) (18). Glomeruli show only mild mesangial hypercellularity.

CNF does not respond to steroids or immunosuppressive agents. Conservative measures include intravenous albumin substitution (20% solution, 3–4 g/kg/day) with frusemide (0.5 mg/kg/day), enteral/parenteral nutritional support (energy 130 kcal/kg, protein 4 g/kg), prevention of thromboses (e.g. warfarin), and aggressive treatment of infections (18). Interventions have been proposed to reduce proteinuria (e.g. enalapril 0.5–1.0 mg/kg/day, indomethacin 1–3 mg/kg/day, unilateral nephrectomy) with a variable success. Dietary control of hypertriglyceridemia and supportive therapy with thyroxine are usually necessary, as well as vitamins, magnesium, and calcium supplementation.

Despite these measures, growth and development may be retarded and the complication rates remain high, to such an extent that bilateral nephrectomy with subsequent dialysis (usually PD) is the currently preferred strategy, as soon as body weight has reached 8–9 kg. RT should be postponed until the NS-associated disorders have been corrected and the nutritional state improved. After RT, 5-year patient- and graft-survival rates reach 98 and 82%, respectively (18). In most children, growth and development further improve, together with quality of life. The reappearance of the nephrotic syndrome in some transplanted patients could be due to the development of anti-nephrin antibodies, just as in AS.

Steroid-resistant nephrotic syndrome   Another kind of familial idiopathic NS is characterized by an autosomal-recessive mode of inheritance, onset between 3 months and 5 years of life, resistance to steroid therapy, rapid progression to ESRD, absence of extra-renal involvement and no recurrence after RT (19). Minimal glomerular changes are observed on early biopsy samples and focal segmental glomerulosclerosis (FSGS) is present at later stages (19). The causative gene, NPHS2, mapped to chromosome 1q25–31, has been identified as an integral membrane protein, only expressed in podocytes, and hence called podocin (20).

Autosomal-dominant FSGS   An autosomal-dominant form of FSGS, characterized by long-standing proteinuria, resistance to steroid therapy, and slow progression to NS in adulthood, is caused by at least three different genes (21). One of them has been mapped to chromosome 19 and identified as ACTN4, a gene encoding α-actinin-4, an actin-binding protein strongly expressed in the foot processes of podocytes (22).

It is likely that mutations in one of these genes will be found in apparently sporadic cases of steroid-resistant NS, both in children and adults. By contrast to the common, sporadic (acquired?) form of FSGS, due to a circulating factor, the above-mentioned hereditary forms do not recur in the graft, at least within 5 years after RT (18, 19, 23). Their recognition should thus encourage opting for RT.

Diffuse mesangial sclerosis (DMS)   DMS is a rare cause of infantile NS, characterized by a fibrillar increase in mesangial matrix without mesangial cell proliferation. It appears either as a primary or a syndromic (see below) condition of probable autosomal-recessive inheritance (24). Proteinuria is usually less severe than in CNF and appears after the neonatal period. Steroids and immunosuppressive drugs are ineffective and the disease progresses towards ESRF within a few months or years. Conservative treatment is that of CNF according to the severity of the NS, aiming to keep serum albumin concentration above 15 g/l. Similarly, bilateral nephrectomy followed by PD and subsequent RT is the optimal strategy. The NS does not recur after RT.

NS and malformation syndromes   1. The Denys–Drash syndrome includes DMS with early-onset NS and progressive kidney failure, male pseudohermaphroditism (XY), and nephroblastoma due to a mutation in the WT1 gene (24). Since incomplete Denys–Drash syndrome may occur, prophylactic bilateral nephrectomy at the time of RRT is mandatory in both isolated and syndromic DMS, because of the risk of nephroblastoma. No recurrence of the NS after RT has been reported.

2. Frasier syndrome includes late-onset NS, due to FSGS, and leads to ESRF, male pseudohermaphroditism (XY), and predisposition to gonadoblastoma. This condition should be suspected in phenotypic females with a history of steroid-resistant NS and primary amenorrhea. Pre-transplant gonadectomy is required (25).

3. FSGS may also be part of other rare malformation syndromes, such as the Bardet–Biedl syndrome, Charcot–Marie–Tooth disease, and mitochondrial cytopathy.

4. Schimke immuno-osseous dysplasia includes spondyloepiphyseal dysplasia, late-onset steroid-resistant NS with further ESRF, growth failure, CD4-lymphopenia, and transient cerebral ischemic attacks (26). The post-transplant outcome depends both on neurological and infectious complications.

Familial hemolytic–uremic syndrome

The hemolytic–uremic syndrome is occasionally inherited in an autosomal-recessive or, more rarely, an autosomal-dominant mode. Mutation in the complement factor H gene has been demonstrated in several families (27). This familial variety recurs in kidney graft in more than 50% of the cases, which is a higher rate than that reported for the sporadic one (27, 28). No predictive marker for recurrence has been identified so far.

Multi-systemic disorders

Tuberous sclerosis

Tuberous sclerosis complex (TSC) is an autosomal-dominant multi-system disorder with a minimal prevalence of 1 in 10 000. It is due to mutation in either the TSC1 gene, located on chromosome 9, or the TSC2 gene, located on chromosome 16 near the PKD1 locus. TSC is characterized by the development of multiple hamartomas in various organs. The most common manifestations are dermatologic (facial angiofibroma, periungueal fibroma) and neurologic (cortical tuber, subependymal tumor). Renal involvement is found in 60% of cases and includes angiomyolipoma, cysts, and, more rarely, renal cell carcinoma and focal segmental glomerulosclerosis (29). ESRF occurs in about 1% of TSC patients at a mean age of 29 years (30); it results from different mechanisms including nephrectomy to treat hemorrhagic angiomyolipomas, replacement of normal parenchyma by cysts, and glomerulosclerosis.

RT has been reported in 34 cases. Results do not differ from those observed in age-matched controls (30, 31). Among five patients with a renal cell carcinoma removed prior to RT, tumor recurred after RT in one (30, 31; personal observation). There is no evidence so far that immunosuppressive therapy has any influence on neurologic involvement (30, 31; personal observation). The risk of hemorrhage and malignancy in native kidneys warrants bilateral nephrectomy at entry of an RRT program.

In summary, TSC patients are excellent candidates for RT. Native kidneys should be removed before (or at the time of) RT.

Von Hippel–Lindau disease

Von Hippel–Lindau disease (VHL) is an autosomal-dominant multi-system disorder with a prevalence rate of 1 in 40 000. The defective gene is located on chromosome 3. VHL is characterized by the development of various tumors involving the cerebellum and spinal cord (hemangioblastoma), retina (angioma), adrenal gland (pheochromocytoma), pancreas (cysts), and kidney (cysts and renal cell carcinoma) (32). Renal cell carcinoma (RCC) develops in about 25% of patients at a mean age of 30 years and is frequently bilateral and multi-centric (32, 33). Despite nephron-sparing surgery, up to 23% of patients treated for RCC will reach ESRF (34) and be candidates to RT.

After RT, the main concern is the risk of tumor recurrence from occult metastasis present at the time of RT. Reassuringly, in a multi-centre review of 32 anephric VHL patients who underwent RT, 5-year patient and graft survival was not statistically different from that of a control RT population. Nevertheless, three VHL patients died from metastatic RCC between 17 and 45 months after RT, raising the issue of a need for surveillance interval dialysis (35). Though there was no difference in the duration of dialysis between these three patients and those who remained tumor-free, the authors suggest reliance on the guidelines established by Penn for sporadic RCC: while no waiting period would be needed for patients with low-stage tumors, an interval of at least 2 years is advocated for those with higher tumor stages (35, 36).

There is no evidence that immunosuppressive therapy has any influence on the progression of extra-renal manifestations of VHL. Among 32 transplanted patients, three developed a cerebellar hemangioblastoma after RT, leading to death in one of them (35). Just as in non-transplanted VHL patients, periodic post-RT examination should include plasma normetanephrine measurement, abdominal and cerebral gadolinium-enhanced magnetic resonance imaging and funduscopy.

In a potential living-related donor at risk for asymptomatic VHL, the existence of the disease should be excluded by genetic testing (32).

In summary, VHL patients reaching ESRF can benefit from RT with a limited risk of recurrent RCC. A waiting time of 2 years on dialysis is recommended for patients with high-grade RCC. Periodic screening of extra-renal manifestations should be pursued after RT.

Metabolic diseases

Cystinosis

Cystinosis is a rare autosomal-recessive disorder (1 : 167 000 live births) characterized by systemic intra-lysosomal accumulation of cystine due to a defective lysosomal membrane protein—cystinosin—whose gene CTNS maps to 17p13 (37). Symptoms may appear as early as the first months of life in the infantile form (nephropathic cystinosis) consisting of failure to thrive, rickets, polyuria/polydipsia, anorexia, and tubular Fanconi syndrome; ESRF and extra-renal involvement occur later. The juvenile form is rather rare and less severe with later onset ESRF. The adult-type form is limited to ocular involvement. Diagnosis is suspected with the recognition of corneal cystine crystals on slit-lamp examination, and ascertained by the measurement of leukocyte cystine concentration. Early oral therapy with the cystine-depleting agent cysteamine delays or prevents renal deterioration, enhances growth, and improves extra-renal complications.

Renal failure   Proximal tubules loaded with cystine exhibit a generalized transport defect characteristic of the Fanconi syndrome. Therefore, in addition to cystine-depleting agents, treatment is aimed at restoring renal losses (38). ESRF occurs at 9–12 years of age in most patients and accounts for less than 1% of ESRF patients younger than 20 years of age (37, 39, 40). RT can be performed without any specific problem; heterozygotes are asymptomatic and may therefore serve as kidney donor.

Cystine crystals may be present in graft-infiltrating cells but there is no recurrence of the disease. Graft- and patient-survival rates do not differ from those of patients with other renal diseases (39).

Extra-renal involvement   Extra-renal involvement continues on RRT, requiring specialized follow-up and maintenance cysteamine therapy. Reassuringly, extra-renal complications do not appear to significantly impact mortality within 10 years of commencing RRT (39).

- Growth retardation remains a major problem: it should be prevented early by pre-transplant conservative treatment, together with aggressive nutritional support. The benefit of recombinant human growth hormone is under evaluation.
- Eye involvement begins during the first months or years of life and consists of cystine corneal deposits leading to severe photophobia, recurrent corneal erosion, and retinal involvement. Blindness occurs after 18 years of age in 15% of the patients (41). A combination of eye drop and oral cysteamine may delay such later complications in compliant patients. Keratoplasty has been performed in some patients but donor keratinocytes are gradually replaced by host keratinocytes and there is a risk of recurrent crystal deposition.
- Hypothyroidism is rather common in patients on RRT. L-thyroxin is usually required from 10–12 years of age.
- A slow, progressive loss of insulin secretion accounts for a 50% risk of developing glucose intolerance by the age of 18 years; some patients require insulin therapy.
- Splenomegaly is often found, sometimes associated with portal hypertension, so that splenectomy or portosystemic shunting might be indicated.
- Muscle and central nervous system involvement may occur by the end of the second decade and may lead to severe mental and/or motor disability.

Cysteamine treatment   Cystine-depleting agents have been shown to improve kidney survival, statural growth, and patient's quality of life. It should, therefore, be started as soon as the diagnosis has been confirmed. It may be given even after ESRF has been reached, in order to limit extra-renal involvement. Cysteamine bitartrate (Cystagon®) is currently given daily at a dose of 40mg/kg divided into four doses; the target leukocyte cystine concentration must be 1nmol half-cystine/mg of protein. Non-compliance is frequently due to the poor taste of the drug.

In summary, patients with cystinosis and ESRF should be offered RT. With prolongation of survival, extra-renal complications dominate the clinical picture, requiring maintenance-cysteamine treatment and specialized surveillance.

Primary hyperoxalurias

Primary hyperoxalurias (PH) are rare autosomal-recessive disorders, which are characterized by over-production and accumulation of oxalate (Ox) in the body. Since Ox cannot be metabolized and is excreted in the urine, the main target organ is the kidney, leading to nephrocalcinosis, recurrent urolithiasis, and subsequent renal impairment (42, 43).

Urine oxalate Hyperoxaluria (normal urinary oxalate, UOx <0.5 mmol/1.73 m^2/day; normal UOx: creatinine ratio <0.10 mmol/mmol) and calcium oxalate (CaOx) crystallization, are the hallmarks of any kind of PH. Monohydrated CaOx crystals in urine or tissues can be assessed by infrared spectrometry or polarized light microscopy. Hyperoxaluria may be associated with increased urinary excretion of either glycolate in type 1 (PH1) or L-glycerate in type 2 (PH2). Diagnosis is accurately established only by enzyme measurement or DNA analysis (43).

Primary hyperoxaluria type 1 (PH1) PH1 is a disorder of glyoxylate metabolism (1:120000 live births) caused by deficiency of the hepatic, peroxisomal, pyridoxine-dependent enzyme alanine: glyoxylate aminotransferase (AGT) whose gene maps to chromosome 2 (43, 44). The disease occurs either because AGT activity is undetectable or because it is mistargeted to mitochondria, leading to considerable phenotypic heterogeneity.

PH1 grossly fits three clinical presentations:

(1) a rare infantile form with early nephrocalcinosis and kidney failure;
(2) a rare late-onset form with occasional stone passage in late adulthood; and
(3) the most common form with recurrent urolithiasis and progressive renal failure leading to a diagnosis of PH1 in childhood or adolescence.

Half of the patients reach ESRF before 25 years of age. PH1 is responsible for less than 0.5% of ESRF in children both in Europe and North America, but for 13% in North Africa due to consanguinity. Along with advancing renal failure, patients experience progressive systemic involvement (bone, joints, retina, heart, vessels, nerves) leading to increased morbidity and mortality. This dismal outcome strongly argues for pre-emptive transplantation in patients with pyridoxine- unresponsive PH1.

An aggressive conservative treatment should be started as soon as the diagnosis has been made (37). When UOx exceeds 0.4 mmol/l, the risk of stone formation is increased, especially if UCa exceeds 4 mmol/l; therefore, supportive therapy should be adapted to keep Uox and UCa below these limits. This can be achieved by a high fluid intake and therapies lowering CaOx crystallization (pyridoxine, potassium/ sodium citrate, orthophosphate, and thiazide diuretics) (42, 43). Restriction of dietary oxalate has very limited influence. Pyridoxine sensitivity is found in 10–40% of patients and must, therefore, be tested with stepwise increase in daily dosage (5–10– 15–20 mg/kg). The effect of such conservative measures may be assessed by serial determinations of crystalluria score and CaOx supersaturation. Obstructive urolithiasis often require extra-corporeal shock-wave lithotrypsy.

In patients who have reached ESRF, a conventional dialysis regimen—either PD or standard and high-flux HD—do not provide sufficient clearance of Ox (45); this would be ideally achieved by daily, 6–8-h duration HD sessions. Clearance of oxalate is mildly higher on hemodiafiltraton than on HD (43).

RT alone provides an efficient removal of soluble Ox. However, because of continuous over-production of Ox, plasma levels remain elevated and Ox re-accumulates in the graft, largely accounting for the poor prognosis of isolated RT: in the European Renal Association data base, 3-year graft survival is only 23% for living-donor and 17% for cadaver-donor grafts.

Since the defective enzyme is only expressed to any significant extent in the liver, liver transplantation represents a biochemical cure. Isolated liver transplantation has been performed in selected patients with PH1 before the onset of chronic renal failure. In patients with PH1 and renal failure, the best option is a combined liver–kidney transplantation. The rate of normalization of plasma and urinary Ox levels after transplantation may be slow, particularly in patients who have accumulated a large burden of tissue Ox. In this setting, the benefit of pre- and post-RT HD to lower Ox levels remains debated. Forced fluid intake, associated with thiazide diuretics and crystallization inhibitors, is indicated. The outcome of combined transplantation is better if patients are transplanted before ESRF.

After a successful transplant procedure, other damaged organs, such as the skeleton or the heart, will significantly benefit from enzyme replacement (43).

Infantile PH1 underlines a worldwide problem: it is a rare disease in developed countries where combined liver-kidney TP is available, but it is more frequent in developing countries (consanguinity) where treatment possibilities are scarce. Its management, as well as that of most recessive inherited diseases with early, life-threatening onset, raises profound ethical and financial issues. Therapeutic withdrawal as a consequence of local conditions in sometimes an acceptable option (43).

Prenatal diagnosis from DNA analysis of chorionic villi or amniocytes can be proposed (44, 45). Such a procedure allows the identification of normal, affected, and carrier fetuses in most families; in the absence of valuable index case, the two most common mutations may be checked.

Non-type 1 PH   Among patients with hyperoxaluria and a typical pattern of urinary metabolites, 10–30% have a normal AGT activity. The urinary metabolic pattern is thus only indicative, and PH1 or PH2 diagnosis requires an enzyme activity measurement in a liver biopsy sample.

Primary hyperoxaluria type 2 (PH2)   Deficiency of glyoxylate reductase/hydroxypyruvate reductase (GRHPR) is believed to be the underlying defect, both in liver and lymphocytes, leading to an elevated urinary excretion of oxalate and glycerate. The gene has been located on chromosome 9. PH2 is less frequent than PH1, although its frequency may be under-estimated. Median age at onset is 15 years, and the classical presentation is urolithiasis, with a lower stone-forming activity and systemic involvement than in PH1.

ESRF occurs in 12% of patients between 20 and 50 years of age (46). RT has been performed in some patients, often leading to recurrence, including increased UOx and glycerate excretion (46). The issue of liver transplantation has, therefore, been approached, but additional enzymatic and biochemical data are mandatory before such a strategy can be recommended.

In summary, the best option for most patients with PH1 and renal failure is a combined liver–kidney transplantation. The outcome is improved when transplantation is performed early.

Fabry's disease

Fabry's disease (FD) is an X-linked disorder with an estimated prevalence of 1 in 40 000. It is characterized by glycosphingolipid accumulation in plasma and tissues as a result of a defective activity of the lysosomal enzyme, α-galactosidase A, due to mutations in the α-Gal A gene located at Xq22.1 (47).

Clinical manifestations, usually manifest in male adolescents, include recurrent painful crises in the palms and soles (acroparesthesia), precipitated by exercise, emotional stress, and changes in ambient temperature, and usually associated with a low-grade fever; angiokeratoma (often confined to the 'bathing trunk'); hypohidrosis; and corneal changes (cornea verticillata). Progressive glycosphingolipid deposition in the cardiovascular system further leads to left-ventricular hypertrophy, valvular, and conduction abnormalities, angina, ischemic or hemorrhagic cerebrovascular lesions, and autonomic neuropathy (47).

Renal involvement is constant in hemizygotes, but present in less than 10% of heterozygote females. Proteinuria may start in late childhood; defective tubular function occurs later, and patients usually reach ESRF around the fourth decade. Histological examination of the kidney shows glycosphingolipid deposits in the endothelial and epithelial cells of the glomerulus, Bowman's capsule, and distal tubule.

HD and PD indications and modalities do not differ from those accepted for other renal diseases. According to an EDTA survey conducted on 83 patients with FD starting RRT between 1975 and 1993, overall 5-year survival is lower (41%) than in patients with standard primary renal disease (68%). However, in the subgroup of 33 patients who were transplanted, survival rates equal those of patients with standard primary renal disease (3-year patient and graft survival: 72 and 84%, vs. 69 and 87%, respectively) (48). Two specific issues regarding RT in FD have been addressed: the risk of recurrence in the graft and the role of the kidney in the correction of systemic enzymatic defect. It is now clear that the engrafted kidney remains histologically free of endogenous glycosphingolipid deposition (47). Although some clinical improvement has been reported in successfully transplanted patients (48), there is no evidence for an increase in the systemic enzyme activity (47). Long-term survivors die mainly from cardiovascular complications (47, 48). Living-donor RT from an unaffected relative may be considered.

Specific post-RT management includes relief of acroparesthesia (by carbamazepine or phenytoin), and control of heart disease and blood pressure (preferably by ACE inhibitors). Heart transplantation has been performed in selected cases.

At present, the most practical and effective therapy is preventive (carrier identification from DNA analysis, genetic counseling, and prenatal diagnosis by α-galactosidase

A determination). Promising preliminary results have been obtained with recombinant human α-galactosidase A. Another approach might be the use of an enzyme inhibitor (1-deoxy-galactonojirimycine) aiming to accelerate both transport and maturation of α-galactosidase A in lymphoblasts.

In summary, FD patients reaching ESRF can benefit from RT without the risk of recurrence into the graft and despite the continuous progression of the disease in the cardiovascular tissues.

Lecithin-cholesterol acetyltransferase deficiency

Lecithin-cholesterol acetyltransferase (LCAT) deficiency is a rare autosomal-recessive disorder characterized by widespread accumulation of low-density lipoproteins in tissues, as a result of a mutation in the gene for LCAT, which is a key enzyme (synthesized by the liver) in the metabolism of cholesterol (49).

In affected patients, the plasma is lipemic and both triglyceride and cholesterol levels are raised, with most of the cholesterol present, not as cholesteryl ester but, as free cholesterol. Plasma lecithin level is increased but lysolecithin is low. Abnormalities of lipoprotein structure and composition (increased VLDL and LDL cholesterol, reduced HDL cholesterol) are commonly observed (49). Diagnosis is confirmed by the absence of LCAT activity.

Clinical manifestations include corneal opacities, hemolytic anemia (due to phospholipid abnormalities in the red cell membrane), and accelerated atherosclerosis. Renal involvement includes proteinuria, hypertension, and progressive impairment, leading to ESRF before the age of 50.

Histologic examination of the kidney shows arteriolar thickening with subendothelial lipid deposits and expanded mesangium containing foam cells (49).

RT has been performed in several patients (49, 50). Despite early re-accumulation of lipids in the graft, graft function has remained satisfactory for more than 4 years after RT (50).

In summary, LCAT deficiency is not a contra-indication for RT, provided there is no severe atheromatosis. Recurrence of the disease is to be expected. No combined liver–kidney transplantation has been reported so far.

Lipoprotein glomerulopathy

Lipoprotein glomerulopathy (LPG) is a rare autosomal-recessive disorder characterized by intraglomerular lipoprotein deposition, most likely resulting from high plasma concentration of apolipoprotein E, due to mutations in the apoE gene (51–53). The majority of the cases reported so far comes from Japan (51).

Clinical manifestations are confined to the kidney, consisting of the nephrotic syndrome leading to ESRF. Glomerular capillary loops are obstructed by lipid deposits. Why such deposits do not appear in other vascular beds remains to be elucidated (51).

Experience of RT is so far limited to four cases. In each of them, early recurrence developed, leading to graft loss in two. Whether lipid-lowering therapy and ACE inhibitors may improve graft outcome is still uncertain.

Disorders of purine metabolism

Adenine phosphoribosyltransferase (APRT) deficiency Adenine phosphoribosyltransferase (APRT) deficiency is a rare autosomal-recessive disorder characterized by the formation of 2,8-dihydroxyadenine stones. In the absence of APRT, adenine indeed accumulates in quantity and is oxidized by xanthine dehydrogenase to 8-hydroxyadenine and then 2,8 hydroxyadenine, which is extremely insoluble in the urine. Intratubular precipitation has led to ESRF in a number of patients in whom the defect was not identified early enough and the highly effective treatment with allopurinol not undertaken (54). As expected, microcrystalline nephritis may recur in the graft if allopurinol treatment is not continued after RT (54).

Familial juvenile hyperuricemic nephropathy Familial juvenile hyperuricemic nephropathy is a rare autosomal-dominant disorder characterized by precocious gout or hyperuricemia, and chronic interstitial nephritis leading to ESRF in adulthood (55). This disorder has striking similarities with autosomal-dominant medullary cystic kidney disease. As expected for a disease that is caused by an intrinsic renal defect, there is no evidence of recurrence after RT (55).

Sickle cell disease

Sickle cell disease is an autosomal-recessive disorder in which the substitution of a single amino acid in the ß globin chain results in a conformational change in the structure of the hemoglobin molecule, producing 'sickling' of red cells, particularly under deoxygenation conditions. This disorder essentially affects people with African ancestry: it occurs at the heterozygote state (sickle cell trait) in 8% and at the homozygous state (sickle cell disease) in 1:400 live births in Afro–Americans (56).

Sickle red cells are destroyed prematurely in the circulation, resulting in hemolytic features. In the kidney, they damage vasa recta, leading to a wide spectrum of functional and pathological changes, culminating, in some patients, in papillary necrosis, focal and segmental glomerulosclerosis, and ultimately ESRF.

The best mode of renal replacement therapy in sickle cell disease has been debated, mainly because affected patients exhibit several co-morbidities, including cardiovascular disease, susceptibility to infections and thrombosis, malnutrition, and persistent anemia. According to a USRDS report, the 30-month actuarial survival of patients with sickle cell disease on dialysis therapy was equivalent to that of other non-diabetic ESRF patients (57). In affected patients on dialysis it is advisable not to increase hemoglobin level above 6–9 g/dl, in order to avoid painful veno–occlusive crises (58).

The outcome of 82 patients with sickle cell disease, who received a kidney transplant, was recently compared with that of kidney-graft recipients with another cause of ESRF and with that of dialysis-treated, wait-listed patients with sickle cell disease. First-year graft survival of patients with sickle cell disease was similar to that of patients with another cause of ESRF (78% and 77%, respectively) but the 3-year graft survival tended to be lower (48% vs. 60%, respectively). Three-year patient survival was significantly lower in patients with sickle cell disease (59% vs. 81% in the control group), which was accounted for by their co-morbid conditions. Transplanted patients with sickle cell disease tended to have a better survival than their dialysis-treated counterparts (56). After RT, the sickling abnormality may be responsible for both the persistence of painful crises and the recurrence of renal involvement.

In summary, the optimal management of patients with sickle cell disease and ESRF remains a challenge. Despite a substantial morbidity and mortality, RT appears to be the best option for those patients with no contra-indications for this treatment.

Renal involvement in rare inherited diseases

Inherited inborn errors of metabolism   Inborn errors of metabolism generally have one or more deficient source organs and several target organs, including the kidney. The most common renal manifestation is the Fanconi syndrome; cysts, urolithiasis, glomerular involvement, and acute or chronic renal failure may also occur. According to the underlying pathophysiology, the ultimate therapy may include, besides RRT, other forms of replacement therapy such as liver transplantation. Gene therapy has not yet entered clinical practice.

Homozygous familial hypercholesterolemia   Homozygous familial hypercholesterolemia is caused by mutations in the LDL-receptor and is characterized by extremely elevated LDL, leading to early cardiovascular complications, including the kidney. Diet and drugs are insufficient; optimal management is currently LDL-apheresis. Only a few patients require liver transplantation.

Glycogen storage disease   Glycogen storage disease type 1 is due to the deficiency of glucose-6-phosphatase activity (type IA) or of its transporter (type IB) in the liver, kidney, and intestine. Renal involvement—including Fanconi syndrome, tubular acidosis with renal calcifications, and glomerular hyperfiltration with subsequent focal and segmental glomerulosclerosis—may lead to ESRF in the third decade; it can be delayed by dietary therapy with cornstarch and/or nasogastric glucose infusion, with the aim of maintaining normoglycemia. Liver transplantation may be considered in some patients, not only as a source of enzyme but also, to eliminate the risk of hepatocellular carcinoma and hepatic failure (59). In patients transplanted with liver alone, it is not yet known whether this treatment is able to reverse renal involvement.

Methylmalonic acidemia   Methylmalonic acidemia is an autosomal-recessive disorder of the metabolism of methylmalonyl CoA. Patients usually present in the first weeks of life with vomiting, neurological distress, failure to thrive, ketoacidosis, and hyperammonemia. Renal manifestations consist mainly of tubular dysfunction and tubulointerstitial lesions, due to both direct tubular toxicity of methylmalonate and hyperuricemia. GFR usually drops slowly, and patients may reach ESRF after puberty (60). Despite its effect on plasma methylmalonate concentration, HD offers no significant improvement in metabolic and nutritional status. Experience with isolated RT, as well as combined liver–kidney transplantation, is limited to a few cases.

Cobalamin C deficiency is characterized by a defect in the synthesis of both adeno-sylcobalamin and methylcobalamin leading to homocystinuria, in addition to methyl-malonic aciduria. Such a defect can be associated with early-onset life-threatening hemolytic uremic syndrome.

Tyrosinemia type 1 Tyrosinemia type 1 is an autosomal-recessive disorder caused by deficiency of fumarylacetoacetase, leading to accumulation of succinylacetone in liver and kidney. Renal involvement consists of the Fanconi syndrome (61). The recent use of NTBC (2-[2-nitro-4-trifluoromethybenzyoyl]-1,3 cyclohexanedione)—a specific enzyme inhibitor—has dramatically improved patient survival, obviating the need for liver transplantation. Though progressive renal impairment has not yet been reported, prolonged survival of NTBC-treated patients could increase the risk for hepatic malignancy and renal complications in non-compliant or poorly responsive patients.

Other forms of inherited diseases

Inherited tubular disorders Due to either a natural late course of the disease or thera-peutic non-compliance, some inherited tubular disorders may lead to ESRF, as result of advanced tubulo-interstitial damage, e.g. familial hypomagnesemia-hypercalciuria syndrome, distal renal tubular acidosis, Bartter syndrome, X-linked hypophos-phatemic rickets, cystinuria, Dent disease. Recurrence of these disorders in the graft has not been reported so far.

Mitochondrial cytopathies Mitochondrial cytopathies are characterized by defects of oxidative phosphorylation, which can affect several organs or tissues. Initial symp-toms occur before 2 years of age in 80% of cases. The diagnosis should be suspected in renal patients with hyperlactacidemia and/or in any unexplained disorder involv-ing two or more organs without apparent link. The number of affected organs increases during the course of the disease, the central nervous system being always involved in late stages. The renal manifestations may consist of Fanconi syndrome, chronic tubulo-interstitial nephritis, and focal and segmental glomerulosclerosis (62). No specific therapy is currently available. RT is questionable when extra-renal involvement is severe and progressive.

Inherited hematological disorders Wiskott–Aldrich disease is a rare X-linked heredi-tary disorder characterized by recurrent infections, thrombocytopenia, eczema, and an increased incidence of malignancies. Progression to ESRF, due to membrano-proliferative glomerulonephritis, is frequent. RT is challenging due to the risk of both infection and malignancy; however, some successful cases have been reported with minimal immunosuppression.

Fanconi anemia is also associated with an increased risk of cancer due to chromo-somal fragility. This should be closely followed as some patients may have renal impairment.

Table 9.2 Malformation syndromes with renal involvement leading to ESRF

Malformation syndrome	Comments
Bardet–Biedl syndrome	Chronic renal failure in 30–60% of patients
Branchio-oto-renal (BOR) syndrome	Chronic renal failure in 6% of patients
Oro-facial-digital syndrome type 1	Polycystic kidneys
Meckel syndrome	Death *in utero* or shortly after birth
Ivemark syndrome	Renal-hepatic-pancreatic dysplasia
Jeune syndrome	Asphyxiating thoracic dystrophy
Williams syndrome	Vascular and tubulointerstitial lesions
Down syndrome	Increased incidence of posterior urethral valves and membrano-proliferative glomerulonephritis

Malformation syndromes

Renal involvement may be part of several malformation syndromes. Management of ESRF depends on the extent and severity of extra-renal manifestations, which may raise an ethical dilemma in the case of severe mental retardation or disability. A selection of malformation syndromes, including renal abnormalities, is listed in Table 9.2.

Congenital malformations of the urinary tract

Congenital malformations of the urinary tract account for 20–30% of all children and 5–15% of all adults admitted for RRT. A large number of these conditions can be diagnosed in utero by ultrasound—mainly those involving dilatation of the urinary tract—and may lead to either pregnancy termination or perinatal death, due to severe oligoamnios and pulmonary hypoplasia. Renal failure affecting the fetus reflects kidney dysplasia, which can be either primary or secondary to early obstruction of the urinary tract. Those children who survive may present with early life-threatening complications, recurrent urinary tract infections, incontinence, growth retardation, and eventually progressive uremia in adulthood. Management of affected patients may be more problematic in developing countries, due to limited access to both prenatal diagnosis and advanced urological and nephrological care, early and late postnatal management, and undertreated recurrent urinary tract infections.

Primary vesico-ureteral reflux and scarring/dysplasia

Primary vesico-ureteral reflux (VUR) results from a congenital deficiency of the normal flap-valve mechanism of the ureterovesical junction, often related to shortening of the intravesical ureter with a laterally located orifice (63). As recently realized, VUR may be a familial disorder, sometimes inherited as an autosomal-dominant trait (64).

Primary VUR has to be distinguished from secondary VUR, which is the consequence of anatomic or functional bladder outlet obstruction (see below).

The mechanism of chronic renal failure in patients with primary VUR is not as clear as previously thought. In a minority of patients, invasion of renal parenchyma by infected urine may cause scarring and progressive renal damage. In most patients with VUR and no history of urinary infection, kidneys are hypoplastic or dysplastic, which may be confused with acquired scars. Patients with VUR may occasionally present with heavy proteinuria, due to focal segmental glomerulosclerosis (65).

The presence of primary VUR is an indication for pre-transplant nephroureterectomy only when there is a hydroureter or when there is recurrent urinary infection.

Congenital urinary tract obstruction

Urinary tract obstruction may cause hydronephrosis leading to progressive renal destruction. Obstruction of the ureteropelvic junction (lesions may be extrinsic, such as aberrant vessels, or intrinsic) or of the ureterovesical junction (megaureter) requires nephrectomy or nephroureterectomy, respectively, before or at the time of RT.

The most common cause of congenital urethral obstruction, occurring only in males, is the existence of posterior urethral valves. Urethral obstruction may also be present in the context of a prune-belly syndrome (abdominal wall distension, muscle defect, and cryptorchidism). In females, urethral obstruction may be related to cloacal anomalies. Severe infantile ureterocoele may also cause obstruction.

In most severe cases, the bladder is thickened and trabeculated; secondary VUR and renal dysplasia are frequently associated. Valves should be ablated, ureterocoele excised, and bladder neck reconstructed. Pre-transplant evaluation should include voiding cysto-urethrograpy and urodynamic tests. Severely damaged, small-capacity, bladders may require reconstruction.

Neurogenic bladder

A normal bladder acts as a low-pressure, adequate-capacity reservoir that is continent, sterile, and empties freely and completely. These functions are controlled by a co-ordinated process involving the brain, brainstem, spinal cord, detrusor muscle, bladder neck, and external sphincter. Dysfunction of any of these components may lead to improper storage of the urine and/or inadequate bladder emptying. Neurologic dysfunction of the bladder is commonly associated with urinary retention and secondary VUR, leading to recurrent pyelonephritis, renal scarring, and ultimately ESRF (66).

The most common congenital cause of neurogenic bladder is myelodysplasia, a group of vertebral column abnormalities of the lumbar and sacral spinal cord, including myelomeningocoele (accounting for 90% of the cases), occult spinal dysraphism (abnormality of the end of the spinal cord associated with a cutaneous lesion such as lipomeningocoele), sacral agenesis, and some rare degenerative affections of the central nervous system (Friedreich's disease).

Evaluation of a transplant candidate with a neurogenic bladder should address both structure and function of the entire lower urinary tract. It includes a detailed medical history (recording previous interventions), a careful physical examination (inspection of genitalia, palpation of lumbar and sacral vertebrae, checking peri-anal and perineal sensation) (66), a voiding cysto-urethrogram (defining bladder volume and wall, existence of a VUR), and a urodynamic evaluation (measurement of bladder residual volume, urethral pressure profile, urethral resistance, and cystometry). An electromyography is required to investigate the external urethral sphincter during the micturation cycle. Patients with a neurogenic bladder often have a combination of several anomalies: reduced bladder compliance, increased residual volume, low bladder capacity, VUR, and urinary incontinence (66).

Intermittent catheterization is recommended in patients with elevated residual post-voiding volume (66). Bladder augmentation may be advocated in patients with reduced bladder capacity and compliance, in order to reduce both intravesical pressure and hyper-reflexic contraction; it can be performed using a segment of ileum or sigmoid, native ureter (ureterocystoplasty), or detrusorrhaphy (auto-augmentation). Bladder augmentation is best performed prior to RT, in order to avoid the negative effect of glucocorticoids on the healing process. Patients with augmented bladder should be told that the procedure often requires intermittent catheterization and prophylactic antibiotherapy after RT.

In the case of high-grade VUR, nephroureterectomy is indicated, whereas only nephrectomy is performed when the ureter is needed for bladder augmentation. In patients with a previous urinary diversion, bladder capacity should be (re)assessed with the aim of reconstructing a competent bladder using one of the techniques described above (66).

RT is also feasible in patients with ileal conduits or continent reservoirs: in a series of 22 such patients, patient- and graft-survival rates were found to be similar to the general kidney transplant population (67).

After RT, a regular urologic evaluation remains mandatory. Self-image, social insertion, and quality of life may be severely impaired by repeated surgery, associated sexual dysfunction, urine, and sometimes fecal, incontinence, requiring appropriate management.

Acknowledgements

To H. Dodat and F. Wese for helpful urological advice, and to K. Voss for secretarial assistance.

References

1. Pirson, Y., Chauveau, D., and Grünfeld, J.P. (1998). Autosomal-dominant polycystic kidney disease. In *Oxford Textbook of Clinical Nephrology* (ed. A.M. Davison, J.S. Cameron, J.P. Grünfeld, D.N.S. Kerr, E. Ritz, and C.G. Winearls), pp.2393–415. Oxford University Press, Oxford.

2. Pirson, Y., Christophe, J.L., and Goffin, E. (1996). Outcome of renal replacement therapy in autosomal dominant polycystic kidney disease. *Nephrology Dialysis Transplantation*, **11**, (Suppl. 6), 24–8.

3. Culleton, B. and Parfrey, P.S. (1996). Management of end-stage renal failure and problems of transplantation in autosomal dominant polycystic kidney disease. In *Polycystic Kidney Disease* (ed. M.L. Watson and V. Torres), pp. 450–61. Oxford University Press, Oxford.

4. Christophe, J.L., van Ypersele de Strihou, C., and Pirson Y. (1996). Complications of autosomal dominant polycystic kidney disease in 50 hemodialysed patients. A case-control study. *Nephrology, Dialysis, Transplantation*, **11**, 1271–6.

5. Thaysen, J.H., Thomson, HS., Sass, A., and Kristensen, J.K. (1985). Volume changes in polycystic kidneys during chronic dialysis and after renal transplantation. *Acta Medica Scandinavica*, **217**, 197–204.

6. Keith, D.S., Torres, V.E., King, B.F., Zincki, H., and Farrow, G.M. (1994). Renal cell carcinoma in autosomal dominant polycystic kidney disease. *Journal of the American Society of Nephrology*, **4**, 1661–9.

7. Kliem, V., Ringe, B., Frei, U., and Pichlmayr, R. (1995). Single-center experience of combined liver and kidney transplantation. *Clinical Transplantation*, **9**, 39–44.

8. Torres, V.E. (1996). Polycystic liver disease. In *Polycystic Kidney Disease* (ed. M.L. Watson and V. Torres), pp.500–529. Oxford University Press, Oxford.

9. Andreoni, K.A., Pelletier, R.P., Elkhammas, E.A., Davies, E.A., Baumgardner, G.L., Henry, M.L. *et al.* (1999). Increased incidence of gastrointestinal surgical complications in renal transplant recipients with polycystic kidney disease. *Transplantation*, **67**, 262–6.

10. Hademeri, H., Johansson, A.C., Haraldsson, B., and Nyberg, G. (1998). CAPD in patients with autosomal dominant polycystic kidney disease. *Peritoneal Dialysis International*, **18**, 419–32.

11. McDonald, R.A., Watkins, S.L., and Avner, E.D. (1999). Polycystic kidney disease. In *Pediatric Nephrology* (ed. T.M. Barratt, E.D. Avner, and W.E. Harmon), pp. 459–74. Lippincott Williams & Wilkins, Baltimore.

12. Roy, S., Dillon, M.J., Trompeter, R.S., and Barratt, T.M. (1997). Autosomal-recessive polycystic kidney disease: long-term outcome of neonatal survivors. *Pediatric Nephrology*, **11**, 302–6.

13. Jamil, B., McMahon, L.P., Savige, J.A., Wang, Y.Y., and Walker, R.G. (1999). A study of long-term morbidity associated with autosomal-recessive polycystic kidney disease. *Nephrology, Dialysis, Transplantation*, **14**, 205–9.

14. Pirson, Y. (1999). Making the diagnosis of Alport's syndrome. *Kidney International*, **56**, 760–75.

15. Peten, E., Pirson, Y., Cosyns, J.P., Squifflet, J.P., Alexandre, G.P.J., Noël, L.H. *et al.* (1991). Outcome of thirty patients with Alport's syndrome after renal transplantation. *Transplantation*, **52**, 823–6.

16. Kashtan, C.E. and Michael, A.F. (1996). Alport syndrome. *Kidney International*, **50**, 1445–63.

17. Kestilà, M., Lennkeri, U., Mannikko, M., Lamerdin, J., McCready, P., Putaala, H. *et al.* (1998). Positionally cloned gene for a novel glomerular protein – nephrin – is mutated in congenital nephrotic syndrome. *Molecular Cell*, **1**, 575–82.

18. Holmberg, C., Jalanko, H., Tryggvason, K., and Rapola, J. (1999). In *Pediatric Nephrology* (ed. T.M. Barratt, E.D. Avner, and W.E. Harmon), pp.765–77. Lippincott Williams & Wilkins, Baltimore.

19. Fuchshuber, A., Jean, G., Gribouval, O., Gubler, M.C., Broyer, M., Beckmann, J.S. *et al.* (1995). Mapping a gene (SRNA) to chromosome 1q2q31 in idiopathic nephrotic syndrome confirms a distinct entity of autosomal-recessive nephrosis. *Human Molecular Genetics*, **4**, 2155–8.

20. Boute, N., Gribouval, O., Reslli, S., Bennessy, F., Lee, H., Fuchshuber, A. *et al.* (2000). NPHS2, encoding the glomerular protein podocin, is mutated in autosomal-recessive steroid-resistant nephrotic syndrome. *Nature Genetics*, **24**, 349–54.

21. Winn, M.P., Conlon, P.J., Lynn, K.L., Nowell, D.N., Gross, D.A., Rogala, A.R. *et al.* (1999). Clinical and genetic heterogeneity in familial focal segmental glomerulosclerosis. *Kidney International*, **55**, 1241–6.

22. Kaplan, J.M., Kim, S.H., North, K.N., Rennke, H., Correia, L.A., Tong, H.-Q. *et al.* (2000). Mutation in ACTN4, encoding α-actinin-4, cause familial focal segmental glomerulosclerosis. *Nature Genetics*, **24**, 251–6.

23. Conlon, P.J., Lynn, K., Winn, M.P., Quarles, L.D., Bembe, M.L., Pericak-Vance, M. *et al.* (1999). Spectrum of disease in familial focal and segmental glomerulosclerosis. *Kidney International*, **56**, 1863–71.

24. Gubler, M.C. (1998). Congenital nephrotic syndrome. In *Inherited Disorders of the Kidney* (ed. S.H. Morgan and J.P. Grünfeld), pp.177–91. Oxford University Press, Oxford.

25. Gubler, M.C., Yang, Y., Jeanpierre, C., Barbaux S., and Niaudet, P. (1999). WT1, renal development and glomerulopathies. *Advances in Nephrology*, **29**, 299–315.

26. Ehrich, J.H.H., Burchert, W., Shirg, E., Krull, F., Offner, G., Hoyer, P. *et al.* (1995). Steroid resistant nephrotic syndrome associated with spondyloepiphyseal dysplasia, transient ischemic attacks and lymphopenia. *Clinical Nephrology*, **43**, 89–95.

27. Warwicker, P., Goodship, T.H.J., Donne, R.L., Pirson, Y., Nicholls, A., Ward, R.M. *et al.* (1998). Genetic studies into inherited and sporadic hemolytic uremic syndrome. *Kidney International*, **53**, 836–44.

28. Kaplan, B.S., Papadimitriou, M., Brezin, J.H., Tomlanovich, S.J., and Zulkharnain. (1997). Renal transplantation in adults with autosomal-recessive inheritance of hemolytic uremic syndrome. *American Journal of Kidney Disease*, **30**, 760–5.

29. Torres, V.E. (1996). Tuberous sclerosis complex. In *Polycystic kidney disease* (ed. M.L. Watson and V. Torres), pp.283–308. Oxford University Press, Oxford.

30. Schillinger, F. and Montagnac, R. (1996). Chronic renal failure and its treatment in tuberous sclerosis. *Nephrology, Dialysis, Transplantation*, **11**, 481–5.

31. Balligand, J.L., Pirson, Y., Squifflet, J.P., Cosyns, J.P., Alexandre, G.P.J., and van Ypersele de Strihou, C. (1990). Outcome of patients with tuberous sclerosis after renal transplantation. *Transplantation*, **49**, 515–8.

32. Neumann, H.P.H. and Zbar, B. (1997). Renal cysts, renal cancer and von Hippel-Lindau disease. *Kidney International*, **51**, 16–26.

33. Chauveau, D., Duvic, C., Chrétien, Y., Paraf, F., Droz, D., Melki, P. *et al.* (1996). Renal involvement in von Hippel-Lindau disease. *Kidney International*, **50**, 944–51.

34. Steinbach, F., Novick, A.C., Zincke, H., Miller, D.P., Williams, R.D., Lund, G. *et al.* (1995). Treatment of renal cell carcinoma in von Hippel-Lindau disease: a multicentre study. *Journal of Urology*, **153**, 1812–6.

35. Goldfarb, D.A., Neumann, H.P.H., Penn, I., and Novick, A.C. (1997). Results of renal transplantation in patients with renal cell carcinoma and von Hippel-Lindau disease. *Transplantation*, **64**, 1726–9.

36. Penn, I. (1993). The effect of immunosuppression on pre-existing cancers. *Transplantation*, **55**, 742–7.

37. Cochat, P., Cordier, B., Lacôte, C., and Saïd, M.H. (1999). Cystinosis: epidemiology in France. In *Cystinosis* (ed. M. Broyer), pp.28–35. Elsevier, Paris.

38. Loirat, C. (1999). Symptomatic therapy. In *Cystinosis* (ed. M. Broyer), pp.97–102. Elsevier, Paris.

39. Rigden, S.P.A. (1999). Data from the ERA-EDTA registry. In *Cystinosis* (ed. M. Broyer), pp.20–7. Elsevier, Paris.

40. United States Renal Data System. (1999). USRDS 1999 annual data report, Pediatric end-stage renal disease. *American Journal of Kidney Disease*, **34,** (Suppl. 1), S102–13.

41. Broyer, M. and Tête, M.J. (1995). Complications tardives de la cystinose, à propos de 33 cas ayant dépassé 18 ans. *Annales de Pédiatrie*, **42**, 635–41.

42. Morgan, S.H. (1998). The primary hyperoxalurias. In *Inherited Disorders of the Kidney* (ed. S.H. Morgan and J.P. Grünfeld), pp.461–75. Oxford University Press, Oxford.

43. Cochat, P. (1999). Primary hyperoxaluria type 1. *Kidney International*, **55**, 2533–47.

44. Danpure, C.J. and Rumsby, G. (1995). Enzymology and molecular genetics of primary hyperoxaluria type 1: consequences for clinical management. In *Calcium oxalate in biological systems* (ed. S.R. Khan), pp.189–205. CRC Press, Boca Raton.

45. Barratt, T.M. and Danpure, C.J. (1999). Hyperoxaluria. In *Pediatric Nephrology* (ed. T.M. Barratt, E.D. Avner, W.E. Harmon), pp.609–19. Lippincott Williams & Wilkins, Baltimore.

46. Kemper, M.J., Conrad, S., and Müller-Wiefel, D.E. (1997). Primary hyperoxaluria type 2. *European Journal of Pediatrics*, **156**, 509–12.

47. Desnick, R.J. and Eng, C.M. (1998). In *Inherited Disorders of the Kidney* (ed. S.H. Morgan and J.P. Grünfeld), pp.355–83. Oxford University Press, Oxford.

48. Tsakiris, D., Simpson, H.K., Jones, E.H., Briggs, J.D., Elinder, C.G., Mendel, S. *et al.* (1996). Report on management of renal failure in Europe, XXVI, 1995. Rare diseases in renal replacement therapy in the ERA-EDTA Registry. *Nephrology, Dialysis, Transplantation*, **11**, (Suppl. 7), 4–20.

49. Harry, D.S. and Winder, A.F. (1998). Lecithin-cholesterol acyltransferase deficiency and the kidney. In *Inherited disorders of the kidney* (ed. S.H. Morgan and J.P. Grünfeld), pp.384–90. Oxford University Press, Oxford.

50. Horina, J.H., Wirnsberg, G., Horn, S., Roob, J.M., Ratschek, M., Holzer, H. *et al.* (1993). Long-term follow-up of a patient with lecithin cholesterol acyltransferase deficiency syndrome after kidney transplantation. *Transplantation*, **56**, 233–6.

51. Karet, F.E. and Lifton, R.P. (1997). Lipoprotein glomerulopathy: a new role for apolipoprotein E? *Journal of the American Society of Nephrology*, **8**, 840–2.

52. Matsunaga, A.K., Sasaki, J., Komatsu, T., Kanatsu, K., Tsuji, E., Moriyama *et al.* (1999). A novel apolipoprotein E mutation, E2 (Arg25Cys), in lipoprotein glomerulopathy. *Kidney International*, **56**, 421–7.

53. Miyata, T., Sugiyama, S., Mangaku, M., Suzuki, D., Uragami, K.I., Inagi, R. *et al.* (1999). Apolipoprotein E2/E5 variants in lipoprotein glomerulopathy recurred in transplanted kidney. *Journal of the American Society of Nephrology*, **10**, 1590–5.

54. Cameron, J.S., Moro, F., McBride, M., and Simmonds, H.A. (1998). Inherited disorders of purine metabolism and transport. In *Oxford Textbook of Clinical Nephrology* (ed. A.M. Davison, J.S. Cameron, J.P. Grünfeld, D.N.S. Kerr, E. Ritz, and C.G. Winearls), pp.2469–82. Oxford University Press, Oxford.

55. Pirson, Y., Loute, G., Cosyns, J.P., Dahan, K., and Verellen, C. (2000). Autosomal dominant chronic interstitial nephritis with early hyperuricemia. *Advances in Nephrology*, **30**, 357–69.

56. Ojo, A.O., Govaerts, T.C., Schmouder, R.L., Leichtman, A.B., Leavey, S.F., Wolfe, R.A. *et al.* (1999). Renal transplantation in end-stage sickle cell nephropathy. *Transplantation*, **67**, 291–5.

57. Nissenson, A.R. and Port, F.K. (1989). Outcome of end-stage renal disease in patients with rare causes of renal failure. I. Inherited and metabolic disorders. *Quarterly Journal of Medicine*, **73**, 1055–62.

58. van Ypersele de Strihou, C. (1999). Should anemia in subtypes of CRF patients be managed differently? *Nephrology, Dialysis, Transplantation*, **14**, (Suppl. 2), 37–45.

59. Chen, Y.T. (1991). Type I glycogen storage disease: kidney involvement, pathogenesis and its treatment. *Pediatric Nephrology*, **5**, 71–6.

60. van't Hoff, W.G. (1999). Renal manifestations of metabolic disorders. In *Pediatric Nephrology* (ed. T.M. Barratt, E.D. Avner, and W.E. Harmon), pp.625–31. Lippincott Williams & Wilkins, Baltimore.

61. Holme, E. and Lindstedt, S. (1995). Diagnosis and management of tyrosinemia type I. *Current Opinion in Pediatrics*, **7**, 726–32.

62. Niaudet, P. (1998). Mitochondrial disorders and the kidney. *Archives of Diseases of Children*, **78**, 387–90.

63. Rushton, H.G., Jr. (1999). Vesicoureteral reflux and scarring. In *Pediatric Nephrology* (ed. T.M. Barratt, E.D. Avner, and W.E. Harmon), pp.851–71. Lippincott Williams & Wilkins, Baltimore.

64. Kaefer, M. and Diamond, D. (1999). Vesicoureteral reflux. In *Pediatric Urology Practice* (ed. E.T. Gonzalez and S.B. Bauer), pp.463–86. Lippincott Williams & Wilkins, Baltimore.

65. Becker, G.J. and Kincaid-Smith, P. (1993). Reflux nephropathy: the glomerular lesion and progression of renal failure. *Pediatric Nephrology*, **4**, 365–9.

66. Ellis, D., Gilboa, N., Bellinger, M., and Shapiro, R. (1997). Renal transplantation in infants and children. In *Renal Transplantation* (ed. R. Shapiro, R.L. Simmons, and T.E. Starzl), pp.427–69. Appleton & Lange, Stamford, Connecticut.

67. Warholm, C., Berglund, J., Andersson, J., and Tydén, G. (1999). Renal transplantation in patients with urinary diversion: a case-control study. *Nephrology, Dialysis, Transplantation*, **14**, 2937–40.

10

Ethical conflicts in renal replacement therapies

J. Cecilia Kjellstrand and Carl M. Kjellstrand

Introduction

The speed of technology in the field of nephrology continues to accelerate, causing unexpected ethical conflicts for physicians. The physician still must balance the four generally recognized ethical principals of beneficence, non-maleficence, autonomy, and justice against each other, but is further called upon to strike this balance in increasingly complex ways. Physicians also have to fulfill an often overlooked ethical obligation, that of advocacy. This is a duty to patient groups, as well as to individuals. For nephrologists it is patients with end-stage renal failure for whom we advocate. Advocacy is necessary to secure enough funds to apply the treatments to all in need and to avoid rationing. It makes physicians compete with the conflicting financial demands of other societal needs, such as defense and education. They also face colleagues who are also advocating for other patient groups for limited funding. The physician–advocate has to harass politicians and bureaucrats and vie with other physicians to secure funds for their patients in need. The opposing force of distant politicians and bureaucrats is powerful and intimidating. There are also enormous for-profit dialysis companies to deal with. They are nor primarily responsible to patients but to their investors, and decisions of treatment are made in distant headquarters by anonymous directors. In general, physicians have not fared well in facing these powers. However, if funding is not secured, the ethical dilemmas faced begin to include uncomfortable and subjective rationing decisions. Thus failing in the duty of advocacy brings in a second ethical conflict, rationing; how to most fairly distribute justice to patients competing for too few dialysis machines or renal transplants. Almost all patients have contributed through in-voluntary tax money to funds for end-stage renal failure. This is through socialized medicine contracts in the law. This exists even in the USA where ESRD patients care is with Medicare; a non-voluntary tax funded program. To ration a life-saving treatment, such as dialysis, is very difficult and emotionally tormenting. It is easiest to pretend it does not exist. The resulting dishonorable fact is that in all countries where studied, the young, the rich, and men receive more dialysis then the old, the poor, and women, and in renal transplants there is also clear evidence of racial discrimination. This is an intolerable injustice for which physicians must bear a heavy burden.

Stopping dialysis is another serious ethical problem facing dialysis-nephrologists. The ethical factors that the physicians' balance are beneficence, non-maleficence, and respect for autonomy. Physicians' reactions to this are mixed, but usually a large element of fear is involved, including fear of persecution, and religious and personal morality conflicts. In some countries, the approach to stopping has been solved, usually through judicial means. In others, the problem is denied and hidden, and patients are left to deal with the decisions without enough information or support in their dying. An open discussion, free from religious, philosophical, and ethical dogma, is necessary to realistically solve this particular problem to the satisfaction of both physicians and their patients.

The source of ethical conflicts

There are three serious and difficult ethical dilemma facing those who treat patients with end-stage renal failure. First, to fight for funds, so that all patients can be treated. As this goal remains distant almost everywhere, the second problem is distributive justice—force, brutality, money, natural law—cannot be allowed to reign. Everyone must be treated equally. Third, to deal with death as the unavoidable result of dialysis discontinuation.

Physicians, through their privileged professional status, have a number of ethical obligations to uphold for their patients. To *individual* patients these are:

1. Beneficence—do what is good for the patient.
2. Non-maleficence—do not do anything harmful to a patient.
3. The principle of autonomy—respect the patient as an individual, with their own distinct beliefs and values, never identical to those held by the physicians and nurses treating them.

To *groups* of patients, the physician owes the fourth obligation:

4. Justice: all must be treated equally.

Very often a fifth principal, advocacy, is forgotten in these discussions (1). Advocacy is the obligation the physician has to speak up on behalf of a group of patients to which he/she is particularly obliged. For nephrology-dialysis and transplanting physicians, this means people who have end-stage kidney disease.

The ethical dilemmas arise when various obligations are contradictory or conflict with a powerful interest that is detrimental to patients' well-being.

In rationing dialysis and transplantation, the advocacy principle brings a physician into conflict with other physicians, such as cardiologists and oncologists, who will also be competing for limited funds. The physician may also be up against powerful state bureaucracies and politicians, who are angry when there are demands that require compromise on their part. If the physician is 100% successful as an advocate, no rationing is necessary and everyone receives treatment. However, if rationing is necessary, another principle—distributive justice—springs to the fore. The physician has to choose from a number of patients and, if perfectly just, no outside influences decide who is lucky. Rationing in dialysis is more important than rationing in transplantation; no dialysis is death, no transplantation is a difference in quality of life. Physicians also have to deal with distant commercial dialysis companies who pay them their salaries. The companies are primarily responsible to their investors, yet anonymous directors make treatment decisions for patients they never see or know.

In dealing with stopping dialysis, the ethical principles governing behavior towards individuals may be in conflict. Beneficence and non-maleficence on one hand conflict with autonomy. If the physician holds very conservative religious views, or is a strict 'right to life' person, then his or her own principles of beneficence and non-maleficence would over-ride the autonomy of the patient who wants the treatment stopped. There are dreadful examples of patients dialyzed against their, and their relatives', wishes. The opposite can occur, patients may be suffering immensely for no good gain, but because of 'right to life' or religious views of one or several family members, the patient's expressed wish to terminate treatment is over-ridden. In either case, the patients own wishes and personality are violated.

Rationing dialysis and transplantation

The rationing of dialysis and transplantation differ in many aspects. Rationing of dialysis could, in theory, be unnecessary. If there is enough money, there should be enough dialysis machines, nurses, technicians, and physicians to care for all. The restriction is thus one of economy and will, we choose to spend the money on something else instead of dialysis. In transplantation, there are a limited number of kidneys available for transplantation and this depends on the public's willingness to donate, not on any economic constraints. For example, in the USA approximately 100 000 patients are accepted for dialysis every year, but only 10 000 transplants are done. Thus, 90% of patients beginning dialysis will never have a chance of receiving a kidney transplant. The situation is different in other countries and, at least in some parts of India, patients are accepted for dialysis only if they have a donor available. Rationing renal transplants is obligatory; there are not enough kidneys for everyone who wants one. Rationing dialysis is facultative—it is a choice we make.

Rationing dialysis

In the early 1960s, the University of Washington in Seattle made a major break-through with the arteriovenous shunt. This invention created an enormous and overwhelming ethical task. They could accept only a few patients out of the tens of thousands in need of chronic dialysis. To select the few from the many, an anonymous selection committee was used to do the rationing based on social worth. Other centers made similar arrangements (2). After a decade or so, it was felt rationing was no longer necessary and the committees were disbanded. What was overlooked was the technical revolution with improvement in blood access, dialysis filters, dialysis machines, and the procedure of dialysis, which suddenly removed all technical restraints that had previously limited dialysis to young and strong patients. Almost anyone can now technically be dialyzed (3). Unwittingly, physicians have since used age as the most important rationing tool. This is proven by the very fact that the mean and medium ages of patients accepted for dialysis is steadily rising everywhere, and that the growth of the yearly incidence of acceptance to dialysis everywhere, far exceeds the population growth (4–7) (Fig. 10.1). The two considerations, the rising mean age and the steeply increasing incidence, and their most perfect regression fit (Fig. 10.2) prove that age was, and is, the tool used for selection.

Detailed examinations of acceptance to dialysis, combined with viewing these in relation to death certificates, also shows that men are favored over women everywhere. In general, in the Western countries, where it has been studied, such as the USA, Sweden, and Canada, women have only 60–70% chance compared with men of being accepted for dialysis (8–11). In the USA, blacks have had higher acceptance rate than whites (8). Perhaps it is in the distrust of the medical system that make blacks not believe a grim prognosis by a white physician as a reason not to start aged relatives on dialysis. They are then more willing than white patients and families to start aged relatives with many co-morbidities on dialysis (8, 12). In Canada, the Native Americans have long been a disfavored group in terms of dialysis acceptance. Their incidence of dialysis acceptance over the years is much steeper and far exceeds that of whites. Asians are in-between (11). All of this indicates that racial rationing has been used in Canada. The most evident sexual discrimination comes from statistics in India, where only 19% of all patients accepted are women (12, 13). Figures from other countries

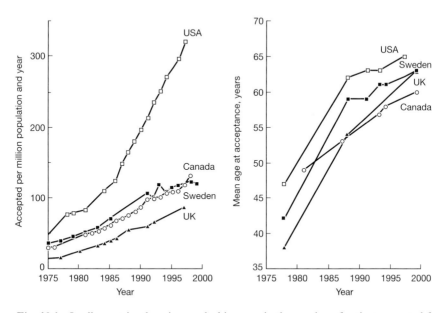

Fig. 10.1   In all countries there is a marked increase in the number of patients accepted for treatment of ESRD failure. In the USA, there has been a more than 30-fold increase over the last three decades. This increase in incidence by far outstrips any explanation by growth or aging of population, and indicates a mixture of an increase in the incidence of serious renal disease, and also the effect of the technological catch up.

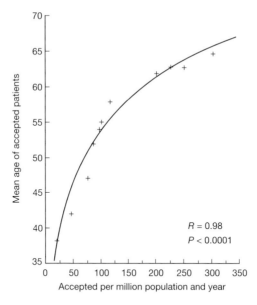

Fig. 10.2 The correlation between acceptance rate and age at acceptance in the USA. There is an almost perfect fit, proving that ageism exists in treatment of end-stage renal failure.

indicate that between 40% and 50% of accepted patients are women. Some of these figures are old and all figures are based on the uncertainty of using death certificates. However, the uniformity of the data indicates that age, racial, and sexual discrimination exist in selection for dialysis everywhere.

There is absolutely no justification for any sexual or racial discrimination in acceptance to dialysis. As age has been the most common tool used, it has been defended by several arguments, none of which hold water when fully analyzed.

One argument has been that older patients have only a short lifespan anyhow and thus in the interest of maximizing the life-years offered by a dialysis machine they should be excluded and young patients favored in the decision to be dialyzed on utilitarian grounds. While it is true that old patients do not live as long as young patients, this argument is flawed as it can be used to justify withholding *any* medical treatment for anyone over a certain age. If one, more realistically, sets the life-expectancy on dialysis in relation to the life-expectancy of an age-matched population, one finds that it is the lifespan of the younger age group that disproportionately is cut short by dialysis. While the death risk in dialysis patients below the age of 20 years is 20 times that of an age-matched person; a patient over the age of 70 on dialysis has only twice the death risk of an age matched not-dialyzed person (14). The argument is groundless. On utilitarian principles, there is further a grotesque equation to consider in age-rationing of dialysis. The older patients do not live as long as the younger ones. A 30-year-old might live 40 years on dialysis, a 70-year-old may not live much more than 5 years. With one dialysis machine, one could thus dialyze eight 70-year-old patients or one 30-year-old. Is one 30-year-old worth eight 70-year-olds? This is not a question in jest, but one that seriously needs to be considered for anyone advocating rationing by age.

A second argument has been that elderly patients are particularly unhappy and miserable, and have low quality of life on dialysis. Careful studies from Sweden (15), Canada (16), England (17), and the USA (18) show the opposite. It is the younger dialysis patients who feel shackled, unhappy, and desperate by the limitations of dialysis, while the older dialysis patients accept the limitations and report having a higher quality of life. This argument is also based on a fallacy.

A third argument has been based on economical constraints. We can not afford to treat everybody and thus the old must stand back. However, nowhere is there an indication that dialysis is causing any strain on societies economic resources (1, 19). As a matter of fact, there is no indication anywhere that medical cost has ruined any country. Bribery, corruption, injustice, abandonment of population groups, and an ever-expanding military machine are the causes of the downfall of nations, not the care of the old.

It has been argued that in the USA, the end-stage renal population, less than 1% of the US Medicare population, consumes 5% of the available resources and that some-how this is not right (20). The argument is spurious and fallacious and ignores the insurance aspects of any medical system. Individuals will have a different need for medical care. Some, even among the young, may need a costly transplant, another lucky individual lives a long life without ever needing any care. There is often no way to predict who will need expensive services, which is why the protection provided by insurance systems were set up initially.

In any system where involuntary payments are made to the medical system, the indi-vidual has a demand for medical care that is accepted and not specifically excluded. There is no justification for using age discrimination in dialysis. The old have contributed much more money than the young, through years of taxes, which built our medical system. We all do so, to secure treatment that we fear we will need later in life. To deny treatment, solely by age, is an insurance fraud. It is immoral, unethical, and unjust.

A peculiar situation has been that some physicians have vigorously defended the low acceptance to dialysis in their population of end-stage renal disease patients when compared to other areas. The most well-known example is the English unofficial age limit of 55 years, which existed for some time as a criterion for acceptance to dialysis (21, 22). It was vigorously defended on the ground 'that everyone who could benefit from dialysis' got it (23), when the number accepted was much lower than in all other wealthy countries and proved the argument wrong. This argument implies that, in other countries with a higher acceptance in the older age groups, physicians are doing something wrong and do not realize the futility and inappropriateness in treating the old with dialysis. Similar arguments have been raised in Sweden and Canada, which have only one-third of the acceptance rate to dialysis of the United States (24).

The argument that everyone 'who benefits' is accepted is backwards. Under this stance, benefit is defined as being accepted and automatically those not accepted are assumed not to benefit from dialysis. It is also a very subjective term, open to any interpretation. The US experience shows that old and sick patients can have the most meaningful existence on dialysis. In Chicago recently, a 100-year-old patient was accepted and lived four full years on dialysis. He elected dialysis in spite of his physicians' strong advice to the contrary.

A second argument often heard by chiefs of nephrology is that everyone who is referred to them gets dialysis, and that the fault is with the referring physicians who stand in the way of referring end-stage renal disease patients to dialysis (25, 26). There are several subtleties involved in this reasoning. When physicians call and try to refer questionable patients, such as very old, diabetic patients with co-morbidity, the patients are not accepted for referral for a variety of reasons. Complicated, conservative management advised and given without follow-up. Thus nephrologists working under lean stars and with insufficient resources put obstacles in the periphery to prevent referral of 'questionable' patients into their already overtaxed dialysis units. It is the obligation of academic centers to remove such obstacles and point out that almost everyone can benefit and have a meaningful time on dialysis before they die. It is also the duty of physicians to speak up. If they do not there cannot be any discussion of the problem. In the UK, there was a 'conspiracy of silence' that infuriated lawyers because it prevented society from the opportunity to address the problem. Physicians, through their special knowledge of what can be achieved by expensive high-technology medicine, have the special, sometimes uncomfortable, duty to advocate and speak up. Silence is the a betrayal of trust to patients. 'They should have acted, but did not.' The sin of omission (St. Augustine).

Dementia, uncertainty, and the need for strict definition of contra-indications for chronic dialysis

From the discussion of rationing of dialysis, it is clear that many bogus reasons for low acceptance rates to dialysis are in circulation. Particularly nefarious is the circular argument that people that do not get dialysis somehow could not possibly benefit from it; also, the erroneous quality of life assumptions that have made people neglect the old. The following are the only three valid medical contra-indications to dialysis.

1. So severe dementia, that the patient does not understand the benefits of the unavoidable discomforts of dialysis: the repeated needle sticks, the disequilibrium or the need for a peritoneal catheter in the stomach, and the fluid exchanges.
2. Short life-expectancy from diseases other than the renal failure; 6 months has been proposed.
3. A wish by the patient not to have chronic dialysis.

It is clear that there are many patients that have so limited an understanding, that they do not understand the inconvenience, pain, and fright that may surround chronic dialysis. It becomes a cruel spectacle to see such patients tied down physically or chemically in order to allow dialysis. For them it is better to live a shorter time without dialysis. Similarly, if the life-expectation is very short, it would be better for a patient to have a limited time at home unencumbered by the need for dialysis, to arrange affairs, say farewell, and die in peace. The problem with expected duration of life on dialysis is that there are no good guidelines. In a Canadian study of 10 centers, approximately 1000 patients who were entered into chronic dialysis were prospectively evaluated, and physicians tried to gauge if the patient would survive for less or more than 6 months. They were wrong in one-half of the cases, or not more accurate than if they had flipped a coin (27). Quality of life is even more difficult to predict. Even well-tested instruments, repeatedly applied, measuring psychological well-being and depression failed to prospectively detect 13 of 235 patients on dialysis who stopped dialysis (28). It is also very difficult to judge, when a confused or apparently demented patient comes for dialysis, how much of the dementia has an organic basis other than the deranged body chemistry of chronic severe renal insufficiency. The solution to these problems, we suggest, is to not start any patient on chronic dialysis, but to start patients on a 1-month trial period of temporary dialysis. The reason for choosing 1 month is that it is the approximate time it takes for a patient to stabilize, and thus learn what chronic dialysis will be for the indefinite future if he/she chooses to continue treatment (29). At the end of the temporary dialysis period, one does not have the decision to stop it, *but to continue it*. If this decision is not made, there is no more dialysis. To make the decision to continue would be self-evident for most patients, but there will also be some patients' families and staff members who can, at that time, have a better basis to decide whether dialysis really is worthwhile to continue. This would overcome the fear of stopping dialysis that will be discussed later. In some instances, dialysis staff appear so afraid of having to stop later, that they would rather not begin many who could benefit.

Just rationing

One of the reasons why physicians so vigorously defend their practices is that there is truly no good way of rationing life-saving treatment. Table 10.1 is an effort to outline all the various possible methods. One would obviously want a value-neutral way of selecting the patients. However, 'first come first serve' is usually a subterfuge for natural selection, as the powerful and the rich easily jump the line to be first. Lottery is a possibility but it is unclear how this should be done, and it has a somewhat grotesque quality. Should all waiting patients draw sticks or be given a number, and when a slot opens a computer chooses them?

Medical values also crumble as sensible rationing tools. Clearly, the medical need for dialysis is independent of age, race, and sex, as death is the only alternative. Similarly, maximizing survival-outcome fails, as shown above. Actually, the older patients have the best outcome if their limited lifespan is set in relation to the lifespan of a matched age group. On the other hand, the total length they will live on dialysis is clearly shorter than that of a younger patient.

Societal, public, and institutional values also tend to be questionable and revert back to natural selection. It was given a worthy try in the first selection committee at Seattle (2). It has been pointed out that middle-class social values carried the day and that neither Henry David Thoreau nor Wolfgang Amadeus Mozart would have had a chance of receiving chronic dialysis in Seattle in the early days.

Much enthusiasm has been generated by 'qualies', (quality adjusted life years) but these tend to reflect societies' prejudice of what is a worthy life. It would perhaps even

Table 10.1 Possible methods for rationing medical life-support treatment

Methods of rationing
I. VALUE NEUTRAL
A. First come, first serve (Usually a subterfuge for natural selection)
B. Lottery
II. MEDICAL VALUES
A. Medical need
B. Maximize outcome
III. SOCIETY/PUBLIC/INSTITUTIONAL
A. Social worth
B. Program policy
C. Public policy
D. Quality of life
IV. MIXED MEDICAL/SOCIETAL
A. Qualies (Quality adjusted life years)
V. NATURAL SELECTION
A. Ability to pay
B. Intellectual capacity—'brains'
C. Squeaky wheel
D. Political power
E. Brutal force

balance the choice between the older and younger dialysis candidates. The old, who accept the limitations of a life on dialysis better than the young, have a higher quality but less quantity, while the reverse is true for the young.

Natural selection needs no further discussion here. Only the most libertarian would be ready to let the brutality of force, money, and power decide how medical resources are distributed.

Thus, there is no easy solution to the rationing problem for physicians, but in light of the shortcomings of the other options, perhaps lottery would be the most likely way to be a just system.

The conflicting interests of finacial incentives and quality of care in dialysis

Financial incentives, particularly in the United States, have made dialysis a very lucrative business and enormous profits are being made by individuals and companies. It is clear that the shorter dialysis is, the higher will be the profit of a company or individual, as time is money. If extra patients can be squeezed in on a shift, then a nurse becomes more 'productive'. Second, very skilled technical personnel are expensive and if they can be replaced by those less skilled, more profit can be made. The USA now has the shortest duration of dialysis among the technically advanced countries and an increasing ratio of patients to skilled nurses. These two facts are most certainly the main contributors to the fact that the USA has the highest death rate on dialysis among the developed rich countries. Originally dialysis lasted for 12 h, three times per week, while now it is down to between 3 and 3.5 h. In Japan, dialysis is paid by the hour of dialysis and, not surprisingly, Japanese patients spend 50% more time on dialysis than their US counterparts. Japan has by far the lowest mortality rate of the developed rich countries, less than one-fourth of USA (4, 7, 30). An increasing ethical dilemma for physicians is the rapid consolidation of dialysis units into a few, gigantic for-profit commercial companies. Presently, almost one-half of all dialysis patients in the USA are 'owned' by two companies: Fresenius and Gambro. Patients are bought and sold like any commodity, without even a chance of expressing their wishes. The sellers, often physicians, make large profits—often in the millions of dollars. The large companies make the dialysis machines and the disposable dialysis equipment, employ the dialysis physicians and nurses, buy and sell patients, and fund the very research that is supposed to be the quality check of their treatment. Distant directors, who are responsible to investors, not patients, dictate detailed dialysis treatment decisions. Both Fresenius and Gambro have been under investigation for Medicare fraud and abuse, and have been, or are, ready to settle these financial shenanigans. Several articles published over the last two decades come to the same conclusion: for-profit dialysis units exclude older or sicker patients but still have the highest mortality rates, the lowest transplant rates, and the lowest CAPD prevalence and home hemodialysis rates, and give the lowest dose of dialysis (31–37).

The implications and the moral judgement are clear. The most common, almost universally present, vice of greed has over-ridden professional obligations and commercialized dialysis at the expense of quality treatment and survival of dialysis patients.

The difficult dialysis patient

How patients and their caregivers get along varies in an infinite number of ways. Dialysis is very intrusive on independence, and compliance with medications, diet, and fluid restrictions difficult. Dialysis personnel sometimes view insufficient compliance as an attack on their professional integrity. Particularly common are sodium and water indiscretions, and the resulting need for extra dialysis, often on weekends and nights, is a source of conflict between staff and patients. Teenagers, trying to establish their independence, and people with a different cultural background than that of the dialysis personnel, are often viewed as 'difficult'.

More serious are the patients who are so disruptive that they threaten and even harm personnel, and the demands they place on personnel decreases the quality of care received by other patients. There is no easy solution to these problems. Our duty is to take care of anyone who needs our care, not only to care for saints. Some extreme situations of violent behavior have lead to physicians dismissing patients from dialysis in the USA. When patients have taken these cases to court, they have universally won their cases, as the courts have reasoned that stopping dialysis is a death sentence that does not fit the crime of harming dialysis personnel. Courts seem to have avoided the other question of how such behavior can decrease the quality of care for other patients by taking away attention and care, as well-trained and skilled personnel leave because of fear and discouragement.

One must analyze why patients are disruptive and violent. Are they psychotic or do they have an organic brain lesion? Is alcohol or drug abuse a factor? Is this a character disorder or are there cultural differences? Often psychiatric and geriatric consultation, or the use of spiritual or cultural counsel, can help. Tranquilizers, restraints, private cubbys for dialysis, and, in some cases, police attention is necessary. Patients can also be rotated between units or transferred to other units where personnel relations may be more favorable. The best available solutions are often unsatisfactory; to some questions, there are no answers.

Rationing renal transplantation

Rationing renal transplant is fundamentally different from rationing dialysis. First, there is no way in which economic or expanding facilities could make rationing of renal transplants unnecessary. It is always going to depend on the public willingness to donate. In many countries, renal donation rates have stalled or fallen, indicating either that all resources for cadaver organ acquisition are depleted or that the public is unwilling to donate to a medical system that is in disrepute, or both. The dreary stories of powerful politicians, sportsmen, and entertainers jumping the queues for renal, cardiac, and liver transplants, make the latter not unlikely. The second difference in rationing renal transplantation is that, while rationing dialysis means death to the one excluded, in renal transplantation it means that a procedure that is more appealing is denied, but it is not a matter of life and death. Although some studies indicate survival advantage of renal transplantation, more careful smaller institutional studies indicate that, when age and disease corrections are done, the survival advantage is non-existent or miniscule.

The first study of distributive justice in renal transplantation indicated discrimination by age, sex, and race (9). Many articles since that time have described the same phenomenon, and a decade after the first paper that did a detailed study of this, the situation remains unchanged (9, 10, 12, 35, 36). The chance to receive a renal transplant falls very steeply with age. Everywhere, women usually have only a 60–70% chance compared with men of receiving a transplant, even when all factors such as differences in cytotoxic enzymes antibodies, co-morbidity, and age are considered (9). Careful studies show that women want renal transplantation every bit as much as men do (38). Similarly, in the USA, blacks receive renal transplants much less often than whites, again even after correcting for differences in age, disease, and co-morbidity. It has also been shown that income influences renal transplant. Wealthy patients have a 50–100% higher chance of renal transplantation than do the poor (39).

While discrimination by race, sex, and income is shameful and immoral, one can defend rationing renal transplantation by age. As long as renal transplants are in short supply, it seems to make sense to put them in the patient where they would last the longest, and age is a very strong determinant of survival after renal transplantation. It is meaningless to do a transplant on an old and very sick patient who will live for a very short time, when it could be put into a younger patient who could live for decades. In the latter case, a dialysis machine would be freed up to treat many other patients. Thus, to ration transplantation very strictly by chance of survival seems both rational, just and ethical.

Ethical conflicts in recruiting donors for renal transplants

Everywhere, kidneys available for transplant are very scarce. In the United States, approximately 100 000 patients begin dialysis every year, but only 10 000 renal transplants are done (4). As many transplants are re-transplants, the chance of receiving the transplant is less than 10%. Over 90% of patients who begin dialysis will remain on it until they die from another cause. The situation has led to a number of tactics to increase available transplants (40).

There are educational efforts to increase the willingness to donate cadaver kidneys and various legislative approaches to do so. One of them is opting out: everyone is presumed to be a willing donor, unless they have expressed a wish not to do so, or unless the family vigorously opposes it. Financial interests, paying for and allowing the sale of kidneys, have been considered. How coercive one would let such a system be, obviously is a societal decision and opinions about this vary greatly (12, 13).

Increasing related-donor donation is a somewhat more risky business. In any family coercion can occur, and particularly children are obviously sometimes poorly equipped to resist coercion or have their wishes over-ridden or inappropriately directed. For all these reasons, increasingly unrelated-living donors are being used, bringing in other ethical conflicts.

One category of unrelated donors, is the 'emotionally related' donor, the other is the unrelated donor donating for a non-emotional reason, money or otherwise. Most common of the emotionally related donors are the wife/husband donations. Almost everywhere, women are more often donors and less often the recipients of kidneys. A careful objective outside evaluation, perhaps by a psychiatrist, is necessary here. Dr Haruki, a psychiatrist on dialysis and serving as a psychiatrist for a transplant team, has pointed out that many Japanese women have felt pressured and even threatened into donating to their husbands. In Japan, over 70% of all transplants are from wife to husband (41). The situation is similar elsewhere (42, 43).

This whole problem of unrelated-living donors is correlated to the sale of kidneys. One can never be quite sure what motivates someone who *claims to be* emotionally related, as in a 'friend'. There are disturbing stories of prisoners being sprung from prison by powerful families working through politicians, and then masquerading as good friends of a potential recipient.

The problem of emotionally unrelated-living donors is closely related to the sale of kidneys. The whole question of the sale of organs at first sight is repugnant; now the rich and powerful who have taken everything else from the poor, will also use their bodies for spare parts. This emotional revulsion has many sources. We fear that the middlemen and the brokers will exploit the defenseless. We hate the greed we all have, but find it particularly repulsive in others. We do not even want to think that there are people so badly off that selling their organs is not only their best option, it is their only option. Radcliff has carefully analyzed this, and disposed of the moral objections (44, 45). To the contrary, she argues that removing the sale of kidneys may remove the best option that very poor people have. It seems clear that the opportunities for abuse are horrible, and that some form of regulation would be necessary (46). Profiteering from the sale of organs should be made a crime against humanity. It is a threat against the altruism that every society needs in order to survive. At the University of Minnesota, an anonymous donation system has been set up to prevent abuses. The only buyer of kidneys should be the government and institutions, and a truly altruistic donor would have no choice in selection of the recipient, but would receive a reward. That way the patient would be released from dialysis, a donor would be rewarded, and abuse, hopefully, prevented. It seems the situation where everyone could benefit, if a thoughtful solution could be found (47).

Can the world afford uremia therapy?

Hemodialysis and transplantation are not cheap treatments. In the USA, one hemodialysis session can be done for approximately $100, as evident of the great profit made by commercial dialysis units charging $125 for dialysis. In the rest of the world, based on observations and discussions in Egypt, the cost is approximately one-third, while it is higher in some European countries. Transplant in the USA may cost approximately $100 000, but can obviously be done much cheaper at other places, where particular physicians and hospitals expect much less (1, 19, 48–50). Nevertheless, the cost for all patients will be many billions of US dollars equivalence. In Table 10.2 is outlined what the cost of dialysis is, and what it would be, if every country had the same number of patients on dialysis per million population as in Japan, which has the highest number: 1 in 800. The total world costs would come to approximately 27 billion dollars. This cost should be set in relation to other costs that societies have, and it is particularly interesting to do so with military cost. As with medicine, there is a lot of disposable equipment in the military and the equipment becomes obsolete very quickly. Overboard arms trade in the world presently amounts to approximately $35 billion US dollars. Less than one-fourth of the overboard trade in arms would cover dialysis for everyone presently on dialysis, and cover 75% of the cost if every 1 in 800 of the worlds' population was dialyzed (51, 52). In every country there is also a large amount of abuse of taxpayers money through waste, bribery, and, in medicine, exorbitant salary expectations and profiteering. In Fig. 10.3 is all the costs in the world for dialysis contrasted both with arms trade and with the USA Savings and Loan scandal of $600 billion. Each physician, each minister of health, and every administrator in each country, has to decide how they want to approach these problems. The whole point is to make clear that one does not necessarily have

Table 10.2 The number of patients on dialysis in various parts of the world 1990 (50), the cost for each dialysis, and the total cost in billion of dollars. Also included is the cost and number of patients that would result if 1 in 800 of the world's population were on dialysis, as now is the case in Japan. The cost is set in relation to the arms trade, and the Saving and Loan scandal in the USA as is graphically illustrated in Fig. 10.3. Two-thirds of the arms cost would pay for dialysis of 1 in 800 people in the rest of the world (Row). (See also references 51 and 52.)

Area	Patients on dialysis (1990)	Cost per dialysis	Yearly cost (billions)	Cost if 1 in 800 were dialyzed	Number of Patients if all were dialyzed
Row	120 000	$40	0.7	27	4 630 000
Europe	145 000	$100	2.0	14	1 015 000
Japan	150 000	$100	2.0	2	150 000
USA	200 000	$100	3.0	4	270 000

Some other costs:
Arms trade   35 Billions
Savings and Loan scandal in USA   600 Billions

to compete with cancer, take the bread out of the mouths of babies, or destroy education, in order to take care of those who need dialysis.

These considerations, and the false belief that the quality of life on dialysis is miserable, are convenient escape lies by physicians, administrators, bureaucrats, and politicians. It is the easy and slick way of getting off the hook. It camouflages the hard moral choices, the tough financial considerations, and leaves a trail of dead patients. A year on dialysis is less expensive than three seconds of the Gulf War. A fraction of the interest of the lost capital of the Savings and Loan scandal would have paid for all dialysis in the USA in perpetuity. (The USA Savings and Loan Scandal was the result of decreasing Federal oversight. Unscrupulous, criminal, and stupid investors over-estimated the value of security for loans, using common peoples' lifetime savings. When the bubble burst, the Federal Government stepped in and used tax-payers' money to cover for the lost and swindled money. Almost none was held responsible. Anyone can find similar waste in his or her country.) Nigeria, known for its exorbitant corruption, recently bought 80 battle tanks from the United Kingdom, and Malaysia bought 40 Mirage fighters from France, each at the cost of tens of millions of dollars (51). Clearly, there are conflicting health needs in many poor nations, and the expense of dialysis and transplantation make application there difficult. The point here is not to throw up our hands in despair, but carefully consider what the cost would be and set them in relation to other purchases society does. No country has gone bankrupt from paying for medicine. Even the wealthiest countries that spend the most on health, use only 7–10% of the gross domestic product on health. The exception is the USA, where 14% of the gross domestic product is spent on medical expenditures. The USA also has by far the highest 'administrative' cost for health, as much money is siphoned off to investors and overpaid executives (19).

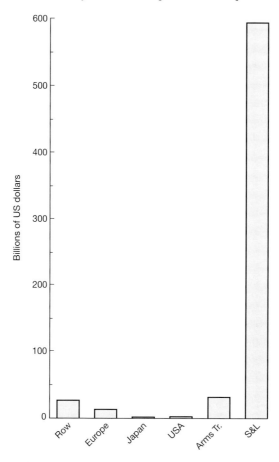

Fig. 10.3 The cost of dialysis in four parts of the world, if 1 in 800 inhabitants was dialyzed everywhere and some and economic relations. The arms trade per year alone would pay for all dialysis in the world, and the Savings and Loan (S&L) dwarf the cost of all dialysis in the USA. Similar scams, bribery, and corruption exist everywhere. The point is not to minimize the difficulties caused by the expense of treating patients dying of renal failure, but to point out that one should not simply accept the argument that it is too expensive to implement, but rather thoughtfully see where the money could be gotten. This is a duty of physicians as advocates for their patient groups. (ROW=Rest of the World).

One peculiar problem in securing funds for end-stage renal failure treatment, is the 'low profile' of kidney diseases when compared to other diseases such as AIDS, cancer, Alzheimer's, and others. It is difficult to understand, as the absence of facilities for uremia has a much starker outcome and so directly leads to death. It is one problem that occurs when politically noisy groups scare the populace, get the attention of mass-media, and thus fear and politics, rather than need, quantity and quality govern how funds are used.

Stopping dialysis

Stopping dialysis involves conflict between the three moral obligations that physicians owe to individual patients: beneficence, non-maleficence, and respect for autonomy. Stopping abuts on assisted suicide, making the problem difficult for many to analyze intellectually. Stopping dialysis frightens physicians because it is surrounded by a whole variety of strongly held and personal religious, philosophical, and ethical beliefs. There is also the fear of shame from the brotherhood in not prolonging life, the fear of litigation, and of public and religious rebuke. Physicians therefore tend to avoid or to lie about the problem. In several articles, Feiffel has described that when he probes the fear of death among various groups in society, physicians always rank as the most fearful (53). Plough and Salem, analyzing 40 deaths of patients on hemodialysis in several different units, found that 22 were due to discontinuing dialysis, suicide, or dialysis accidents. Only in one case was the cause of death correctly described, 21 were due to 'cardiac arrest' (54). Some dialysis registries still do not have a heading for stopping dialysis. For example, in Canada it is due to 'social cause' and in the USA stopping as a cause of death is not included in the collapsed death rates, although it is the fourth most common of the 19 causes of death included (4, 5).

At a recent conference on ethical problems in dialysis held in Yokohama, Japan, several speakers still voiced their opinion that participating in stopping is similar to homicide and that the patients are performing suicide, although the major religions tend to view it in a more merciful way (55). Thus there swirls a controversy around the stopping of dialysis that involves religious, ethical, philosophical thoughts, and bigotry, as well as rational and irrational fear. Once it is acknowledged that death from stopping occurs, and it is tracked, there is a rapid increase in stopping reported as a cause of death in dialysis patients.

How common is stopping?

There are multiple reports, both from registries and individual dialysis units, which show that in Australia, Canada, New Zealand, and the United States, stopping is very common and it is now the second leading cause of death in dialysis patients, following cardiovascular causes of death. Stopping causes approximately 20% of all deaths in these countries. Stopping is less often described from Europe, where it causes approximately 4% of all deaths. It shows rising incidence in all other countries. It is uncommon in Japan, causing approximately 1–2% of all deaths (4–7, 12, 13).

The first duty that a physician has in dealing with stopping is to try to prevent it from occurring. The second one is to smooth the avenues of death once dialysis has been stopped.

Preventing stopping

In order to prevent stopping, one needs to know which patients are at risk and why patients stop. There are several detailed analyses of the patients at risk. In general, these analyses find that stopping increases steeply with age. The exception to this is Japan, where stopping actually declines with rising age and is much more common in the younger than in the older age group (Fig. 10.4e). Another factor is race. White patients stop twice as often as black patients in the USA. Perhaps this reflects the distrust that black patients have in the medical system, often directed by white personnel, which is disproportionately prevalent. They may not believe a hopeless prognosis by a white physician and thus insist on continued treatment. Third, patients with diabetes and patients with co-morbidity stop twice as often as patients with other diseases and no co-morbidity. Fourth, patients on home hemodialysis and CAPD stop much more often then those on in-center dialysis, when age differences are corrected for. This perhaps reflects the absence of a neutral support outside of the family. In home dialysis, a patient and his/her family have to deal alone with the problems and tribulations of dialysis. Thus old age, white race, diabetes, and home patients and patients with other diseases besides their renal failure, are at risk (12, 56–63).

In the only prospective study of the risk of stopping, 235 hemodialysis patients were followed for over 4 years (28). Out of 100 patients' who died, 13 died from stopping. In univariate analysis, old age, loneliness, nursing-home living, unemployment, never going outdoors, high co-morbidity, low activity on the Karnofsky scale, and severe pain, were all significantly more common in patients who stopped. However, when these factors where made to compete in a multivariate analysis, only three factors were significant. Severe pain in a patient increased the risk of stopping by a factor of three. Becoming alone through divorce or widowhood doubled the risk, as did each co-morbidity. Thus, it is not the fact that patients are old or have diabetes, but the fact that they have pain and other diseases to contend with, and that they come home to a lonesome house with no one to support them, that sets the stage for stopping. Thus, to prevent stopping our skills in dealing with pain needs to be sharpened; co-morbidity one can deal with only by prevention long before dialysis becomes necessary. Once co-morbidity exists, it is unavoidable. Support for the lonely would also be an important factor and voluntary organizations can have a big role to play, as busy dialysis personnel hardly have time to take care of the patients at home.

Smoothing the avenues of death

Once the question of stopping dialysis comes up, a whole number of ethical, religious, legal, and practical matters come to the fore. In Table 10.3 are outlined the factors and preparation necessary to deal well with stopping.

Everyone dealing with patients on chronic hemodialysis need to have contemplated his or her ethical framework, unshakable moral beliefs, and, if religious, the religious implications. This will help prepare one to deal with these matters in a thoughtful, respectful way, with the main goal being to assist the patient based on their belief system. Religious considerations are obviously very important. Both Catholics and major Protestant groups allow stopping. They do so by allowing the weighing of benefits versus the burden of pain, discomfort, and, somewhat surprisingly, the economic burden. If these weigh in favor of stopping, this is allowed. It is not

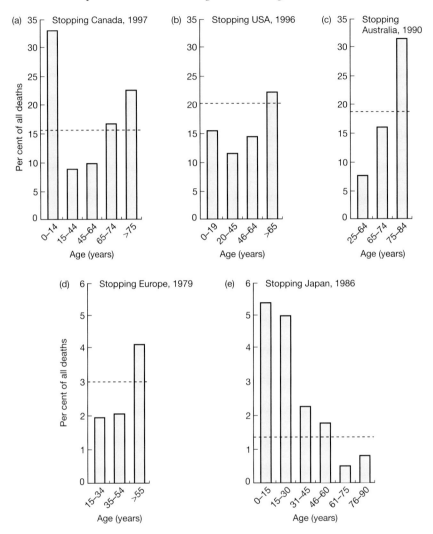

Fig. 10.4 The percentage of death caused by stopping versus age in different parts of the world. (a)–(c) are at the same scale, while (d) and (e) are scaled together, but the scale is six times larger than (a)–(c). It is clear that in all countries, except Japan, stopping increases markedly with the age of the patients. There is some tendency in Canada and the USA that it also occurs more commonly in the very young. In Japan, the reverse is true, stopping falls steeply with increasing age of the patients. There are many explanations. Perhaps in the very young, at least in Japan, there is no way out of dialysis to transplantation, as this procedure is almost never performed there. Thus, a young patient cannot look forward to a transplant as a release from dialysis and it is the young patients who find dialysis particularly difficult. Different cultural views of aging may explain the increase of stopping with increasing age in the west and decrease in the east.

Table 10.3 Philosophical, moral and practical considerations necessary for a dealing with patients who decide to stop dialysis to die

---

I. Ethical framework—Kantian deontology

    Beneficence—Sanctity of life
    Non-maleficence—Do not cause suffering
    Autonomy—Respect dignity and difference

                    None has Absolute Priority

II. Intellectual/emotional analysis—existentialism

    Weigh burden vs. benefit: suffering vs. life gain
    Non-maleficence and autonomy vs. beneficence

III. Practical analysis 1—classical utilitarianism

    What are the alternatives?

    Act   Consequences
      Do everything   Analyze and predict
      Change course
      Do less
      Stop everything

IV. Practical analysis 2—common sense

The circumstances:	Patient competent
	Temporary mental or physical stress over-ride decision
	If incompetent, who decides?
Medical aspects :	Disease understood
	Prognosis known
	Maximal care tried
	Do experts agree?
Why do you want to stop:	Patient's best interest
	Family desperate
	Friends squeamish
	Team discouraged
	You depressed and tired
	Administrative power pressure
Making the decision:	Be prepared for the unexpected

                  Discuss—Listen—Document

Insoluble situations:	Religious imperative
	Patient undecided or periodically lucid
	Family feuds
What do you plan to do:	Do not kill
	Do not practice medical scrupulosity

V. After stopping   Visit patient daily, listen to chest, converse
                              Do no tests
                              Comfort medications only—fluid restriction
                              Visit family

VI. After patient is dead   Follow-up with family?
                                Consequences for family?

---

regarded as suicide and personnel involved with the care of the patients are blameless. There are no official statements from Coptic Christians, Muslim, Buddhists, and the Shinto religion. The Jewish religion remains divided by liberal and conservative Jews, who would allow it, and orthodox Jews, who think that this is a non-question that does not even need discussion, it is prohibited (12, 52). Thus, although stopping has been known to occur for over two decades and was frequently debated, it was not until the late 1990s that such a case arose in Israel. In this case, the patient had to go to the Israeli Supreme Court to be allowed to discontinue dialysis, because of orthodox Jewish opposition. In Egypt, there is no preparation by the Coptic Christians or the Muslims. When questioned how stopping was dealt with, it was stated that the wish was that the patient would not show up for dialysis when they became so desperate. This clearly prevents physicians and other personnel from helping the dying patients, and leaves them and their families to deal with this alone.

The legal aspects arise in very litigious societies such as the USA. Somewhat astonishingly, out of at least six known litigation's surrounding stopping dialysis, five of them involved families who went to court to force reluctant hospitals and frightened physicians to stop treatment of their loved ones (55). Only once was there a court case where a physician and a hospital were sued for stopping. Two children, not known to the dialysis unit, sued for abandonment 2 years after their mother had died from stopping. The decision to stop was made by her husband, who died shortly after, and the treating physician. The case was decided in favor of the physician and the hospital. A lengthy review of religious and legal aspects has recently been published (55).

There may be unavoidable conflicts between patients' families and physicians based on religious, ethical or philosophical *convictions*. A devout Orthodox Jewish physician obviously cannot take care of the emotional well-being of a staunch Shinto Japanese samurai who has decided that enough is enough. The duty of a physician in such impossible conflicts is to withdraw and transfer care to someone who can speak to the patient on her or his terms. Religious bigotry must never be allowed to stand in the way of a patient's true wishes. For those physicians who plan to deal with patients in regards to discontinuing life-support, there is need for a secular moral system. Of the three major Western philosophical systems, Kantian deontology, utilitarianism, and existentialism, that could be considered as guides, .existentialism seems an unreliable guide with its 'gut-reaction' to an infinity of different problems and will most certainly lead to unprincipled *ad hoc* decisions, if used as the first approach. Its main use is an existential view of burden versus life gain, and considers non-maleficence and autonomy versus beneficence. The decision to stop is not only a matter of intellectual analysis, but also a reflection on one's emotional response. 'The heart knows matter that the mind does not' (B. Pascal).

Similarly, classical utilitarianism, with its weighing of contradictory factors, appears too un-sophisticated to solve so spiritual a decision as to hasten death. It can serve as a useful tool for the consideration of alternatives, what are the different acts and what are the consequences of each of them, but not as the primary ethical guide to action.

Kantian deontology seems the best load-star to follow: do your duty, listen to the inner moral compass, and act towards other as you want them act to you. It reflects the most fundamental principle of the world's major religions: do unto others what you want done to yourself. This principle seems the best and most ethical approach. One problem in using the Kantian approach is that some people let beneficence or non-maleficence trump and have absolute priority over autonomy. This could than be used to deny stopping to anybody. In reality one has to give different weight to these principles in different circumstances. A hasty, irrational decision to stop because of temporary physical, or psychological, or social problems, can be over-ridden as described by Kaye (64, 65). One lets beneficence carry the day. On the other hand, a mature decision by an aged patient with multiple illnesses, or untreatable pain, or a decline in dignity, must be respected and thus autonomy over-rides beneficence and non-maleficence.

Practical approach

As discussed, the first duty of a physician is to establish an ethical framework to deal with stopping. Once the question is brought to the fore, a number of practical considerations are necessary. A practical approach to stopping is outlined in the second half of Table 10.2. The circumstances that need to be considered are:

1. Is the patient competent?
2. Does he/she have temporary and physical stress that should be over-ridden due to its temporary nature, a necessary but ethically difficult and risky undertaking (64, 65).
3. If the patient is incompetent, is it clear who the decision-maker is, and are all involved present, or is there an important family member not there?

A conference involving nurses, social workers, and family members, is necessary on behalf of the incompetent patient. It is important to involve social workers, who almost always know most of the family members and family dynamics, and they are usually the best ones to ferret out the dissenter that has difficulties in dealing with stopping dialysis. It has been cynically stated that the force with which relatives demand unnecessary or harmful treatment is directly proportional to the distance between that member and the patient. Physicians must ask: are the medical aspects in the case fully known? Why does the patient want to stop? Is it truly the best solution in a situation where all options are so poor? The decision should never be one of an emergency, but one of deliberation. Being pushed into a hasty stopping is never a good thing, as it almost assures an unnecessary stress level in the final and crucial decision process, as well as potential long-term questioning of the decision made.

Care of the dying patient after stopping RRT

The most thorough analyses of what happens to a patient after stopping RRT are those by Cohen and his team (66–70). They grade the quality of death according to three factors: the presence of pain and discomfort, the presence of support by family and loved ones, and the time it takes to die. Out of approximately 150 patients followed prospectively by Cohen and his co-workers, 75% of the deaths were graded by the above factors as very good or good; about 25% were regarded as bad. It is sad to notice that pain was present in 42% of the patients after they had stopped dialysis. Pain management is often not well handled in the acute-care hospitals where most of these patients are. The duties are crystal clear: we must prevent pain, nausea, vomiting, diarrhea, and other sources of discomfort. Therefore, pain medication should be timed, not given only when pain occurs, and not dictated by our fear of 'giving too much' medication based on fear of addiction, etc. We can combat loneliness and a sense of abandonment in the final hour of need. Visiting patients, which admittedly can be an uncomfortable and scary duty of physicians, is greatly appreciated by patients and relatives, and makes for a sense of better care, compassion, and empathy, and dispels much loneliness (71).

One need not fear metaphysical and impossible discussions about the existence of God, the meaning of life, and the presence of Hell, and so forth. My personal experience, based on many such cases, is that this never comes up. Patients discuss it with family and spiritual advisors, not their physicians. Patients' conversations with physicians are neutral, about such things as weather, or expressing pride in past accomplishments or family members. Visit often and follow through carefully with questions about nausea, shortness of breath, and other problems. Stop all diagnostic tests, such as potassium measurement, and unnecessary uncomfortable therapy, such as phosphate binders. If the patient develops incipient pulmonary edema, perform ultra-filtration *without* dialysis. Through these measures, a physician can help both with the physical dimension of preventing discomfort and the psychological dimension of being present and supporting. Family members should also be encouraged to be there often, and there should be no restrictions to their visits. Comfortable lounge chairs for sleeping and permission for relatives to stay the night are important to remember.

Cohen and his co-workers also found that patients who died in hospices or homes, always had a better death than those who died in the hospital. Therefore, going home or to a hospice should be encouraged and appropriate support arranged.

The duration of death has been studied by several authors, all showing the same results: death as a mean occurs 8–10 days after the last dialysis (56) (Fig. 10.5). There are some patients that live for several weeks after stopping. This brings up the question of shortening the patient's dying period actively by hypnotics, muscle relaxants, and IV potassium; assisted suicide as advocated by Dr Kevorkian (72). The debate over actively helping a patient to pass away continues to rage in most places. However, it is allowed by legislation only in a few places, such as Bolivia, Switzerland, and the state of Oregon. Like the debate over abortion rights, this question is presently hopelessly stuck in irrevocable positions, and there is no immediate or universal solution available (55, 73, 74).

For the future

For a better future, physicians and others involved with the care of patients with end-stage renal disease, have many obligations. The first is to stand up for their patients and seek out opportunities to ensure funds so that all patients needing care can receive it.

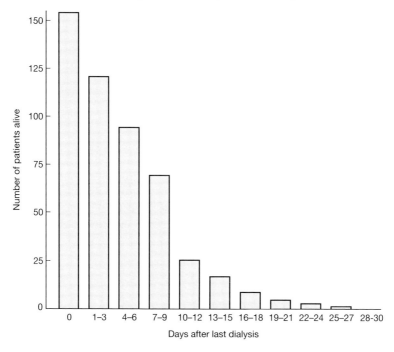

Fig. 10.5 Number of patients alive out of 155 after stopping dialysis. As a mean, death occurs 8 days after stopping dialysis, but a few patients will live for 3 or 4 weeks after stopping. There is no known formula to pin-point these patients that live for a long time after their last dialysis. Families of patients should be aware of these rare occurrences.

One must bravely face the pressure from powerful special interests in the form of politicians, bureaucrats, and competing financial temptations.

Until that goal has been achieved, we must ensure that a system of justice and accountability to humane standards is upheld, which will help us make just decisions in distributing the too few treatment opportunities. We must guard against unhappy choices based on forces that promote inadequate medical management in order to make a profit.

When dealing with stopping dialysis, we all have the duty of learning how to prevent it when humanely that is best, and to learn how to smooth the avenues of death when stopping is the best alternative. We all must try to contribute to an impartial debate. The goals are to formulate an acceptable and workable ethical framework, to decide what the patient's religious belief supports, and to make sure that pain, discomfort, and loneliness is never visited upon the dying patient.

The patient's responsibility is to give advance directives. These should be simple and state what the patient wants done, if they are no longer in charge. They should specify whom they trust to make decisions, and with what leeway such decisions should be made. Finally, what factors are important to those involved? Religious beliefs? Hope of other treatment? Their idea of dignity? Financial considerations?

We can assist patients and their loved ones greatly in experiencing the last days of life, not as a final tempest, but in tranquility, dignity, and often also, some somber joy. As physicians, it is not only the responsibility of participating in a patients death, but also a privilege entrusted in us by our patients to help them transition comfortably into the final hours of life.

References

1. Kjellstrand, C. (1996). High technology medicine and the old, the dialysis example. *J Intern Medicine*, **239**, 195–210.
2. Darrah, J.B. (1987). The committee. *Trans Am Soc Artif Intern Organs*, **33**, 791–3.
3. Kjellstrand, C. (1997). All elderly patients should be offered dialysis. *Geriatric Nephrol Urol*, **6**, 129–36.
4. Excerpts from the United States Renal Data System (1999). Annual data report. *Am J Kid Dis* 1999, **34**(2), (Suppl. 1), pp. S1–S176.
5. *Report, Vol. 1, Dialysis and Renal Transplantation, Canadian Organ Replacement Register* (1999). Canadian Institute for Health Information, Ottawa, Ontario.
6. *ANZDATA Registry Report* (1999). Australia and New Zealand Dialysis and Transplant Registry, Adelaide, South Australia.
7. Shinzato, T., Nakai, S., Akiba, T., Yamagami, S., Yamazaki, C., Kitaoka, T. *et al.* (1999). Report on the annual statistical survey of the Japanese Society for Dialysis Therapy in 1996. *Kid Inter*, **55**, 700–12.
8. Kjellstrand, C.M. and Logan, G. (1987). Racial, sexual and age inequalities in chronic dialysis. *Nephron*, **45**, 257–63.
9. Kjellstrand, C.M. (1988). Racial, sexual and age inequalities in renal transplantation. *Arch Intern Med*, **148**, 1305–9.
10. Kjellstrand, C.M. and Tyden, G. (1988). Inequalities in dialysis and transplantation in Sweden. *Acta Med Scand*, **224**, 149–56.
11. Kjellstrand, C.M. and Hasinoff, D. (1993). Exclusion of old patients from dialysis in Sweden, Canada and USA. In *Nephrology and Urology in the Aged Patient*, (eds. Oreopoulos, D.G., Michelis, M.F., Herschors, S.) pp. 569–84. Kluwer Academic Publishers, Dordrecht.
12. Kjellstrand, C.M. (1988). Giving life-giving death. Ethical problems with high technology medicine. Ph.D. thesis. Karolinski Institute, Stockholm. *Acta Medica Scandinavica*, (Suppl. 725), pp. 1–126
13. Kjellstrand, C.M. and Dossetor, J. (1992). *Ethical Problems in Dialysis and Transplantation*. Kluwer Academic Publishers, Boston.
14. Hellerstedt, W.L., Johnson, W.J., Ascher, N., Kjellstrand, C.M., Knutson, R., Shapiro, F.L. *et al.* (1984). Survival rates of 2728 end-stage renal disease patient. *Mayo Clinic Proc*, **59**, 776–83.
15. Theorell, T., Konarski-Svensson, J.K., Ahlmen, J., and Perski, A. (1991). The role of paid work in Swedish chronic dialysis patients—a nation-wide survey, paid work and dialysis. *J Intern Med*, **230**, 501–9.
16. Moody, H., Moody, C., Szabo, E., and Kjellstrand, C.M. (1992). Are old dialysis patients happy, and can they fend for themselves? *Abstr ASAIO*, **39**, 54.
17. Auer, J., Gokal, R., Stour, J.P., Hillier, V.G., Kincey, J., Simon, L.G. *et al.* (1990). The Oxford–Manchester study of dialysis patients. *Scand J Urol Nephrol*, **131**, (Suppl.), 31–7.

18. Westlie, L., Umen, A., Nestrud, S., and Kjellstrand, C. (1984). Mortality, morbidity, and life satisfaction in the old dialysis patient. *Trans Am Soc Artif Intern Org*, **30**, 21–0.

19. Kjellstrand, C., Kovitavongs, C., and Szabo, E. (1998). On the success, cost and efficiency of modern medicine—an international comparison. *J Intern Med*, **243**, 3–14.

20. Collins, A.M.D. (2000). *Director Coordination Center USRDS*. Lecture Nephrology Renal Administrators Association.

21. Berlyne, G.M. (1982). Over 50 and uremic-death. The failure of the British Health Service to provide adequate dialysis facilities. *Nephron*, **31**, 189–90.

22. Berlyne, G.M. (1985). The British dialysis tragedy revisited. *Nephron*, **41**, 305–6.

23. Medical Services Study Group of the Royal College of Physicians (1981). Deaths from chronic renal failure under the age of 50. *Br Med J*, **283**, 283–6.

24. Kjellstrand, C.M. and Moody, H. (1994). Hemodialysis in Canada—a first class medical crisis. *Can Med Assoc J*, **150**, 1067–71.

25. Challah, S., Wing, A.J., Bauer, R., Morris, R.W., and Schroeder, S.A. (1984). Negative selection of patients for dialysis and transplantation in the United Kingdom. *Br Med J*, **288**, 1119–22.

26. Anonymous (1981). Audit in renal failure, the wrong targets? (Editorial). *Br Med J*, **283**, 261–2.

27. Barrett, B., Parfrey, P., Morgan, J., Barre, P., Fine, A., Goldstein, M. *et al.* (1997). Predictions of early death in endstage renal disease patients starting dialysis. *Am J Kidney Diseases*, **29**, 214–22.

28. Bajwa, K., Szabo, E., and Kjellstrand, C. (1996). Stopping dialysis: a prospective study of risk factors and decision making in stopping dialysis. *Arch Intern Med*, **156**, 2571–7.

29. Rosa, A.A., Fryd, D.S., and Kjellstrand, C.M. (1980). Dialysis symptoms and stabilization in long-term dialysis, practical application of the CUSUM plot. *Arch Intern Med*, **140**, 804–7.

30. Held, P.J., Pauly, M.V., and Diamond, L. (1987). Survival analysis of patients under going dialysis. *JAMA*, **257**, 645–50.

31. Plough, A., Salem, S., Shwartz, M., Weller, J., and Ferguson, W. (1984). Case mix in end-stage renal disease. Differences between patients in hospital-based and free-standing treatment facilities. *N Eng J Med*, **310**, 1432–6.

32. Schlesinger, M., Clearly, P., and Blumenthal, D. (1989). The ownership of health facilities and clinical decision making, The case of the ESRD industry. *Med Care*, **2**, 244–57.

33. Delmez, J.A. and Windus, D.W. (1992). Hemodialysis prescription and delivery in a metropolitan community. *Kid Int*, **42**, 1023–8.

34. Collins, A.J., Ma, J.Z., Constantini, E.G., and Everson, S.E. (1998). Dialysis units and patient characteristics associated with reuse practices and mortality, 1989–1993. *J Am Soc Nephrol*, **9**, 2108–17.

35. Garg, P., Frick, K., Diener-West, M., and Powe, N. (1999). Effect of the ownership of dialysis facilities on patients' survival and referral for transplantation. *N Engl J Med*, **341**, 1653–60.

36. Ayanian, J., Clearly, P., Weissman, J., and Epstein, A. (1999). The effect of patients' on racial differences in access to renal transplantation. *N Engl J Med*, **341**, 1661–9.

37. Levinsky, N.G. (1999). Quality and equity in dialysis and renal transplantation. *N Engl J Med*, **341**, 1691–3.

38. Kjellstrand, C.M., Lins, L.E., Ericson, F., Traeneus, A., and Noree, L.O. (1989). On the wish for renal transplantation. *Transactions ASAIO*, **35**, 619–21.

39. Held, P.J., Pauly, N.V., Bovbjerg, R.R., Newmann, J., and Salvatierra, O. Jr. (1988). Access to kidney transplantation. Has the United States eliminated income and racial differences? *Arch Intern Med*, **148**, 2594–600.

40. Gridelli, B. and Remuzzi, G. (2000). Stategies for making more organs available for transplantation. *New Engl J Med*, **343**, 404–10.

41. Haruki, S. (1998). *Psychological and Psychiatric Aspects of Renal Transplantation between Spouses in Japan—from the Point of View of the Consultation Psychiatrist.* Lecture International Psycho-Nephrology Conference, New York.

42. Singh, P., Kumar, A., Bhandari, M., Sharma, R.K., and Gupta, A. (2000). *Kidney Donation From Wives, an Exploitation or Social Complusion.* The XIIth International Congress on Psychonephrology Abstracts Yokohama, Japan.

43. Zimmerman, D., Donnelly, S., Miller, J., Stewart, D., and Albert, S. (2000). Gender dispaity in living renal transplant donation. *Amer J Kid Disease*, **36**, 534–40.

44. Richards, J.R. (1992). From him that hath not. In *Ethical Problems in Dialysis and Transplantation* (eds. Carl M. Kjellstrand and John B. Dossetor), pp. 53–60. Kluwer Academic Publishers, Dordrecht, Boston, London.

45. Radcliffe-Richards, J., Daar, A.S., Guttmann, R.D., Hoffenberg, R., Kennedy, I., Lock, M., *et al.* (1998). The case for allowing kidney asales. *Lancet*, **351**, 1950–2.

46. Levinsky, N.G. (2000). Organ donation by unrelated donors. *New Engl J Med*, **343**, 430–2.

47. Matas, A.J., Garvey, C.A., Jacobs, C.L., and Kahn, J.P. (2000). Nondirected donations of kidneys from living donors. *New Engl J Med*, **343**, 433–6.

48. DeVecchi, F., Dratwa, M., and Wiedemann, M.E. (1999). Healthcare systems and end-stage renal disease (ESRD) therapies—an international review, costs and reimbursement/funding of ESRD therapies. *Nephrol Dial Transplant*, **14**, (Suppl. 6), 31–41.

49. Horl, W.H., de Alvaro, F., and Williams, P.F. (1999). Healthcare systems and end-stage renal disease (ESRD) therapies—an international review, access to ESRD treatments. *Nephrol Dial Transplant*, **14**, (Suppl. 6), 10–15.

50. Gurland, H.J. and Lysaght, M.J. (1993). Future trends in renal replacement therapy. *Artif Organs*, **17**, 267–71.

51. Sidel, V.W. (1995). The international arms trade and its impact on health. *Br Med J*, **311**, 1677–80.

52. Judd, F. (1995). Conflicts, famine and the arms trade. *Med War*, **11**, 99–104.

53. Feiffel, N.H. and Branscomb, A.B. (1973). Who's afraid of death? *J Abnorm Psychol*, **81**, 282–8.

54. Plough, A.L. and Salem, S. (1982). Social and contextual factors in the analysis of mortality in end-stage renal disease patients, implications for health policy. *Am J Public Health*, **72**, 1293–5.

55. Kjellstrand, C., Cranford, R., and Kaye, M. (1996). Stopping dialysis, practice and cultural, religious and legal aspects. In *Replacement of Renal Function by Dialysis*, (4th edn). (eds. J. Winchester, C. Jacobs, K. Koch, and C. Kjellstrand), pp. 1480–1501. Kluwer Academic Publishers, The Netherlands.

56. Neu, S. and Kjellstrand, C.M. (1986). Stopping longterm dialysis. an empirical study of withdrawal of life supporting treatment. *New Engl J Med*, **314**, 14–20.

57. Husebye, D. and Kjellstrand, C.M. (1987). Denial of and withdrawal from dialysis in the old. *Int J Art Organs*, **10**, 166–172.

58. Roberts, J. and Kjellstrand, C.M. (1988). Choosing death, withdrawal without medical reason from chronic dialysis. *Acta Med Scand*, **223**, 181–6.

59. Kjellstrand, C. (1993). Stopping dialysis—different views. In *Nephrology and Urology in the Aged Patients* (eds. D. Orcopolous, M. Michelis, and S. Herschorn), pp.563–8. Kluwer Academic Publishers, Dordrecht.

60. Port, F.K., Wolfe, R.A., Hawthrone, V.M., and Ferguson, C.W. (1989). Discontinuation of dialysis therapy as a cause of death. *Am J Nephrol*, **9**, 145–9.

61. Rothenberg, L.S. (1992). Withholding and withdrawing dialysis form elderly ESRD patients, Part 1: A historical view of the clinical experience. *Geri Neph Urol*, **2**, 109–17.
62. Rothenberg, L.S. (1993). Withholding and withdrawing dialysis from the elderly ESRD patients, Part 2: Ethical and policy issues. *Geri Neph Urol*, **3**, 23–41.
63. Nelson, C.B., Port, F.K., Wolfe, R.A., and Guire, K.E. (1994). The association of diabetic status, age, and race to withdrawal from dialysis. *J Am Soc Nephrol*, **4**, 1608–14.
64. Kaye, M., Bourgouin, P., and Low, G. (1987). Physicians' non-compliance with patients' refusal of life-sustaining treatment. *Am J Nephrol*, **7**, 304–12.
65. Kaye, M. and Lella, J.W. (1986). Discontinuation of dialysis therapy in the demented patient. *Am J Nephrol*, **6**, 75–9.
66. Cohen, L.M., Germain, M., Woods, A., Gilman, E.D., and McCue, J.D. (1993). Patient attitudes and psychological considerations in dialysis discontinuation. *Psychosomatics*, **34**, 395–401.
67. Cohen, L.M., McCue, J.D., Germain, M., and Kjellstrand, C.M. (1995). Dialysis discontinuation. A 'good' death? *Arch Intern Med*, **155**, 42–7.
68. Cohen, L.M., McCue, J.D., Germain, M., and Woods, A. (1997). Denying the dying. Advance directives and dialysis discontinuation. *Psychosomatics*, **38**, 27–34.
69. Cohen, L.M., Fischel, S., Germain, M., Woods, A., Braden, G.L., and McCue, J. (1996). Ambivalence and dialysis discontinuation. *Gen Hosp Psychiatry*, **18**, 431–5.
70. Cohen, L.M., Germain, M., Poppel, D.M., Woods, A., and Kjellstrand, C.M. (2000). Dialysis discontinuation and palliative care. *Am J Kid Dis*, **36**, 140–4.
71. Larson, D.G. and Tobin, D.R. (2000). End-of-life conversations—evolving practice and theory. *JAMA*, **284**, 1573–8.
72. Cohen, L.M., Steinberg, M.D., Hails, K.C., Dobscha, S.K., and Fischel, S.V. (2000). Psychiatric evaluation of death-hastening requests. Lessons from dialysis discontinuation. *Psychosomatics*, **41**, 195–203.
73. Kevorkian, J. (1988). The last fearsome taboo, medical aspects of planned death. *Med Law*, **7**, 1–14.
74. Wilson, K.G., Viola, R.A., Scott, J.F., and Chater, S. (1998). Talking to the terminally ill about euthanasia and physician assisted suicide. *Can J Clin Med*, **5**, 68–74.

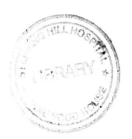

11

Treatment strategies for end–stage renal failure in developing countries

Alex M. Davison, Rashad Barsoum, Kar Neng Lai, M.K. Mani, Zaki Morad, and Boleslaw Rutkowski

Introduction

Hemodialysis was first introduced for the treatment of acute renal failure but it soon became obvious that a number of patients did not have a satisfactory return of renal function and so the clinician was faced with the decision of stopping further dialysis or finding a satisfactory method of providing long-term therapy. In addition, it also became obvious that treatment suitable for acute renal failure could be applied to patients with end-stage irreversible renal failure. The major obstacle to overcome was the development of a means of achieving repeated vascular access and, had it not been for the Teflon–silastic® shunt, and subsequently the subcutaneous arteriovenous fistula, it is doubtful whether long-term hemodialysis would ever have become a viable long-term treatment. The remarkable success of dialysis is now obvious, with more than one million people world-wide depending on dialysis for survival. This success, however, is not enjoyed with equity around the world because of the cost-implications of providing such treatment and the differing healthcare priorities that exist in the various communities of the world.

The pattern of diseases encountered has marked geographical variation around the world. In developed countries, the major emphasis is on degenerative diseases and conditions associated with affluence, such as diabetes mellitus, and cardiovascular diseases, such as hypertension, coronary artery disease, and peripheral vascular atherosclerosis. In the developing world, infectious diseases and nutritional problems are of much greater importance. This presents a problem for those involved in the allocation of scarce resources for healthcare, where it is of paramount interest to ensure that the finances available obtain the maximum benefit for the community. In the developed countries, there is an increasing awareness that in treating end-stage renal failure a small number of patients consume a significant share of the allocated financial resource; in Europe 1–1.9% of the healthcare budget is allocated to the 0.005% of the population who have end-stage renal failure. The annual increase in the number of patients receiving dialysis in Europe, Japan, and North America is in the region of 7–10% and it is difficult to see how this can be sustained at this rate of growth, which results in a doubling of the dialysis population every 7–8 years. There is, at present, no indication that the number of patients on dialysis therapies is stabilizing in developed countries, and this is because of a number of different factors. Survival on dialysis is increasing due to greater experience, better equipment (both machines and dialyzers), and an increased awareness of the complications of uremia, coupled with therapeutic advances such as the introduction of erythropoietin to relieve anemia and alfacalcidiol to maintain calcium homeostasis. In addition, greater experience and improved technology have resulted in dialysis is being offered to more and more elderly people. Finally, the number of patients undergoing successful cadaveric transplantation is not increasing in proportion to the increase in the dialysis population. In several Western European countries, the number of cadaveric renal donors has declined by approximately 20% in the last ten years due to a decline in the number of fatal road traffic accidents and improvements in the rapid diagnosis of intracerebral vascular events. In spite of optimistic predictions, it would appear that the provision of organs for transplantation, by either xenotransplantation or cloning, remains a hope rather than an expectation for the foreseeable future. Although it is well-recognized that prevention is better than cure, it is unlikely that any non-specific preventive measures will have an impact on the requirement for renal replacement therapy for many years. It would seem, therefore, that dialysis, either hemodialysis or some form of peritoneal dialysis, will remain for some time the only treatment option available to the majority of patients with end-stage renal failure.

Internationally, there are wide differences in the way that communities are provided with treatment for end-stage renal failure. The reasons for this are diverse and are sometimes difficult to understand. A major factor is finance, but in addition there are other variables such as the availability of consumables (e.g. CAPD fluids). This chapter explores the situation in a number of geographical areas: Central and Eastern Europe, where in the last ten years there has been dramatic changes; Africa and India, where the scale of the problem is considerable and other healthcare needs are pressing; Malaysia, which has experienced unprecedented growth followed by a serious economic downturn; and the Asian Pacific countries, with particular reference to Hong Kong.

Causes for differences in practice in renal replacement therapy

The incidence of end-stage renal failure in Europe is in the region of 100–120 pmp/year and it is recognized that the incidence in the developing world may be in excess of twice this number. The prevalence of patients on renal replacement programs in Europe, Japan, and North America increases at about 7–10% each year. It is interesting to note the diversity of practice that exists from country to country, and between the industrialized and developing world. It would appear that each community has evolved its own particular practice, and although it is tempting to compare, and as a consequence criticize, it is a fruitless exercise unless a very comprehensive evaluation is undertaken to understand all the factors influencing the provision and development of a particular service.

Almost every country has evolved an unique response to providing renal replacement therapy. Economic factors seem to be the major influence in the provision of an end-stage renal failure program. It has been estimated that world-wide there are more than 500 000 cases of incident end-stage renal disease annually, and that more than 75% of these occur in the Third World (1). The provision of healthcare in any community is dependent upon the wealth of the nation (2) and, in both the developed and developing world, there is a close correlation between the number of patients sustained on a renal replacement program and the gross national product (3). However, the economic state of a country is not the only factor to play an important role, because, even in industrialized nations, there are marked differences in practice (4).

In Scandinavian countries, for example, there is considerable reliance placed on transplantation, particularly from related donors; whereas transplantation is less common in countries such as Italy, and in Japan the contribution of transplantation is virtually zero. Dialysis regimens also vary from country to country, with total treatment times being generally less in the United States of America when compared to Europe. The contribution of CAPD is greater in the United Kingdom than almost any other country. These wide divergencies and practice are not easy to explain, and are clearly multi-factorial. In considering options in renal replacement therapy, the management plan for any particular patient will depend on available resources and local expertise. The over-riding principle must be to make the best use of the available resource to the maximum benefit of as many patients as possible. Choices have to be made because it is highly unlikely that any society will ever be able to finance the treatment of all patients with uremia without some restrictions.

Central and Eastern Europe

Current status and prospect for renal replacement therapies.

Historical background

Central and Eastern Europe consists of 19 very heterogenic countries, in which important differences exist—not only in population, country area, and ethnic groups, but also, what is more important, in economic development. There is one common denominator—after the Second World War, all became members of the so-called Socialistic Bloc. For more than fifty years they were affected by a very inefficient economic system and expenditure on health was very low. Nevertheless, even in this field there were important differences between countries, e.g. the situation was much better in the former Yugoslavia, much worse in the former Soviet Union, and intermediate in such countries as Hungary and Poland. These differences affected the care of patients with ESRF and the development of renal replacement therapy (RRT) programs (5, 6). In former Yugoslavia, where some elements of a free market economy were present, development of dialysis therapy was satisfactory and comparable to many Western European countries. It was moderate in former Czechoslovakia and Hungary, less satisfactory in such countries as Poland and Bulgaria, and very bad in

Romania and Albania (5, 7). Information about RRT in the Soviet Union was considered as strictly secret and thus details are not available for international comparisons; but from personal observations it was quite obvious that the situation of ESRF patients was tragic in this huge and very potent country. In 1989–90, the political and economic liberation of the countries located in this region took place, starting in Poland with the Solidarity Movement and expanding throughout the whole of Central and Eastern Europe. As a result of these movements, a number of new countries gained independence following the dissolution of the Soviet Union and disintegration of former Yugoslavia. Economic differences and difficulties in many became more visible, with the introduction of democracy and an open information policy. On the other hand, the economic situation of some of the countries in Central and Eastern Europe became worse as a result of intrinsic or ethnic conflicts. Those located on the Balkan Peninsula, such as Yugoslavia, Macedonia, and Croatia, were deeply affected by these disturbances. These trends are clearly visible in Fig. 11.1, where information concerning gross domestic product (GDP) in US $ per capita and annual health expenditure

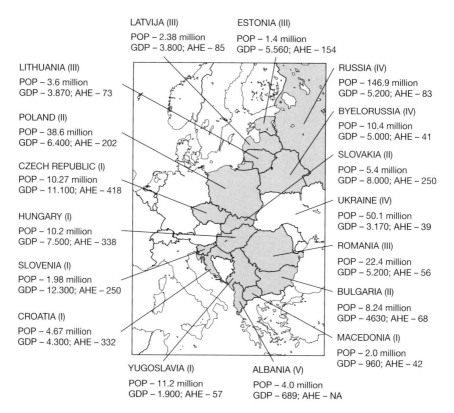

LATVIJA (III)
POP – 2.38 million
GDP – 3.800; AHE – 85

ESTONIA (III)
POP – 1.4 million
GDP – 5.560; AHE – 154

LITHUANIA (III)
POP – 3.6 million
GDP – 3.870; AHE – 73

POLAND (II)
POP – 38.6 million
GDP – 6.400; AHE – 202

CZECH REPUBLIC (I)
POP – 10.27 million
GDP – 11.100; AHE – 418

HUNGARY (I)
POP – 10.2 million
GDP – 7.500; AHE – 338

SLOVENIA (I)
POP – 1.98 million
GDP – 12.300; AHE – 250

CROATIA (I)
POP – 4.67 million
GDP – 4.300; AHE – 332

RUSSIA (IV)
POP – 146.9 million
GDP – 5.200; AHE – 83

BYELORUSSIA (IV)
POP – 10.4 million
GDP – 5.000; AHE – 41

SLOVAKIA (II)
POP – 5.4 million
GDP – 8.000; AHE – 250

UKRAINE (IV)
POP – 50.1 million
GDP – 3.170; AHE – 39

ROMANIA (III)
POP – 22.4 million
GDP – 5.200; AHE – 56

BULGARIA (II)
POP – 8.24 million
GDP – 4630; AHE – 68

MACEDONIA (I)
POP – 2.0 million
GDP – 960; AHE – 42

YUGOSLAVIA (I)
POP – 11.2 million
GDP – 1.900; AHE – 57

ALBANIA (V)
POP – 4.0 million
GDP – 689; AHE – NA

Fig. 11.1   Information concerning gross domestic product (GDP) in US $ per capita and annual health expenditure (AHE) per person for central and East European countries.

(AHE) per person is shown. However, RRT does not always correspond to the present economic situation.

Current status of renal replacement therapies (RRT)

At the end of the twentieth century, four groups of countries presenting with different levels of RRT development could be defined in the region of Central and Eastern Europe. The first group (I) consisted of six countries: Croatia, Slovenia, Czech Republic, Yugoslavia, Macedonia, and Hungary, with the highest rate of patients on RRT, over 400 per million population (pmp). Three other countries formed a second group (II) with an RRT rate of more than 200 but not exceeding 400 pmp (Slovakia, Bulgaria and Poland) and a third group (III) of four countries (Lithuania, Latvija, Estonia, and Romania) with a RRT rate between 100 and 200 pmp. Most tragic was the situation of patients with terminal renal failure in the fourth group (IV) of countries (Byelorussia and Russia), which treated less than 100 pmp. In the remaining countries, the situation of RRT is unknown because such information is not available at present. Nevertheless based on rare personal experiences one can determine that the Ukraine has to be located in the latter group, together with her yesterday hegemon—Russia. Additionally, members of an ERA-EDTA and ISN delegation found that in Albania RRT is practically non-existant despite, a small group of patients being dialyzed in one unique center in the capital—Tirania (7). The exact numbers characterized above are presented in Fig. 11.1 and Table 11.1.

Modality of treatment

Altogether, excluding Russia, Ukraine, and Albania, 38 860 patients were on RRT at the end of 1998 in 14 Central and Eastern European countries, which amounts to 296 pmp (together with Russia: 46 759 patients or 166 pmp). Of these, 78% were treated with different modalities of dialysis and 22% had a functioning graft.

Renal transplantation

Renal transplantation is a much cheaper treatment than any other form of maintenance dialysis. This economic factor has to be taken into account in this economically under-developed part of the world. The transplantation rate differs between countries: the percentage is lowest in Slovenia, Bulgaria, and Yugoslavia; intermediate in Russia, Croatia, Byelorussia, and Macedonia; good in the Czech Republic, Hungary, and Poland; and, surprisingly, best in Estonia, Latvija, and Lithuania. (Table 11.1). The very poor status of renal transplantation in the whole of the Balkan region is probably caused by a number of reasons, such as custom and religion, but also because of the impact of the lack of peace and domestic war. The number of transplant units has increased during the last decade significantly but the increase in renal transplantation has not been satisfactory, in view of the still increasing number of patients on the waiting-list. It is worth mentioning that renal transplantation is probably best-organized in the Czech Republic, where more than one-third of the patients on

Table 11.1 Status (1998) and development of the renal replacement (RRT) in Central and Eastern Europe

Country	Prevalence (pmp)		Incidence (pmp)	Modality (%)			Diabetic patients (%)	EPO treatment (%)	Development 1990–98 (%)	
	RRT	DT	DT	RT	HD	PD			Δ RRT	Δ DT
Bulgaria	298	287	80	9	87	4.0	7.4	50	58	49
Byelorussia	65	52	30	19	77.9	3.1	6.5	65	112	126
Croatia	643	522	102	20	76	4.0	9.5	40	13	50
Czech Republic	545	344	126	34	62.7	3.3	31	63	148	176
Estonia	157	65	54	58	21.4	20.6	NA	39	159	226
Hungary	439	307	128	30	67.8	2.2	7.4	79	273	228
Latvija	157	90	52	43	34.2	22.8	16.8	65	73	188
Lithuania	160	78	70	38	58.7	3.3	14	90	NA	105
Macedonia	461	427	60	17	82.1	0.9	11.3	19	NA	NA
Poland	252	178	52	30	61.8	8.2	11.7	69	164	194
Romania	139	127	40	9.4	79	11.6	8.3	30	913	835
Russia	53	41	NA	23	72.9	4.1	2.0	20	NA	NA
Slovakia	363	334	108	8	85.6	6.4	11	55	166	160
Slovenia*	571	500	110	13	77.1	9.9	11	63	39	51
Yugoslavia	435	399	108	9	76.4	14.6	10	15	40	39

RRT: renal replacement therapy; RT: renal transplantation; DT: dialysis therapy; HD: hemodialysis; PD: peritoneal dialysis; EPO: erythropoietin treatment; NA: Data not available; pmp: per million of population.
* Data available from 1997.

RRT are living with a functioning graft (201 pmp). On the other hand, despite all the economic and social disturbances after liberation from the Soviet Union, renal transplantation is also relatively well-developed in all three Baltic countries: Latvia, Estonia, and Lithuania (8, 9). In the majority of countries, the triple drug (cyclosporin, azathioprine, and corticosteroids) immunosuppressive regime is used, and long-term results are comparable to those obtained in developed countries.

Dialysis therapy

The main advance observed in Central and Eastern European Countries is the availability of dialysis therapy. The most striking and spectacular increase in the number of dialyzed patients was achieved in Romania, despite very poor economic conditions (Fig. 11.1). Hungary, Poland, Czech Republic, and the Baltic countries, once again are among the states intensively developing their dialysis possibilities. In most of them the majority of patients are treated by hemodialysis as the basic modality but there is a significant increase in the number of patients treated with peritoneal dialysis, especially in the last few years. The progress achieved in hemodialysis has not only been quantitative but also has a qualitative dimension: most hemodialysis units are currently equipped with new and modern machines. Also, the number of units able to use such techniques as controlled ultrafiltration and sodium modeling, have recently increased dramatically. There are still differences in the technological possibilities among the countries in Central and Eastern European region, but, despite economic shortages in Bulgaria during the last three years, nearly all dialysis units are equipped with reliable water-treatment systems. This is a great achievement because, until 1996, nearly 85% of centers in that country used tap-water for hemodialysis (6). The introduction of modern hemodialysis machines, and step-by-step a wider choice of different, more biocompatible, dialyzers and concentrates, have permitted individualization of dialysis procedures.

For many years, peritoneal dialysis was almost non-existant as a dialysis modality in patients with ESRF in Central and Eastern Europe. Only small numbers of children, and a limited number of adult patients, were treated using this technique. During the past few years its use has increased dramatically (8). The availability of peritoneal dialysis differs among Central and Eastern European countries (Table 11.1) but the number of patients treated with this modality has increased in the whole region by 306%. It has to be noted that in some countries automated peritoneal dialysis (APD) has also been introduced. The most spectacular progress in peritoneal dialysis has occurred in Poland, where the number of patients on peritoneal dialysis has increased from 31 in 1990 to 795 in 1999 (2464% increase). Nearly 11% of adults, and most children, with ESRF are treated by peritoneal dialysis (6). Amongst adults, this modality is used mainly in diabetic patients, elderly people, and patients with cardiovascular instability. It is worth also mentioning that in Estonia and Latvija a striking development of the peritoneal dialysis program has been observed in the last few years (9) Nearly half of dialyzed patients in Estonia, and 40% in Latvija, are maintained using peritoneal dialysis. The situation is a little different in the third Baltic country—Lithuania, nevertheless, one has to remember that 4 years ago in this state only a few patients were treated using this modality, supported by charity organizations.A comprehensive program financed by a central budget started in 1998. A similar situation has been observed in Macedonia.

Development of RRT modalities in Russia is a very special issue. In 1999, for the first time, it was possible to collect reliable data concerning treatment possibilities for patients with ESRF. It became clear that ESRF care is still problematic in this huge and potent country, although within Russia the availability of RRT is not uniform. In the big, rich agglomerations, such as Moscow and St Petersburg, the situation of ESRF patients is much better than in the poor rural areas (8).

Erythropoietin availability

Erythropoietin is one of the important factors influencing the quality of life in ESRF patients. This important drug is available for nearly half of the ESRF patients in the region. However, the availability of erythropoietin always corresponds strictly with the economic situation of the country. Surprisingly, the greatest percentage of ESRF patients treated with erythropoietin is noted in Lithuania. A satisfactory situation is observed in Hungary, Poland, Czech Republic, and Slovenia, but in Yugoslavia, Russia, and Romania the situation is poor. At present there are differences in the dosage of erythropoietin between Central and Eastern Europe and more developed countries. The recently performed European Survey for Anemia Management (ESAM) has shown that the doses used in our region, and the predicted target hemoglobin, are slightly lower than in the rest of Europe.

Changes in ESRF epidemiology

In the majority of Central and Eastern European countries, RRT for many years was available mainly for patient with primary (i.e. non-systemic) renal diseases. There also existed age-limitations in the qualification of patients to any RRT modality. During the last decade, the number of patients with diabetic nephropathy is still increasing, despite different levels of RRT availability (8). The most dramatic increase was noted in the Czech Republic, but in Poland—and even in countries with lower acceptance rates, such as Romania or Byelorussia—a sharp increase was observed. Also the number of patients with hypertensive nephropathy has increased significantly in our region. It has to be underlined that a dramatic increase in the number of elderly ESRF patients has been observed in Central and Eastern Europe (Fig. 11.2). The most pronounced increase was noted in the Czech Republic. All these changes are in parallel with the observations in Western Europe, USA, and other developed parts of the world.

Future perspectives of RRT in Central and Eastern Europe

Further development of RRT possibilities will be strictly dependent on the economic progress of the individual countries. Nevertheless, the prognosis for the future is good in that all the positive changes mentioned above were achieved despite the existing economic constraints. Data presented in Fig. 11.3 show that the whole re-imbursement system is changing step by step in our region, with the increasing introduction of insurance systems, which are already well-developed in such countries as Slovenia, Czech Republic, Hungary, or Slovakia, but only started very recently in Poland, Estonia, Latvija, and Lithuania. Other countries, such as Bulgaria, Byelorussia, Yugoslavia, Macedonia, Romania, or Russia, are still waiting to change their whole healthcare system. Together with the introduction of insurance systems, partial privatization of dialysis units started in some countries a few years ago (Hungary, Czech Republic, Slovenia).

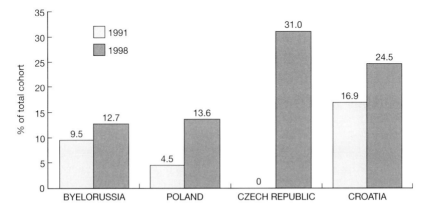

Fig. 11.2 Changes in the percentage of elderly patients being dialyzed in countries representing Central and Eastern Europe. Four levels of dialysis availability are shown: poor, Byelorussia; moderate, Poland; good, Croatia; very good, Czech Republic.

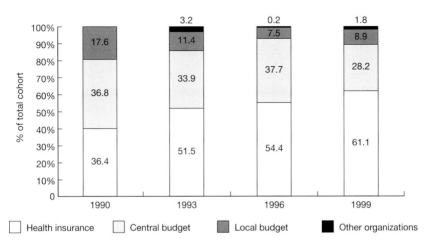

Fig. 11.3 Providers of the total re-imbursement budget for renal replacement therapy in Central and Eastern European countries.

There is a great probability that further spreading of privatization, with the introduction of necessary funds, will have a positive impact on the development of dialysis facilities (mainly hemodialysis), especially in countries with an established re-imbursement system. Hungary is a good example because hemodialysis units were privatized, with Euro Care, organized by the Braun Company, as the main investor. On the other hand, a slight but obvious decrease in CAPD patients in Hungary has been observed since privatization (8). Fresenius Medical Care is mostly involved in privatization procedures in the Czech Republic, Slovakia, and Slovenia. Other countries await their turn but stable and adequate re-imbursement systems are necessary to attract investment from industry. Even in Poland, where the economy appears to be relatively stable, the first private hemodialysis units started only in 1999, with a few developing in 2000. All have been organized by small local companies, the larger international companies are probably waiting for improvements in the economic conditions. Nevertheless, it is probably only a matter of time before these providers start having an important role in the privatization of dialysis services in Poland. In many countries in Central and Eastern Europe, the development of renal replacement therapies is based, not only on regional or local budgets but, on national government-funded programs. It will be an important issue to increase the awareness of local, regional, and central authorities to the problem of patients with end-stage renal failure through publicity and pressure from the whole nephrological community of patients and their staff. These measures are necessary for the further development of all modalities of renal replacement therapy, in order to achieve acceptance rates comparable to those of the developed world. It is clear that some countries have to focus attention on progress in renal transplantation (Slovenia, Yugoslavia, Macedonia, Croatia, Bulgaria) but there are countries where the development of all modalities in renal replacement are required (Byelorussia, Romania, Russia). Special effort from the international nephrological community will be required to improve renal replacement treatment in countries with a very poor economic situation, such as Albania and the Ukraine.

For the five countries mentioned above and for the Baltic States (Estonia, Latvija, Lithuania), the educational needs of the medical staff is particularly important. The programs organized by ERA-EDTA, EDTNA, ISN, and other international associations and institutions play a crucial role in the development of medical and nursing staff. In addition, participation in international congresses and symposia provide, for all nephrologists in the region, the opportunity of obtaining information regarding new technology and treatment strategies. Support from medical and pharmaceutical companies is essential. However, there are obvious differences between countries concerning access to these facilities. In 1999, nearly 70 nephrologists from Poland participated in the ERA-EDTA Congress, while many physicians from Russia were unable to take part in their National Nephrology Congress because of economic constraints. In the Czech Republic, Hungary, Slovakia, the Balkan Countries, and Poland, educational programs are part of postgraduate medical education. In Poland, parallel to the needs of developing dialysis facilities, an educational program has been intensified in recent years. Several professional courses and meetings have been organized, supported by scientific societies and by medical and pharmaceutical companies. In particular, a series of manuals has been prepared and edited for physicians, nurses, and patients. In the last decade, more than 200 physicians have completed specialist training in nephrology and, very recently, a special program of training in dialysis for nurses has been prepared.

It is worth mentioning that exchanges of expertise between different countries in our region is very important, especially for physicians from less-developed countries. Apart from updating medical and technical knowledge, it is of the utmost importance in guiding nephrologists on how to establish and realize successful programs of renal replacement therapy, even in unstable political and economic circumstances.

Africa

End-stage renal failure: epidemiology, management, and outlook

Humans made their first foot-steps in Africa. The heights, falls, and lakes of sub-Saharan Africa have witnessed the creation of *Homo sapiens*, as the final stage in the evolution of the animal kingdom. It must have been there and then that technology was born, in the form of the wheel (transport technology) and fire (energy technology). The know-how must have been dispersed all over the globe as successive generations of *Homo sapiens* migrated. Given the appropriate conditions, technology has developed to amazing horizons in Europe, America, and Japan, while certain remote areas in Africa remain with the wheel and fire. However, many African populations, privileged by better education, economy, or civilization, have no choice but to import technology with all its complexity and cost.

The result is frustrating, particularly when the technology in question relates to health. Taking end-stage renal disease management as an example, dialysis technology was introduced in many areas without adequate training leading to disastrous morbidity and mortality. The enormous expenditure on chronic dialysis encroached on the other much more important programs of prevention and primary care. Establishment of dialysis units and patient selection was often based on political rather than medical or social grounds, thereby raising serious questions about equity and justice.

The introduction of renal transplantation as a viable option resulted, surprisingly, in even more damage, owing to a lack of national policies in most African countries. Cadaveric transplantation, being unacceptable in most communities due to religious or social constraints, gave way to paid organ donation. In such communities, only the rich can afford to be treated; the poor being left with the scars of lumbar incisions. The social turmoil so generated is self-explanatory.

This socio-economic impact, however negative, must not over-ride the great potential benefits of adopting medical technology in the management of ESRD. If optimization is required elsewhere, its need in Africa is most pressing. Its meaning in this continent extends beyond technology, into organization, cost-effectiveness, and even social and political aspects. In order to address the issue of optimization, it is mandatory to understand the current situation in different African territories. For this purpose, I have chosen the 'KAP' methodology, referring to Knowledge, Attitude, and Practice.

Socio-geographical background

Africa is the second largest of the earth's seven continents, covering about 22% of the world's total land area. It may be divided into three major regions: the Northern Plateau, including the great African Sahara; the Central and Southern Plateau; and the Eastern Highlands.

About 12% of the world's population live in Africa. The Sahara serves as a dividing line between the peoples of northern Africa, mostly Caucasoid of Egyptian, Arab, and Berber origin constituting 25% of the total population, and those of sub-Saharan Africa, who are black Bantu-speaking peoples, constituting 70%. Pockets of Khoisan peoples are located in Southern Africa, and Pygmies in the Congo basin. Scattered throughout Africa, but primarily concentrated in Southern Africa, are some 5 million people of European descent. An Indian population, numbering some 1 million, is concentrated along the eastern coast and in Southern Africa. Within this broad classification, there are more than 3000 ethnic groups in Africa.

This unique background, and the resulting contrasts in political systems and national economies, explain the wide diversity in culture, heritage, disease prevalence, and standard of medical service in the continent, which are factors of direct relevance to the issue of renal replacement therapy.

Sources of information

It is hard to gather reliable information on renal disease in Africa, owing to the lack of adequate reporting systems. The information provided in this section has been assembled from the following sources:

1. *Registries*. There is a pan-African registry that belongs to AFRAN, the African Association of Nephrology. So far, this has been only concerned with members and dialysis units, but no patient data appear in either of its two published reports. The EDTA-ERA registry contains some information about certain countries in North Africa, but the data provided are incomplete and under-representative. The UNO and CTS registries provide some information on the transplant activity in Africa, but they also suffer similar problems. On the other hand, there are three fairly reliable national registries in Egypt, Tunisia, and South Africa, which constitute a major source of information for this review.

2. *Statistical series*. Reports appear from time to time in local or international periodicals or conferences about the breakdown of hospital admissions, outpatient visits, analysis of mortalities, or autopsy series. As many as possible of these reports were used to collect information about countries that do not have registries, particularly Kenya and Nigeria from English-speaking Africa and the Cote d'Ivoire and Burkina Faso from the French speaking territories.

3. *Personal communication*. A statistical questionnaire was sent out to about 50 leading renal physicians all over the continent. About one-third replied, providing more or less personal estimates about the prevalence and causes of renal diseases, as well as

of the available therapeutic modalities. This information has been used with caution, being unsupported by documented data.

Prevalence of renal disease

The reported prevalence of ESRD in Africa varies from 89 pmp in Kenya to 225 pmp in Egypt. Figures as low as 34 pmp have been reported in the Northwest, but this may represent an under-reporting error. Data about the annual incidence of new cases are lacking, but an old study based on the analysis of mortalities in Egypt suggests a figure of 192 pmp. The proximity of incidence to prevalence figures reflects the poor acceptance rate on renal replacement therapy, as well as the high mortality on dialysis.

Principal causes of renal failure

Glomerulonephritis remains the leading cause of chronic renal disease, with a general average of about 45%. Figures as low as 16.6% are reported in better-developed countries in the Northern Plateau, and as great as 58.4% in the Eastern Highlands. This seems to reflect the richness of the microbiological environment, including, for example, streptococcal infections of the skin (complicating scabies in Central and Eastern Africa), quartan malaria in the West, schistosomiasis and hepatitis C in the North, and hepatitis B in the South. Focal segmental glomerulosclerosis (23–34%) and proliferative glomerulonephritis (10–32%) are the most common histological types. Steroid-sensitive nephrotic syndrome is relatively rare, even in children (20–30% among black children).

Hypertensive nephrosclerosis is the major rival etiology. Its proportional contribution amounts to 28% in the Egyptian registry and even to 43% in a series from the Benin City, Nigeria. Figures around 25% are reported from many sub-Saharan countries. The South African registry suggests a figure of 15.9%, but also highlights the all-important aspect of ethnic susceptibility, whereby hypertensive nephrosclerosis was responsible for ESRD in 34.6% of blacks, 20.9% of coloured populations, 13.8% among Indians, and only 4.3% in whites. These data match with the known aggressive course of essential hypertension among African Americans, and with a local study in sub-Saharan Africa, that showed that 38.2% of black hypertensive patients ultimately develop renal failure.

Chronic interstitial nephritis comes next on the list, with a general average of about 15%. In Egypt, Tanzania, and Nigeria, schistosomal ureteric obstruction is the major cause (20–33% of all renal failures). Calcular obstruction is of considerable importance in the rural areas of most sub-Saharan Africa. The role of mycobacterial infections is prominent among the poor classes, and is further augmented with the epidemic dimensions that AIDS has attained among the blacks. The proportional contribution of chronic interstitial nephritis is increasing in many large African cities, where the tendency to industrialization is growing rapidly, which may reflect a significant role of occupational and environmental exposure to nephrotoxic agents.

Ochratoxin-associated interstitial disease has been sporadically reported in the rural areas of the Northern Plateau. The potential role of other toxins of plan origin remains obscure.

The role of diabetes mellitus is still marginal, usually accounting for less than 10% of renal failures in most series. Its contribution is increasing in more industrialized and urbanized areas, reaching almost 25% in a university hospital series in Egypt. This relatively low profile is due to the high prevalence of other causes of renal failure. Diabetes in Africa is as aggressive as elsewhere, as shown in a recent study from Zambia, where the overall prevalence of proteinuria among patients with type 2 diabetes was 23.8%. The same study has also shown that the course of overt diabetic nephropathy in blacks is notoriously progressive.

Other causes of chronic renal failure in Africa are not substantially different from those in the rest of the world. Amyloidosis remains fairly common, chronic suppuration and tuberculosis being the most common underlying causes. Schistosomiasis, kala-azar, hydatid disease, and familial mediterranean fever, are important etiologies. Sickle cell disease is a relatively common cause of glomerular disease in Northwest Africa and in the Eastern Highlands. Polycystic disease and other hereditary disorders account for less than 5% of cases.

Attitude

Although the incidence of ESRD in Africa is among the highest in the globe, the disease accounts for only 1–3% of the total mortalities. However, the availability of costly methods of treatment, and the moral issues that this raises with respect to priorities in healthcare, patient selection, changes in the conception of death, and the introduction of commercial organ transplantation, have made ESRD a topic of extensive public debate.

Four parties are involved in this controversy, namely the patients, their treating physicians, the health authorities, and the public.

Patients

As in other developing countries, the social stratification of people in Africa is too acute. On one end of the spectrum are the powerful. These include the rich, the politicians, the media leaders, and religious avant-garde. If they develop renal failure, they automatically have a top priority in dialysis and transplantation; they can afford five-star treatment in first-class private centers, and are able to buy the best-matching kidneys. If they are not satisfied, they can readily receive treatment overseas, where they can always find listening ears to their business language.

At the other end of the spectrum are the overwhelming majority of illiterate, extremely poor citizens, who receive their medical care by sangomas, magicians, and quacks. These patients may never find their way to proper renal replacement therapy, and often die unreported.

In all African countries, there is a varying proportion of middle-class citizens, who know, demand, and argue. It is this class that constitutes the motivating force in favor of adequate, candid, and affordable renal failure management. Any real advances towards optimization of ESRD therapy are directly proportionate to the size and effectiveness of this class in a particular country.

Physicians

As mentioned earlier, renal failure patients in Africa may never be referred to a renal physician. Even if they are, they are often taken care of by internists rather than nephrologists. Although the former may be quite efficient in clinical nephrology, their experience in renal replacement therapy is limited. Accordingly, they are not sufficiently motivated to claim budgets and equipment to deal with ESRD.

In less than half a dozen African countries, there are well-trained nephrologists, who implement state-of-the art technology to a minority of patients. The ability of these physicians to recruit adequate staff, equipment, and funding, largely depends on their political or social standing, rather than their patient data. Hence, a striking feature of African hospitals is the bizarre distribution of facilities, totally unrelated to patient load or staff abilities. Duplication of expensive equipment in neighboring capital hospitals is typical, while remote hospitals in heavily populated areas may be totally deprived of the simplest diagnostic or therapeutic facilities. Collaboration of influential physicians with industry may exceed ethical norms. Involvement of leading physicians in private practice, which is inevitable in view of the very modest fees they get from public hospitals, may color their practice with a commercial tinge.

Health authorities

The health budgets in most African countries are extremely limited, varying from 0.5% to 3% of the gross national income, which in turn is quite limited. Accordingly, the health authorities are usually frustrated between patients' and physicians' demands on one hand, and the necessity of fairly distributing the budget on the other. There is a lot to do in prevention and primary care programs, and in secondary care for more common diseases that are less expensive to treat. In fact, the decision to support ESRD management is, to a large extent, political rather than rational.

In an attempt to compromise, the health authorities tend to be too concerned with cost-containment, even at the expense of cost-effectiveness (see later). Experience from all over the world has shown that this attitude often leads to a disastrous increase in morbidity and mortality. When this happens, the blame falls on the treating physicians!

The public

As mentioned earlier, the propaganda propagated by different media has significantly magnified the size of ESRD as a health problem. Expectedly, the public reacted by fear, blame, and concern. The reaction to fear from acquiring the 'deadly' disease varies from panic to neglect to generous financial donation. Blame again falls to the physicians, who are unable to prevent or treat the disease with drugs, as well as on the health authorities that do not support active national treatment programs. The public is often concerned about the injustice of providing treatment to a selection of patients, and the social turmoil generated by the trade of organs. The average middle-class citizen is often suspicious about ulterior motives in changing the concepts of brain death that permit cadaver-donor transplantation, with all the current question marks about patient-selection criteria. It is always possible, in every religion, to find support for turning down the concept of brain death.

Practice

While acute dialysis is available in the majority of African capitals, regular dialysis is only sporadic. One can speak of renal replacement programs only in the Northern Plateau, South Africa, and Kenya. A few of those countries have a committed political system that takes population kinetics into their consideration while planning for ESRD management (*vide infra*).

Hemodialysis is the principal modality used for more than 90% of cases all over the continent. Intermittent peritoneal dialysis is used when the facilities for hemodialysis are not available. CAPD has, for long, stumbled due to the high incidence of infection, yet the newer techniques have encouraged an increasing number of centers to use it as a first choice in Egypt, Tunisia, and South Africa.

Basic dialysis machines are the core of hardware equipment. Locally constructed dialysis systems have been successfully implemented in Egypt and South Africa. The newer volumetric, variable sodium, bicarbonate-supporting systems are also available in the larger centers, particularly in private practice. Cellulose-based dialyzers are used routinely, though the African market share in synthetic membrane dialyzers is rapidly growing. Dialyzer re-use is common, though adequate precautions, as regards safety and efficiency, are limited. Re-use is illegal in Egypt. Water treatment is rather optional in many African countries, leading to a high prevalence of aluminium and other heavy metal intoxication. However, it is compulsory in the more developed countries.

Supportive treatment is often neglected by the physicians, as well as the patients, or is financially unaffordable when it comes to expensive medications as erythopoietin or alfacalcidol.

The mortality rate on regular hemodialysis remains high. In the few reliable reports, the average first-year mortality ranges from 35% to 50%, reflecting the late referral of patients. In subsequent years it ranges from 25% to 30%, reflecting dialysis inefficiency, toxicity, and associated morbidity. The question of efficiency has been addressed in several Egyptian studies that showed a considerable inter-center variation in favor of private dialysis, where the facilities are more optimal, the staff better motivated, and the medical and administrative supervision adequate. Expectedly, a close correlation was found between survival and the dose of dialysis, the number of weekly sessions as an independent factor, and the implementation of urea kinetic modeling for monitoring dialysis efficiency. The issue of toxicity with aluminium, copper, lead, and strontium has received attention as a cause of increased morbidity and even mortality in a number of African studies.

Co-morbidity is an important factor in the high mortality among regular dialysis patients. Many patients already have associated bacterial, viral, or parasitic infections at the start of dialysis therapy. Many others acquire such infections while on treatment, notorious being the hepatitis viruses. Hepatitis B (HBV), which used to be a major problem over the past decades, has now regressed in most units to less than 10% of patients. On the other hand, Hepatitis C (HCV) has increased dramatically, particularly in Egypt, where an average of 50% of patients have evidence of past or present infection. In some centers, the proportion of infected patients is almost 100%. It is interesting that neighboring countries, with similar socio-economic standards, have a much lower prevalence of HCV. The reason why Egyptians are so vulnerable is unclear, but a suggested symbiotic relation between the virus and schistosomiasis may have some relevance.

Despite all these limitations, regular dialysis poses an unbearable load on the national economy of countries where the service is offered free or partially subsidized. Patients in Egypt, Tunisia, South Africa, and other countries, may be fully covered by a national fund. However, private dialysis has emerged and flourished in those countries, attracting many patients by the better service and outcome. Patients treated in those centers are partially refunded.

Owing to technical and financial limitations, renal transplantation is even less accessible. It is available only in the North, Kenya, and South Africa. The Egyptian transplant pool is the largest in relation to the total inhabitants, accommodating about five patients per million population. Cadaver-donor transplants are most widely used in South Africa, but occasionally in the Northwest countries. Legal difficulties still hamper the transplant programs in many countries, particularly Egypt, where unrelated living-donor transplantation accounts for more than two-thirds of the pool.

Restriction of transplant activity to the larger centers has certainly helped to build a fair experience, that is reflected in the improved outcome. In most of the reported series, graft survival matches with international standards, particularly in the early years. Patient survival is a bit lower, owing to the increased infection-related mortality.

Suggested optimization strategy

Nothing in medical planning needs to be more regionally oriented than the development of an optimal strategy for managing ESRD. As shown in different chapters of this monograph, the focus for optimization is quite variable. While technical improvement and individual patient care are the main concerns in the developed world, national planning, cost-consciousness, and proper administration are the major foci in Africa. Within such an optimal system, technical and individual improvement becomes inevitable.

National planning

An accurate estimate of the ESRD population kinetics is essential for development of a national strategy. The best known method is the 'Stock-and-Flow' scheme adopted by the EDTA for several decades (Fig. 11.4). In essence, all patients who develop renal failure, as well as those who do not, will ultimately die! The different therapeutic modalities can only prolong their survival and/or improve their quality of life. These two are therefore the only objective parameters of success or failure, and they serve as the basic information upon which cost-effectiveness is calculated.

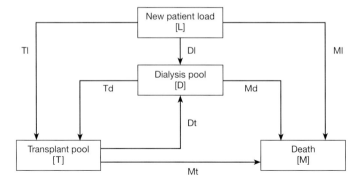

Fig. 11.4   Stock and flow population kinetic model. Upon reaching mathematical equilibrium, L must equal Ml + Md + Mt. With optimal healthcare development, Ml must be reduced to a negligible fraction, while the dialysis and transplant pools must be large enough to permit acceptable mortality rates (Md and Mt, respectively) to compensate. They have to grow even larger as experience improves and mortality rates decline. M: mortality; T: number of transplant patients; L: new patient load; T1: number of patients transplanted prior to dialysis; M1: number of patients dying prior to the start of end stage renal failure therapy; D1: number of patients commencing dialysis; Td: number of patients transplanted from dialysis; Md: number of patients dying on dialysis; Dt: number of patients returning to dialysis following transplantation.

Prevention

The Stock-and-Flow chart provides objective evidence that reduction of the new patient load (L) is the most effective way of handling the optimization issue. In addition to obvious individual health and productivity advantages, it permits keeping the dialysis (D) and transplant (T) 'stocks' within reasonable reach, and saves the available budgets for improving quality. It has been shown earlier on in this chapter that much can be done in preventing renal disease in Africa. It was shown that infection and hypertension are the major two ultimate causes of ESRD all over the continent. Control of bacterial and parasitic infection is underway in many countries. Most impressive results have been obtained with the malaria-eradication programs in Nigeria and Uganda, which were already rewarded by a sharp decline in the prevalence of glomerulonephritis. Schistosomiasis-control programs in Egypt have achieved a two-thirds reduction in the prevalence of the disease, and were associated with a remarkable decline in the contribution of related glomerulonephritis to dialysis unit admissions over the past 10 years. Similar experiences are expected with the control of scabies, and hepatitis B, and, hopefully not too long in the future, HCV.

Early detection and control of essential hypertension is the second cornerstone in reducing the incidence of ESRD. There are some logistic problems with early detection, including the vast rural communities that have their own 'medical' algorithms, and the heavily populated urban communities with their relative shortage of primary medical care. Here is an area where adequate national planning is needed.

Management of essential hypertension in the black population is a problem: they tend to respond poorly to beta blockers and ACE inhibitors; they often cannot afford the expense of continuous therapy with costly medications. Hence the high incidence of treatment non-compliance. Here is an area where well-planned clinical research can identify relatively inexpensive but effective medications, and where the media can help to spread the concept of persistent control of blood pressure.

Other preventable causes of renal failure in Africa include environmental pollution and the inappropriate use of certain medications. Adequate legislation and environmental control regulations should help in this respect.

Patient priorities

These have always been the most difficult questions to answer throughout the history of dialysis. Ideally, all patients should be given the same chance. When this is not possible, some selection takes place, either (inevitably) when there is no more space for new patients, or (deliberately) when there is a scheme of selection. Unfortunately, Africa, similar to other developing parts of the world, tolerates a lot of irregularities in keeping a rigid system of patient selection (*vide supra*). Here there is a place for national intervention through implementing a rigid and fair system by which free or subsidized treatment is offered only to patients who are most likely to benefit from renal replacement therapy. The spectrum can be very dynamic, shrinking or enlarging according to the available funds and facilities. Implementation of such a transparent system may restore the confidence of people in their health politicians, which would ultimately mirror on their willingness to co-operate, for example, in a national transplant program.

Modality priorities

Taking all factors into consideration, the ultimate goal in renal failure management in Africa should be renal transplantation. According to local experience, the median survival on dialysis is about 2 years, compared to 7 years following transplantation. Quality of life is much superior in transplanted patients. The absolute cost is comparable, but given the remarkable increase in survival, transplantation expenses are much more cost-effective.

However, transplantation needs an optimal set-up of knowledge, training, legislation, and modulation of public opinion and funding. If the choice is made, it should take many years to establish the proper medical and surgical teams, train technicians and nurses, and establish a reliable laboratory and imaging backup. It would need lengthy negotiations with opinion leaders, usually religious, to accept the concept of brain death, thereby paving the way for adequate legislation. During this period, there must be a relentless media campaign to convince the public to donate their organs. No large-scale national transplant program can be established without cadaver donors.

Although pre-emptive transplantation has proven its long-term benefits, it is difficult to accept it as a national choice while patients are accumulating in the dialysis pools waiting for the suitable donors. Dialysis will, therefore, remain as the cornerstone in any strategy for renal failure management. It may be the ultimate choice for patients who are unfit for transplantation.

The choice between hemodialysis and peritoneal dialysis is a difficult issue. It seems irrational that the latter is more expensive in Africa, as well as in most other developing countries that have to import the fluid. Furthermore, there are many questions about the efficiency of CAPD in the absence of appreciable residual renal function. The improper handling of the catheter, bags, and connections, often leads to recurrent peritonitis, which is an additional morbidity, costs money, and eventually destroys the peritoneum as a dialyzing surface. However, the Mexican experience is worth mentioning, where the local manufacture permitted the proportional contribution of CAPD to reach 90% of the total dialysis population with good clinical results. Additional advantages of CAPD must also be taken into consideration, and although hemodialysis remains the gold standard of life support in ESRD, technical improvements in CAPD practice will continue and will be eventually acquired in Africa. At present, staff training and adequate administration are more urgently needed.

Cost-consciousness

Cost-consciousness is of vital importance for the wide implementation of an ESRD treatment strategy, particularly in an underdeveloped community such as Africa. However, it is essential to understand that cost-consciousness is not a synonym of cost-containment. Although the issue of how much is spent is important, it is much more meaningful to weigh how much is gained for what has been spent. Unfortunately, health politicians are more concerned with cost-containment, and tend to disregard the true expenses of good dialysis (Table 11.2). Experience from all over the globe has shown that undue budget cuts inevitably increases morbidity and mortality on dialysis.

Physicians should be more interested in a specific aspect of cost, which is cost-efficiency. It is their duty to decide whether they need, or can effectively use, very highly sophisticated equipment. Does the performance of a synthetic compared to a cellulose-based dialyzer justify the difference in cost? Does re-use of dialyzers cut down the running expenses without undue encroachment on dialysis adequacy or introduction of new risk factors? Does every transplanted patient need expensive prophylactic anti-rejection therapy? The answer to all these questions, and many others, must vary from one community to the other, but they should be put on the table and considered in the light of objective evidence before claims are made to the health politicians for increasing funds.

Patients are interested in a third aspect of cost evaluation, namely cost–benefit. What they hope to see is that what is spent on whatever items must result in a better quality of life and improved survival. These outcomes are not only functions of technical performance. Indeed, making a patient feel better can cost very little, if adequate care is given to nutrition, control of anemia, acid–base balance, and bone problems. Care of dialysis patients tends to shift from physicians to nurses, which is acceptable

Table 11.2 Items of dialysis expenditure

Predialysis preparation	Dialysis procedure
Fistula	Supplies
Other temporary access	Dialyzers
Medications	Fistula needles
Auxiliary investigations	Dialysate concentrate,
Interdialytic medications	Disinfectants
Erythropoietin	Syringes, infusion sets, etc.
Active vitamin D	Infusions and medications
Anti-hypertensive medications	Gloves, towels, etc.
Aluminum chelators	Unit disinfection and sterilization
Other	Wages and insurance
Hospital admissions	Water treatment
Administrative and financial fees	Hardware depreciaton
Stocks	Maintenance
Transportation	Overhead expenses
Patient's absence from work	Secretarial work
	Administrative expenses

in the dialysis ward, but certainly not outside it. The role of interdialytic therapy on the patient's well-being is an integral part of dialysis therapy, which can only be fulfilled by the proper physician–patient interaction.

Administration

A national ESRD strategy must be planned, conducted, and audited by a comprehensive network, which includes physicians, nurses, technicians, psychiatrists, financial specialists, directors, politicians, and media representatives. Figure 11.5 shows a suggested scheme for providing a comprehensive administrative service, based on a three-level system: national, regional, and local. The national administrator should consider needs versus abilities, define patient and modality priorities, negotiate a re-embursement plan, organize a registration system, and supervise the performance audit. The regional administrator should be executive, taking care of the appropriate selection of renal unit locations, defining their size, staffing, equipment and supplies according to a general plan. Adequate designing at this level can avoid a lot of waste in terms of occupancy, staff-to-patient ratios, staff and patient transportation, and

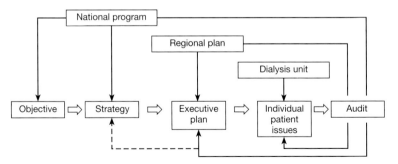

Fig. 11.5 Suggested scheme of the levels of planning for cost-conscious dialysis therapy.

may lead to better purchase bargains. Local renal unit administration should focus on individual patient issues. The unit's policy should be prospective and realistic, and should address the ultimate details with regards to the acceptable norms of consumption per dialysis session or transplant operation.

Summary

End-stage renal disease has a higher prevalence in Africa compared to most other parts of the world. The available experience, facilities, and funds do not permit adequate handling of this problem. A strategic national plan is suggested to optimize ESRD management in the continent, based on the mathematical model of 'Stock-and Flow' population kinetics. It was shown that prevention is the most effective strategy to deal with the problem. Fortunately, the two most common causes of renal failure, namely infection and hypertension, are either preventable or controllable. It was shown that renal transplantation should be the ultimate choice of therapy, on the basis of survival, quality of life, and cost–benefit. However, reaching this goal requires a lot of preparation concerning staff training, legislation, and modulation of public conceptions. Dialysis remains as the cornerstone of ESRD management. Although CAPD would have been the best alternative, cost, inefficiency, and complications still limit its widespread use in Africa. Organization of hemodialysis services is therefore mandatory at the present stage, as well as in the future. The current status shows a high mortality and morbidity due to inadequacy, toxicity, and co-morbidity, all of which are subject to technical improvement. What is even more important is to develop a cost-conscious national administration system that stratifies responsibilities into central, regional, and local, each with well-defined targets. An audit system would then integrate the activities of all levels. Emphasis should be to recognize the difference between cost-consciousness and cost-containment, and to focus on cost-efficiency and benefit. Excessive budget cuts are dangerous and defeat their objective by increasing the cost–benefit ratio. The physician's role is important in selecting appropriate equipment, and focusing on an adequate doctor–patient relationship, that can improve quality of life and reflect on the patient's perception of cost–benefit.

India

End-stage renal failure: socio-economic profile and management

India is a nation with in excess of one-thousand million people, the second most populous country in the world. It is also one of the poorest, with per capita income now at approximately $US225 a year. Just 1.3% of the population earns more than $US975 a year, and 37% of us lie below the poverty line, which has been drawn at $US32 a year. The bulk of our earnings goes to providing a bare minimum of food, shelter, and clothing. The average Indian cannot afford to pay for medical relief and depends on the Government to look after his/her health.

Facilities for medical care

Despite the abject poverty, the country has a tradition of learning and scholarship. Many medical colleges in the country are of a very high standard, and produce outstanding medical men and women. There are excellent hospitals, some run by the Government as teaching facilities for medical colleges, and many in the private sector. However, all of these are in cities, while 70% of the population lives in villages. The Government runs primary health centers (PHCs), each of which is staffed by two doctors and some preventive and social health workers. Each center has responsibility for a population of 25000. Medical care is provided free of charge; the patient pays for neither consultation nor medicines. The average expenditure of the State and Central Governments together per head of population per year amounts to $US3.20. This meagre sum covers immunization, family planning, water supply, and sanitation, in addition to the relief of illness. The budget for medicines works out to approximately 30 cents per person per year.

There is another problem in the delivery of medical relief. The PHC gives a week's supply of medicine at a time. Since every village has a population of around 3000, the majority of villagers have to travel some distance to reach the PHC—often a distance of 10 km. This is negligible in a city, but the villages often lack good roads and the sick villager must trek across the fields to see his doctor. Where a bus service is available, they lack the money to pay for it. A visit to the PHC takes at least half a day. For a laborer on daily wages, this means the loss of a day's income, and therefore he goes to the PHC only if his illness is such that he cannot work, and cannot earn a wage that day anyway. Chronic ailments are neglected by the patient, and there is no maintenance therapy. The PHC lacks laboratory facilities, and cannot diagnose renal failure. The best a well-informed doctor can do is to strongly suspect that it exists. Diagnostic aids are restricted to examination of the urine and a blood smear. The doctor could refer the patient to the nearest secondary health center for further investigation but it is unlikely that the patient will go there. While the hospital would be better equipped and could make the diagnosis, and might offer some treatment without cost, the patient would have to bear the cost of travel to the town, and the cost of their stay there. Given that 37% of Indians make less that 6 cents daily, and it might cost

36 cents to take the bus to town, and they rarely have that much money saved, then the vast majority of the rural poor, have no access to treatment. They take whatever the PHC can offer, or resort to practitioners of indigenous systems of medicine, of whom there are many in the villages.

Traditional systems of medicine are well developed. The ancient Indian science of health is called Ayurveda. Its weakness is that dissection of the body was not performed in ancient times, and knowledge of anatomy and physiology was rudimentary. On the other hand, the ancient Ayurvedic texts have excellent descriptions of disease, and there are many effective remedies, some of which, including *Rauwolfia serpentina*, have entered modern medicine. However, there are no remedies for renal diseases and the Indian villager with renal failure dies untreated. In the southern parts of India, the science of Sidda is practised, and a peculiarly Indian brand of homeopathy has developed all over the country. They have similar strengths and weaknesses.

Facilities for the treatment of renal failure vary from state to state. The eastern region and Central India lag behind in this respect. The Southern States have the best network of dialysis centers and trained nephrologists are available in many of the larger towns. Acute renal failure is well looked after, but the treatment of end-stage renal disease is not one of the priorities of the Government. Some of the leading medical colleges train nephrologists and run transplant programs to provide material for their students. These programs, like the rest of the work in the colleges, are free of cost to the patient, but even the busiest units can do no more than two transplants a month.

Most of the burden of end-stage renal disease is, therefore, borne by the private sector. There are a number of well-equipped private hospitals all over the country, many of which treat end-stage renal disease. Patients at these hospitals have to pay, and expensive treatment is beyond their means. However, State and Central Governments, the Armed Forces, and the Railways pay for treatment of their employees in private hospitals if their own hospitals lack the facilities, and many businesses offer similar care to their staff. This enables many from the lower economic strata to benefit.

The burden of renal disease in the community

There are no reliable statistics of disease prevalence or of causes of death, and it is thus necessary to rely on data from renal units, which can give the causes of end-stage renal disease but not the numbers in the community. Diabetic nephropathy is the most common, accounting for 30% of all chronic renal failure. The incidence of this disease is rising with the increase in diabetes associated with changes in the life-style and food habits of the people. Around 25% of patients have chronic interstitial nephritis, the cause of which has not been established, and 20% have chronic glomerulonephritis. About 10% each have hypertensive nephropathy and chronic pyelonephritis related to infections of the kidney. While there are no figures for the burden of renal failure in the community, it is known from some surveys that 10–15% of city dwellers have diabetes and a similar number have hypertension. In rural areas, 6% have hypertension and 4% diabetes. While the city dweller is likely to take some treatment, the villager neglects any chronic disease since they cannot go to the PHC every week to take medicine.

Renal transplantation

The average Indian nephrologist is trained in all modalities of treatment of ESRD. However, economic considerations make transplantation the first choice. A renal transplant costs around $US4875 including investigations of donor and recipient, around two months of dialysis, and surgery on both. Immunosuppression is usually with cyclosporin, azathioprine, and prednisolone, but many patients withdraw cyclosporin after the first year, and 35% in this author's program use only azathioprine and prednisolone. Azathioprine costs around $US245, and cyclosporin $US2450. There is no significant difference between results with cyclosporin and azathioprine in this author's related donor program.

Family ties in India are strong, and most patients are able to obtain a kidney from a related donor. Kidneys are accepted from the extended family, including second-degree relatives. However, the country actively promotes family planning, and the people are abjured to adhere to a one-child norm. The availability of related donors is, therefore, systematically being reduced, especially among the more educated classes who are likely to seek treatment for end-stage renal failure. A large number of poor are willing to donate a kidney for a consideration, and this has led to a thriving commercial unrelated-donor program. A personal objection to this type of transplant is that it exploits the poor, who are unaware of the value of their kidneys. The recipient takes cyclosporin, which costs $US2450 a year, but the donor of the kidney receives only $US500–750. The availability of a poor man's kidney militates against the development of a cadaver-kidney program, since the rich and influential are the ones who can afford to buy a kidney. If they could not buy a kidney, they would use their influence to motivate the public to accept the idea of donating organs after death.

Cadaver transplantation was permitted by the passage of the *Transplantation of Human Organs Act 1994*. This act also accepts the concept of brain death. Since that time, a few cadaver-donor renal transplants have been done, though by no means enough to satisfy the need. Government has been conspicuous by its inaction on this front. There has been no attempt to persuade members of the public to donate organs. One drawback of the Act is that it accepts the concept of an emotionally related donor. An Authorisation Committee appointed by the Government has to interview every patient and donor in such cases, to determine that the emotional relationship is genuine. Unfortunately, the committees have displayed a tendency to accept every such case uncritically, thereby permitting commercial unrelated-donor transplantation. The only difference from the days before the Act came into force, is that foreigners can no longer buy kidneys in India.

Despite the drawbacks, a few hospitals with a commitment to cadaver-organ donation have been able to perform a significant number of cadaveric renal transplants, and some cardiac and liver transplants as well. It is clear that the better informed the members of the family are, the more likely they are to donate organs, and this offers hope for larger numbers of cadaver donors in the future, as awareness spreads.

Hemodialysis

Hemodialysis is largely done in preparation for renal transplantation. Only a small number of patients opt for maintenance dialysis. Since dialysis is a costly procedure, it is an option only for the very rich. Even those Government hospitals that perform renal transplants, do not offer their patients maintenance dialysis, since the cost is unrealistic in relation to the national income. It is possible to maintain a patient on dialysis at home for less than the cost of transplantation with cyclosporin, when the patient learns to make their own dialysis concentrate and re-uses tubing and dialyzers, but home hemodialysis has not proved popular. One of the reasons may be the unreliability of the power supply in many parts of the country. Even in hospital-based dialysis, re-use of dialyzers and tubing is universal for economic reasons.

Continuous ambulatory peritoneal dialysis

Unlike the situation in other countries, this procedure is more costly than hemodialysis. Till recently, CAPD fluid was not available in the appropriate bags, and all supplies were imported. The bulk and weight of the consignment contributed to the cost. One Indian manufacturer has just marketed CAPD fluid at a lower price, and the bags are being evaluated. If they are found satisfactory, CAPD will be cheaper than hospital based hemodialysis, as it is elsewhere.

Before CAPD was implemented in India, there were fears that the infection rate would be unacceptably high because of dusty conditions and the hot weather making people sweat excessively. Nevertheless, it has been possible to maintain a rate of infection comparable to good units elsewhere. Another fear was of albumin levels being too low, as Indians consume less protein than Westerners, and much of that is of vegetable origin. However, experience has shown that albumin levels are acceptable, and therefore CAPD can be done if the patient can afford it.

ESRD: an approach we can afford

Effective treatment can be offered to patients with end-stage renal disease, but only a minuscule minority of Indians can afford to pay for it, and the State cannot afford to provide this treatment in our present economic conditions. Our only hope is to prevent the disease. Indians living in rural areas do not receive treatment for diabetes and hypertension. Diabetes is the major cause of chronic renal failure in the country, and hypertension, while directly causing 10% of renal failure, contributes to rapid progression in all other renal diseases. The Kidney Help Trust of Chennai has set up a project to detect and treat diabetes and hypertension, providing domiciliary care using trained paramedical workers. Only the cheapest medicines are used: reserpine, hydralazine, and hydrochlorothiazide for hypertension; and glibenclamide and metformin for diabetes. Fortunately, more than 99% of Indian diabetics have NIDDM. Excellent control of blood pressure has been achieved in the program. While there is some improvement in diabetic control, it is still far from ideal. Encouraging reports show that any reduction of glycated hemoglobin, even if not to normal levels, results in a reduction in the incidence of the vascular complications of diabetes. Since prevention is the only feasible option for the treatment of renal failure, the hope remains that the experiment will prove a success.

Malaysia

Renal replacement therapies for end-stage renal failure

Although issues of costs and economics of RRT are as relevant to developed countries as to developing ones, they are more apparent in the latter. Most countries in the Asian region spends between 3% and 6% of their GDP on healthcare, much of which is spent to combat communicable diseases, develop preventive healthcare, and provide basic clinical services. Renal replacement therapy thus does not receive the priority that renal physicians wish and is perceived as a costly intervention consuming a disproportionate share of the healthcare budget.

Malaysia currently has a population of 21 million, with an annual population growth rate of 2.3%. Its gross national product per capita in 1997 (before the onset of the financial crisis affecting Asia) was estimated at US$4466. The country spent 6.17% of its budget in 1996 on healthcare, this amounted to about 3% of the national GDP. About 57% of the healthcare budget went to clinical services. The renal replacement program thus comes under constant scrutiny as it competes for limited funds. The situation has been made more acute for Malaysia and other East Asian countries due to the recent financial and economic crisis affecting the region.

Development of RRT in Malaysia

Hemodialysis was first introduced in Malaysia in the late 1960s, primarily for the treatment of acute renal failure. It was only in 1975 that hemodialysis became organized as a treatment modality for end-stage renal disease (ESRD). In the same year, the first renal transplantation was performed. By 1984, when CAPD was introduced, it was possible to provide an integrated service.

From these beginnings, the RRT program in Malaysia has grown rapidly—particularly in the last ten years (Fig. 11.6) In 1998, data from the sixth report of the National Renal Registry showed a dialysis acceptance rate of 44 per million population per year and a transplantation rate of 3 per million. The year 1998 was the first to show a negative growth, reflecting the impact of the financial crises in the country. More than half of the patients receiving RRT are on programs run by the Ministry of Health, which are heavily subsidized by the government.

Renal replacement therapy, almost exclusively hemodialysis, is also provided in the private sector by 'for-profit' institutions, where patients either pay out of pocket or have their employers pay for the treatment. These for-profit institutions are found in the more affluent parts of the country and their development was primarily market

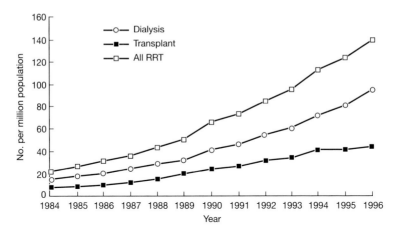

Fig. 11.6   Renal replacement therapy prevalence rate in Malaysia 1984–96.

driven. There were also non-profit organizations, including service clubs such as the Rotary, which provide heavily subsidized hemodialysis treatment. Many of these charitable organizations do not have proper professional services support. The subsequent growth of the various treatment modalities depended on a number of factors including funding, availability of trained personnel, and familiarity of non-renal physicians with the particular modality.

Strategies in the development of RRT

Dialysis

Hemodialysis facilities in the public sector were initially confined to the big general hospitals with resident nephrologists, and many patients had to relocate themselves to be near the facility. The major limitations were lack of skilled staff and funds. However, with the involvement of general physicians in the care of dialysis patients, and an increase in funding in the last ten years, it was possible to extend the hemodialysis services to even smaller district hospitals. Nephrologists from the nearby major hospitals visit these smaller centers regularly to supervise treatment of dialysis patients, see general nephrology cases, and at the same time conduct teaching sessions for the general medical doctors and paramedical staff. Another strategy to extend hemodialysis services was the empowerment of nurses and paramedical staff to take a major share of the responsibility of patient care. All the nursing staff in the hemodialysis units have undergone centralized training at the main hospital center in Kuala Lumpur for 6 months. The centralized training enables them to follow standard practices, which are regularly reviewed and updated. There are regular continuing education programs for the staff.

The element of costs and the need for its control were considered from the very beginning in the planning and development of the dialysis program in the country. This led to certain biases in the approach to dialysis treatment. In the early years, due to the limited funds and lack of skilled personnel, acceptance of patients for dialysis was restricted and there was major emphasis on patient selection. Only the younger and potentially more rehabilitable patients were accepted. In recent years, with increasing affordability, more and more patients were selected for dialysis and, although emphasis was still placed on rehabilitation, more elderly patients and patients with diabetes mellitus were accepted.

A number of measures were introduced in the dialysis practice to contain cost. These include:

(1) self-care dialysis;
(2) dialyzer and bloodline re-use;
(3) use of cellulosic membrane as the main membrane type;
(4) progressive increase in the use of bicarbonate buffer; and
(5) appropriate use of erythropoietin.

Self-care dialysis, apart from decreasing the staff costs, enabled patients to be involved in their treatment and many felt a sense of fulfilment in doing so. The level of self-care dialysis has, however, declined from more than 90% in the early years to 70% in 1996, due to the intake of elderly and patients with some co-morbid conditions. The introduction of erythropoietin increased costs considerably. In the initial years, there were stringent criteria to be fulfilled before a patient could be started on erythropoietin. In recent years, guidelines on the use of erythropoietin, including management of iron stores, have been developed. With this, it has been possible to increase the number of patients on erythropoietin to the current level of about 33%.

Two other initiatives have helped the development of dialysis and transplantation in the country. These were:

(1) the development of practice guidelines in all aspects of patient care in dialysis; and
(2) transplantation and the development of the Dialysis and Transplantation Registry.

The guidelines, which are reviewed every 2–3 years, have helped to reduce variation in practices, especially in dialysis, and also have enabled staff to keep abreast of contemporary practices. The data from the Dialysis and Transplantation Registry have been used by both clinicians and managers. While the latter found useful information for planning of new facilities, the clinicians have used the data for quality assurance activities amongst others.

CAPD has developed rapidly over the last 15 years. About 45% of new patients accepted for dialysis are started on CAPD. This was facilitated by the minimal start-up costs and the short duration of training for both staff and patients. However, direct costs of CAPD solutions and disposables are more expensive than hemodialysis disposables, and this has limited the intake of patients.

Renal transplantation

The major source of kidneys for transplantation has been the live-related donor. From 1975 till the end of 1998, the number of transplantations performed in the country was 709, of which only 37 were from cadaveric donors. The average rate for renal transplantation performed in the country was two per million population per year. There were more patients who had transplantation undertaken overseas, mainly in India and China. They constituted about four per million population per year. While the government does not condone commercial live-unrelated or commercial cadaveric transplantation, it cannot stop its citizens from going overseas for transplantation. There is an ongoing effort to promote cadaveric organ donation but it has not borne the desired results. A survey of the population on their attitude towards cadaveric organ donation showed that only less than 20% were willing to donate their organs upon death. An 'opting in' legislation—the *Human Tissues Act 1974*—is currently being reviewed to enhance its effectiveness in promoting cadaveric organ donation. The major religions in the country, including Islam, do not prohibit cadaveric organ donation.

Patient outcome in RRT

The overall death rate on dialysis is 8%, the death rate on CAPD is 11%, and that on hemodialysis 8%. Patient survival on hemodialysis is 93% and 86% at 1 year for patients less than 40 years and 55 years and greater, respectively. The corresponding figures for 10-year survival are 66% and 14%. Survival on CAPD for patients less than 40 years at 1 and 5 years are 94% and 80%, respectively. In renal transplantation, the patient and graft outcome at 1 year are 97% and 88%, respectively.

In a resource-intensive program, such as renal replacement therapy, gross outcome is not the most important measure; other measures that reflect cost-effectiveness are probably more important and relevant. The rehabilitation rate amongst patients receiving dialysis is high: 72% of the patients are able to do full- or part-time work, including housework. Quality of life was regularly assessed amongst dialysis patients using a summated score. In 1996, 71% of the patients reported a normal quality of life.

Impact of the economic slowdown

In 1997, a financial crisis, which started initially in a few countries, engulfed most of East Asia. Malaysia was amongst the countries affected. Currencies were effectively devalued, making imported materials more expensive. Except for blood-lines and dialysis concentrates, most other dialysis-related disposables were imported. Similarly, dialysis machines and immunosuppressive drugs were imported. Apart from this there was a cut-back on expenditure as part of general measures to combat the financial and economic crisis. Renal replacement therapy programs were affected by this crisis. Planned expansion had to be deferred and thus intake of new patients was restricted. Hemodialysis practices had to be reviewed to keep costs within the new reduced budget. These included: increasing the frequency of re-use of dialyzers; judicious use of expensive drugs, such as erythropoietin; and reducing the number and type of 'routine' investigations. The impact of these new measures on adequacy of dialysis and patient outcome has not been fully assessed.

Summary

The RRT program of the Ministry of Health, Malaysia generally has been successful. From a very limited beginning in 1975, it has achieved a prevalence rate of 34 patients per million population in 1996. The program, however, has been heavily dependant on dialysis and renal transplantation, and this has not changed over the last 20 years. Efforts at promoting cadaveric organ donation have been intensified. Patient outcomes have generally been satisfactory, with many returning to full- or part-time work and enjoying a normal quality of life. As in many other countries, cost-containment and funding issues continue to receive attention and the continued growth of the program will depend on a demonstration of its cost-effectiveness. The current financial crisis affecting the region, including Malaysia, has affected the program, necessitating further cost-cutting measures.

Asian Pacific countries

End-stage renal disease: epidemology and management

Asia comprises a vast number of countries with diverse cultures, socio-economic statuses, and different ethnic populations. Chronic renal failure remains an important cause of death in this region but, not surprisingly, the pattern of renal diseases differs from that of the Western countries (10). Furthermore, the diverse cultures and socio-economic statuses pose a major impact on the choice of treatment for end-stage renal failure (ESRF), and the availability of different treatment modalities in this region. The choice of treatment modalities is greatly influenced by non-medical factors, which include education deficits, financial reimbursement, physical bias, resource availability, and cultural habits (11). Unfortunately, published data on the renal replacement program in Asian countries is limited. This text examines the treatment strategies for end-stage renal failure in representative countries in the Asian Pacific regions, namely, China, Hong Kong, Japan, Korea, Singapore, Malaysia, Thailand, and Taiwan. Some of these clinical data were compared with those from representative dialysis centers in selected Western countries.

Health economics in the Asian Pacific countries

A close correlation is demonstrated between the dialysis treatment rate for ESRF and the gross domestic product (GDP) per capita income (Fig. 11.7). Furthermore, the financial support, or the re-imbursement policy, also presents a non-medical influence on the choice and utilization of different treatment modalities for ESRF. Table 11.3

summarizes the renal re-imbursement systems in these Asian Pacific countries. Full comprehensive coverage of dialysis expenses by Government resources is not often available in these countries. Not infrequently, treatment cost is met by patients' earnings or by charity, best illustrated in the cases of Hong Kong, Singapore, and Thailand.

Despite the economic growth in most Asian Pacific countries over the last three decades, the resource spent by government in health service is less than other developed countries (Fig. 11.7). As illustrated in Hong Kong and Singapore, not infrequently a two-tiered system comprising a national health system and a private health system function in parallel. In Hong Kong, only 10% of the population have health insurance or receive health benefits from their employment. The Government spends 2.97% of GDP for public health service covering 92% of all hospital admissions, while the general population spends 1.8% of GDP for private health service that covers 8% of all hospital admissions. With few exceptions, medical staff in public and private hospitals are distinctly separated in these Asian Pacific countries. Hence, the actual health-spending in most Asian Pacific countries is greater than the government budget, as self-payment is not uncommonly practised for admission to a private hospital.

Pattern of renal diseases in Asian Pacific countries

The differences between the general pattern of renal diseases in Asian countries and that observed in the Western world are decreasing. With increased survival of the population (e.g. 76 years for male and 82 years for female in Hong Kong, Japan, Singapore, and Taiwan), renal diseases are more commonly encountered in the

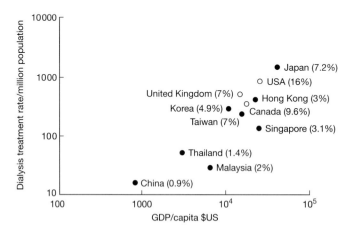

Fig. 11.7   The relationship between dialysis treatment rate and gross domestic product (GDP) per capita in different Asian Pacific countries in comparison to United Kingdom, Canada, and USA. The percentage of GDP spent by individual governments are shown in parenthesis.

Table 11.3 The renal re-imbursement systems in the Asian Pacific countries

Country	Eligibility for re-imbursement		Type of re-imbursement				Source of financial support		
	Civil servant	General public	HD	CAPD solution	CAPD tubing	APD machine	Government	Charity	Self paid/ insurance
China	Depends on the work unit	Depends on the work unit	Yes	Yes	No	No	Depends on the work unit	No	Yes
Hong Kong	Yes	Yes	Yes	Yes	No	Limited	Yes	Some	Yes
Japan	Yes	Yes	Yes	Yes	Yes	Yes	Yes	No	No
Korea	Yes	Yes	Yes	Yes	No	No	80%	No	20%
Singapore	Yes	Limited	Yes	No	No	No	Limited	Some	Yes
Taiwan, China	Yes	Yes	Yes	Yes	Yes	Limited	Yes	No	No
Malaysia	Yes	No	Yes	Yes	No	No	Yes	Yes	Yes
Thailand	Yes	No	Yes	Yes	No	No	Yes	Few	Yes

HD: hemodialysis; APD: automated peritoneal dialysis; CAPD: continuous ambulatory peritonieal dialysis.

elderly (such as diabetes mellitus and renovascular diseases) and contribute significantly to the general nephrology practice and the maintenance dialysis program.

Four renal disorders are of particular interest in populations from the Asian Pacific regions, namely: IgA nephropathy, hepatitis B virus (HBV) associated glomerulonephritis, diabetic nephropathy, and Takayasu arteritis, with IgA nephropathy and diabetic nephropathy being the two most common disorders leading to ESRF. Chronic hepatitis B virus infection poses a difficult problem in both hemodialysis and renal transplantation. Aggressive treatment of these conditions should be practised in order to prevent or delay the development of ESRF.

IgA nephropathy

This glomerulonephritis accounts for 30% of renal biopsies in all primary glomerulonephritides in this region (12). The classical synpharyngitic macroscopic hematuria is the present symptom in less than 20% of patients (13, 14). Not infrequently, the diagnosis is made by renal biopsy for investigation of asymptomatic microscopic hematuria or proteinuria. Nephrotic-range proteinuria usually signifies a poor prognosis (14). This disorder runs a relentless and slowly progressive course leading to end-stage renal failure in about 25–30% of patients over a period of 20 years. A genetic predisposition (15) and abnormality in IgA synthesis (16) have been demonstrated, and these immunological abnormalities could be of pathogenic importance.

Hepatitis B virus-associated glomerulonephritis

Glomerulonephritis is not infrequently detected in chronic HBsAg carriers. Some of the association may be coincidental as 2–12% of the adult population in this region are HBsAg carriers, with infection acquired in the neonatal period or early in childhood (17, 18). The renal pathologies that have been shown to have an etiological association with hepatitis B virus (HBV) infection include: membranous nephropathy; mesangiocapillary glomerulonephritis; and mesangial proliferative glomerulonephritis with predominant mesangial IgA deposits. Recently, the detection of HBV DNA and RNA in glomerular cells and renal tubular epithelia in renal tissues from these patients support the presence of viral transcription and the development of immune-complex information *in situ* (19). Treatment with interfon α in chronic HBV carriers is not always effective, as the infection has been acquired early in childhood (18). Prevention by vaccinating all newborns in endemic areas should be encouraged. This was practised in Hong Kong for the last 10 years and the incidence of HBV-associated glomerulonephritis in the pediatric population has markedly declined.

Diabetic nephropathy

The incidence of insulin-dependent diabetes mellitus (IDDM) in children is less in the Asian Pacific region than in European countries. It is not unusual to see non-insulin dependent diabetic mellitus (NIDDM) present in the second decade of a child's development in Asia, whereas in Caucasian countries, where IDDM is prevalent in children, NIDDM is usually present in the fifth or sixth decade of life, or thereafter (20). Interestingly, there appear to be more cases with a slow onset IDDM in the young than in Caucasian countries (20). The overall incidence rate of IDDM for children 0–14 years of age at diagnosis in Japan is 1.65–2.07 per 100 000, and the corresponding incidence of NIDDM is 2.80–4.61 per 100 000 (21). In a Japanese survey of more than 2000 adult diabetic patients (60% were aged 55–74 years), only 7% had IDDM (22). Hypertension was present in 39%. Proteinuria was present in 20%, and 29% had visual disturbance. Micro-angiopathies are generally more frequent and more severe in IDDM than NIDDM. Macro-angiopathies, including coronary artery disease, cerebrovascular infarction, and peripheral vascular disease, are less frequent than figures from the United States. Similarly, NIDDM is common among Chinese, despite some of the patients being relatively young. Contrary to the white population, in which 8–10% of the NIDDM develop uremia due to diabetic nephropathy, this figure increases to 15% in Chinese patients in Hong Kong. Nephropathy is frequently part of the triopathy involving the nerve and retina.

Takayasu arteritis

Takayasu arteritis is a panarteritis that may affect the aorta, pulmonary arteries, and other major arteries of the body. It commonly affects young females and may lead to hypertension, due to renal artery involvement. In selected regions, it is the most common cause of renovascular hypertension, accounting for 60% of such patients in North India (23). The natural history of the disease has two phases. The acute phase is characterized by systemic symptoms of inflammatory disorders; fever, weight loss, malaise, and arthralgia. Late phase occurs after an interval of 6–8 years, leading to vascular occlusive disease. The kidneys are affected mainly by renal artery stenosis but various glomerulonephritides have been reported (24). The long-term prognosis is dependent upon the presence of aortic incompetence, severity of hypertension, and arterial aneurysm formation. Renal failure is one of the main causes of death.

Dialysis treatment in Asian Pacific countries

Most of the Asian countries (with only a few exceptions) have a lower gross domestic product (GDP) per capita income than that in North America or Western Europe. Similar to our survey in 1998, another survey of 11 representative Asian countries in 1995 (25) revealed a close correlation between the treatment rate for ESRF and the GDP per capita income. Chronic glomerulonephritis remains the most important cause of renal failure. With the exception of China (26), diabetic nephropathy has emerged as the second cause of renal failure in this region. Similar to that now reported from Caucasian populations, non-insulin dependent diabetes mellitus (NIDDM) is more common than insulin-dependent diabetes mellitus (IDDM) in most Asian dialysis populations. The pattern of dialysis prescription in Asian Pacific countries is summarized in Table 11.4. Hemodialysis is the preferred dialysis modality in this region, except in Hong Kong and Malaysia, where 79% and 63% of uremic patients, respectively, are treated with continuous ambulatory peritoneal dialysis (CAPD). Nevertheless, the pattern of peritoneal dialysis (PD) utilization in different Asian countries is likely to change in the future as nephrologists and nurses become more experienced with this treatment modality and the economic status of their countries improves progressively. That such a trend is present is supported by the observation that most Asian countries have recorded a growth rate that is greater for PD than hemodialysis (25).

Peritoneal dialysis treatment in Asian Pacific countries

A previous survey of 11 representative Asian countries (25) found a biphasic relationship with the GDP per capita income and PD utilization rate, in that countries with the highest and lowest treatment rates tend to have lower PD utilization rates, whereas countries with modest treatment rates tend to have higher PD utilization rates. Our present data, collected 3 years after Cheng's initial study (1996), reveal that this pattern of PD utilization remains unchanged (Fig. 11.8a). The low PD utilization in countries with the high GDP per capita income is related to the lack of physician incentive to introduce CAPD as an alternative form of ESRF treatment in the presence of full Government re-imbursement for hemodialysis treatment. At the same time, CAPD is also less preferred in countries with low GDP per capita income due to the complete lack of Government re-imbursement.

Conventional straight-line systems used to be the dominant PD system in some countries, such as Korea and Hong Kong. Over the last 2 years, a rapid shift from straight-line systems to disconnect systems is evident. In countries where PD has been introduced only recently (e.g. China), the disconnect systems are used almost exclusively.

The average number of daily CAPD exchanges varies between different Asian Pacific countries, although most use 8 l/day. Dialysis centers in Hong Kong and China

Table 11.4 The pattern of dialysis treatment in the Asian Pacific countries

Country	Dialysis patient per million general population	Percentage of hemodialysis	Percentage of CAPD treatment	Average volume of CAPD exchange (l/day)	Percentage of straight-line CAPD system
China	20	94	6	7	0
Hong Kong	378	21	79	6.4	30
Japan	1328	94	6	8	10
Korea	270	63	37	8	40
Singapore	125	83	17	8	2
Taiwan, China	240	94	6	8	3
Thailand	50	60	40	7	65
Malaysia	28	37	63	7	25

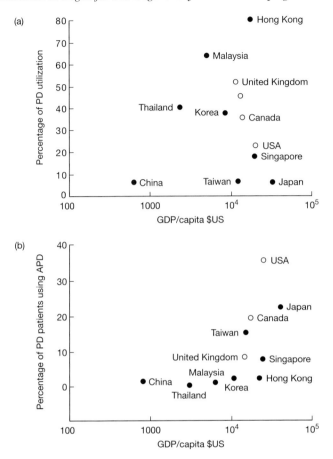

Fig. 11.8 (a) The relationship between peritoneal dialysis (PD) utilization (as a percentage of all dialysis patients) and gross domestic product (GDP) per capita in different Asian Pacific countries in comparison to the United Kingdom, Canada, and the USA. (b) The relationship between the percentage of PD patients using automated peritoneal dialysis (APD) and GDP per capita in different Asian pacific countries in comparison to the United Kingdom, Canada, and the USA.

tend to use small-volume CAPD exchanges. Three 2-l daily exchanges has been the standard CAPD regime in Hong Kong over the last 10 years due to budgetary constraint (27). This dialysis prescription would be considered as sub-optimal by Western standards but the survival of these patients is comparable to, or even better than, other areas despite a lower Kt/V (mean 1.65) (28). The reported 5-year and 10-year survival rates under such a dialysis regimen were 79% and 55%, respectively, despite the lower Kt/V. Notably, the protein catabolic rate of these patients in Hong Kong was greater than that in Western patients with Kt.V<1.7, and this could be attributed to dietary difference and nutritional status. The proportion of patients working full-time with good rehabilitation was similar between patients with Kt/V < 1.7 and those with Kt/V > 1.7. These preliminary studies suggest small-volume dialysis may be an acceptable alternative in an Asian population with smaller body size, given the financial constraints (27, 28). These issues are especially important in Asia where financial resources for renal replacement therapy are still limited in most countries and many patients have to continue working to pay for their ESRF treatment. Furthermore, if the practice is an acceptable compromise for patients awaiting renal transplantation, more patients can be treated with the limited financial resources available in some Asian countries.

Automated peritoneal dialysis treatment in Asian Pacific countries

With the exception of China, the practice of automated peritoneal dialysis (APD) in Asian Pacific countries totally contrasts that of CAPD. Countries with high CAPD-utilization rates have the lowest APD-utilization rates (< 2% of patients on PD) (Fig. 11.8b). The low APD-utilization rate is due to the fact that, in most Asian Pacific countries, the APD machine has to be purchased by the patients themselves. Such machines are expensive, ranging from $US4500 in Korea to $US18 500 in Japan—a sum equal to at least 45% of yearly income of an average individual. In contrast, the cost of APD machines in North America is lower ($US500–6000). Renting of APD machines is not a common practice in most Asian Pacific countries.

Due to the late introduction of APD in Asia, APD machines with pneumatic-pressure systems are used in most Asian Pacific countries, except China (10%) and Malaysia (50%). This contrasts with the USA and the United Kingdom, where APD machines with volumetric systems are predominantly used. Of the four different modes of APD treatment, namely intermittent peritoneal dialysis (IPD), continuous cycling peritoneal dialysis (CCPD), nocturnal peritoneal dialysis (NPD), and tidal peritoneal dialysis (TPD), CCPD is most frequently practised (Fig. 11.9a). Tidal peritoneal dialysis is not practised in any Asian Pacific countries and IPD remains the main mode of PD treatment in China.

The indications of APD utilization over CAPD utilization are depicted in Fig. 11.9b. The findings differ widely between countries but, generally, convenience for employment is the main indication for the utilization of APD. Other important indications are the convenience of treatment in young or elderly uremic patients. Re-use of tubings is practised in China, Singapore, and Malaysia, but not in other Asian Pacific countries. Unlike North America and the United Kingdom, low-calcium dialysate is only used in a small percentage of patients on APD. The addition of bicarbonate, amino acid supplement, or growth hormone is not practised in APD.

Hemodialysis dialysis treatment in Asian Pacific countries

With the exception of Hong Kong and Malaysia, hemodialysis remains the main dialytic treatment modality (> 50%) in most Asian Pacific countries. The utilization rate of hemodialysis (> 90%) occurs in Japan, Taiwan, and China. High-flux short

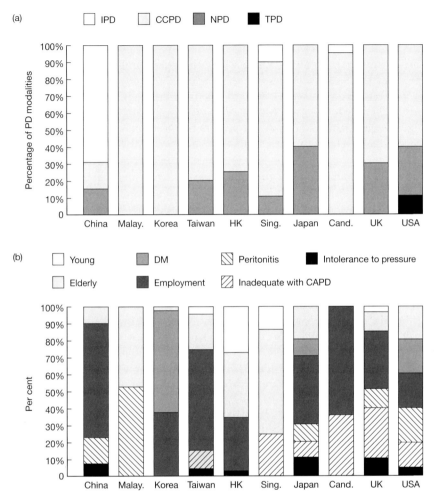

Fig. 11.9 (a) The utilization of different modes of peritoneal dialysis in different Asian Pacific countries. IPD, CCPD, NPD, and TPD represent intermittent peritoneal dialysis, continuous cycling peritoneal dialysis, nocturnal peritoneal dialysis, and tidal peritoneal dialysis, respectively. (b) The indications for the utilization of APD in different Asian Pacific countries. DM and CAPD denote diabetes mellitus and continuous ambulatory peritoneal dialysis, respectively.

hemodialysis is not commonly practised in Asian Pacific countries. Due to the smaller body mass, better patient compliance, and budgetary constraints, twice instead of thrice weekly hemodialysis is practised in some countries with longer dialysis lasting 5–6 h per treatment. There is a growing tendency towards the use of low calcium and bicarbonate dialysate. Re-use of dialyzers and tubings is frequently practised.

Renal transplantation in the Asian Pacific countries

The kidney transplantation rate in these Asia Pacific countries is low. The yearly transplantation rates for Japan, Korea, China, Singapore, Taiwan, and Hong Kong are 5, 16, 2, 21.5, 4.5, and 13/million general population/year, respectively (26, 29, 30). The percentages of cadaveric transplantation for Japan, Korea, China, and Hong Kong are 27%, 5%, 90%, and 64%, respectively. Different factors are responsible for the low transplantation rate in these countries but the traditional belief of burial with an intact body in these cultures definitely negates the practice of organ donation. Some issues are unique in individual countries. Japan only introduced a law on brain death in 1997. On the contrary, the higher transplantation rate in Singapore can partly be explained by the enactment of an opt-out law for organ donation. There is a high incidence of non-related donors (41%) or parents as donors (24%) in Korea. The low transplantation rate in China is partly attributed to the high cost of transplantation, compared with the average earning of the general population (26).

The immunosuppressive regimens in these Asian Pacific countries are similar, although the graft-survival rates vary. In Hong Kong, 64% of cases are cadaveric transplantation. The 1-year survival rate is 92% with a 5-year graft-survival rate of 75%. Similar figures for Japan are 84% and 60%, respectively (29). It is not certain whether the difference may be related to the longer 'warm ischemic period' of the graft with the practice of cardiac death in Japan. The 1-year survival rate in China is 85% but the long-term results are still not optimal (26). Most renal transplants in China were performed without HLA matching, and infection, particularly pulmonary, is the most important post-operative complication (26, 31).

Hepatitis B and hepatitis C infection in the renal replacement program

Chronic hepatitis B virus infection is endemic in Asian Pacific countries, affecting 2–12% of the adult population in this region (16, 18). Hemodialysis or renal transplant facilities are inadequate for these HBsAg carriers. Not infrequently, HBsAg carriers with uremia are treated with CAPD. The results of renal transplantation are not satisfactory, as the clinical course is frequently complicated by 'flare-up' of hepatitis following immunosuppressive therapy. In isolated centers, antiviral therapy, such as lamivudine, has been administered to HBsAg carriers following renal transplantation. The long-term benefit is not clear and the length of antiviral treatment may well be life-long. Their immunosuppressive therapy is frequently tapered to avoid deterioration of hepatic unction due to reactivation of hepatitis. The ultimate target is to prevent transmission by vaccinating all newborns in endemic areas, and medical personnel and patients at risk.

The other emerging cause of chronic liver disease in renal units of this region is hepatitis C virus (HCV) infection. Spontaneous clearance of HCV is unusual. The clinical course and response to treatment may vary according to the HCV genotypes. The high prevalence of HCV infection among hemodialysis patients (30%), as compared to patients on CAPD (<5%), is largely attributable to their greater transfusion requirements (32).

Renal registry in the Asian Pacific countries

Accurate data are essential for the strategic planning of a treatment program for end-stage renal failure. This also provides direction for preventive medicine. Even more importantly, healthcare budgeting can be accurately projected from data of the renal registry. With the exception of China, the Philippines, Vietnam, and Myanmar, other countries in the Asian Pacific region, namely, Hong Kong, Japan, Korea, Singapore, Malaysia, Thailand, and Taiwan, have developed a national renal registry. China is planning to launch a renal registry in 1999. A report on the status of nephrology, dialysis, and transplantation in Shanghai (the largest city in China), based on the interim results of a survey carried out in 1999, has been recently published (33). As of May 1999, there were dialysis facilities available in 59 city hospitals, about 3000 patients were treated with hemodialysis, and about 500 with peritoneal dialysis. In 1998, 300 patients had undergone renal transplantation. Published data of renal services in the Philippines, Vietnam, or Myanmar are scarce.

Summary

End-stage renal disease has a growing prevalence in Asia. With increased survival of the population, renal diseases more commonly encountered in the elderly (such as diabetes mellitus and renovascular diseases) contribute significantly to the general nephrology practice and the maintenance dialysis program. Despite the economic growth in most Asian Pacific countries over the last three decades, the resources spent by Governments on health services are less than in other developed countries. Generally, the dialysis treatment rate for ESRF correlates with the gross domestic product per capita income. Furthermore, the financial support, or the re-imbursement policy, also presents a non-medical influence on the choice and utilization of different treatment modalities for ESRF. With the financial crisis affecting most countries in the Asian Pacific region since 1997, further expansion of the renal replacement program is likely to be limited due to budgetary constraints. This may, in turn, influence the treatment modalities, with the predicted growth of peritoneal dialysis and satellite hemodialysis centers. The universal problem of renal replacement programs in all Asian Pacific countries is the low transplantation rate. The traditional belief of burial with an intact body, in certain cultures and religions, definitely negates the practice of organ donation. Enactment of an opt-out law for organ donation may need to be considered till other solutions, such as animal organs from genetic engineering, are available. These issues should be carefully addressed, so that a cost-effective renal replacement program can be implemented extensively in Asia.

Conclusions

The five contributions to this chapter illustrate the problems that have been overcome and those that remain in providing services for renal failure and renal replacement treatment in countries of the developing world. The major limitation identified is financial, although there must be a serious shortage of trained medical, nursing, and technical staff in many areas of the developing world. As has been well described, it is not a problem for wealthy patients, who can afford treatment or afford to travel to a country in the developed world for their care. The expanding middle class have increasing expectations and will be a powerful force in pressing for the continued development of local services. It is the poor, who are generally accepting of their lot, who will miss out for the foreseeable future. Throughout the world, the allocation of resources for renal replacement programs is closely related to the gross domestic product of the country, and, thus, expansion of services will, to a large extent, be dependent on increasing prosperity. It has also been demonstrated that developing countries have very different healthcare priorities, than the industrialized parts of the world, and priority has to be given to obtaining the maximum benefit for the community from that which is spent on healthcare.

The causes of renal failure from the five areas discussed in this chapter seem to vary considerably. Infection and related renal disease are more common in Africa and India, whereas glomerulonephritis and hypertension are more common in Central and Eastern Europe, Malaysia, and the countries of the Pacific rim. This would seem to reflect the overall wealth of the countries, which indicates that, in poorer areas, infections, particularly malaria, tuberculosis, and schistomosiasis, remain a major problem. Significant health gains will arise from effective programs aimed at controlling such conditions. In many ways, this reflects the experience of the developed world, where a century ago— in a completely different economic climate—infections were a serious health problem. This has changed considerably due to improved nutrition and improved healthcare, such that now the major problem in such countries is degenerative disease.

The results reported in those patients who received treatment on an end-stage renal failure program are very impressive, and, in the main, compare very favorably with that achieved in developed countries. Renal registries are in existence, or are being formed, and these will be powerful tools to persuade politicians that a renal replacement program can be successful in rehabilitating patients and returning them to gainful employment. The experience reported from Malaysia and the countries of the Pacific rim are most impressive and demonstrate the value to be obtained from an effective program.

The pattern of renal replacement therapy is biased towards hemodialysis, with a view to subsequent transplantation. This seems to be predominantly financially driven because, at present, the cost of CAPD fluids is prohibitive. There is clearly scope for the local production of fluids, as indicated from India. The fear that CAPD would not be particularly successful, due to the possibility of high infection rates, seems to be disproven. There is, thus, potential for expansion of this mode of therapy, to bring treatment to a greater number of patients. As has also been indicated, there are a number of measures that can be taken to limit this cost of hemodialysis, such as increasing the concept of self-care, re-use of dialyzers and blood lines, and the use of cheaper cellulosic membranes. The introduction of high-technology medicine for political gain is to be deplored, and every effort should be made to ensure that the maximum is gained for the investment made—even if this includes the use of technology that is not state-of-the-art but is still functionally effective in providing appropriate care. Initiatives leading to the local production of equipment are to be welcomed.

The development of transplantation has been slow for a number of reasons. Although nearly all religious groups support the concept of cadaveric and living-related transplantation, few actively promote this treatment. This is not a problem confined to the developing world but is also present in industrialized societies. It has taken many years to overcome the natural reluctance to accept the principle of brain death and, in many ways, the general population is at present ahead of the religious leaders in accepting this concept. In addition to religious beliefs, there are cultural traditions to be overcome, as well as the superstitious fears that many hold avidly. It is only with time that there will be an increasing acceptance of cadaveric transplantation, and until then we are likely to have to face the commercialization that currently exists in some countries. Education is very much needed if the rate of transplantation is to increase significantly. Legislation can help but until there is more widespread acceptance by the community, little progress will be made.

Prevention of renal disease receives scant attention in most countries but there are encouraging reports from India, where control of blood pressure and diabetes mellitus with simple medications are having a significant influence. It is likely that, if similar measures are applied to the control of major infectious diseases, then there will be a further reduction in the incidence of renal failure. This could have as much, if not more, beneficial effect than expanding dialysis facilities in certain areas.

Strategies for the development of end-stage renal failure services in developing countries is clearly an important issue. It is clear from the presentations in this chapter that there is no single solution, and that each community has to develop a program that addresses the needs particular to that community. Dialysis, whether hemodialysis or CAPD, is expensive and clearly not affordable for all, in much of the developing world. It is inevitable that some selection will take place, thus raising problems of equity and justice. These issues have to be solved locally, because it would seem to be better to treat some patients than not to offer treatment to anyone. Initiatives to reduce costs and thereby bring treatment to a larger number of patients are to be encouraged. Campaigns to increase awareness of renal failure and the potential treatment options are required and, in particular, the benefits of transplantation need to be more widely advertised. The advances of the past two decades have been considerable, and there is every reason to believe that advances will continue and thereby bring benefit to those in developing countries who are unfortunate enough to suffer from end-stage renal failure.

References

1. Woods, H.F. (1993). Perspectives on dialysis in the third world, a problem of economics. *Contribut Nephrol*, **102**, 237–47.
2. Poikolainen, K. and Eskola, J. (1988). Health services resources and their relation to mortality from causes amenable to healthcare intervention, a cross-national study. *International Journal of Epidemiology*, **17**, 86–9.

3. Valek, A. and Wing, A.J. (1984). Development of dialysis and transplant activity in the world in the seventies of the 20th century. *Zeitschrift Experimentelle Chirurgie Transplant Künstliche Organe*, **17**, 69–78.

4. Fassbinder, W., Brunner, F.P., Brynger, H., Ehrich, J.M., Geerlings, W., Raine, A.E., *et al.* (1991). Combined report on regular dialysis and transplantation in Europe, XX, 1989. *Nephrology, Dialysis, Transplantation*, **6**, (Suppl. 1), 5–35.

5. Rutowski, B., Ciocalteu, A., Djukanovic, L., Kiss, I., Kovac, A., Krivoshiev, S. *et al.* (1998). Evolution of renal replacement therapy in Central and Eastern Europe 7 years after political and economical liberation. *Nephrology, Dialysis, Transplantation*, **13**, 860–64.

6. Rutkowski, B., Ciocalteu, A., Djukanovic, L. *et al.* (1998). Treatment of end-stage renal disease in Central and Eastern Europe. Overview of current status and future needs. *Artificial Organs*, **22**, 187–91.

7. Zucchelli, P. (1997). Report on a fact-finding mission on nephrology in Albania. *Nephrology, Dialysis, Transplantation*, **12**, 159.

8. Rutkowski, B. On behalf of the CEE Advisory Board in CRF (2000). Changing pattern of end-stage renal disease in Central and Eastern Europe. *Nephrology, Dialysis, Transplantation*, **15**, 156–60.

9. Kuzminskis, V., Bumblyte, I.A., and Surkus, J. (1999). Development of nephrology and replacement therapy in Lithuania since 1989. An update. *Nephrology, Dialysis, Transplantation*, **14**, 2846–8.

10. Lai, K.N., Li, C.S., and Chan, D.T.M. (1998). End-stage renal disease amongst Asians. *International Journal of Artificial Organs*, **21**, 67–71.

11. Nissenson, A.R., Prichard, S.S., Cheng, I.K., Gokal, R., Kubota, M., Maiorca, R., *et al.* (1993). Non-medical factors that impact on ESRD modality selection. *Kidney International*, **43**, (Suppl. 40), S120–7.

12. D'Amico, G. (1987). The commonest glomerulonephritis in the world, IgA nephropathy. *Quarterly Journal of Medicine*, **245**, 709–27.

13. Lai, K.N., Lai, F.M., Li, P., Chan, K.W., Au, T.C., and Tong, K.I. (1988). The clinico-pathological characteristics of Iga nephropathy in Hong Kong. *Pathology*, **20**, 15–8.

14. Kobyashi, Y., Tateno, S., Hiki, Y., and Shigamatsu, H. (1983). IgA nephropathy, prognostic significance of proteinuria and histological alteration. *Nephron*, **34**, 146–53.

15. Li, P.K.T., Poon, A.S.Y., and Lai, K.N. (1994). Molecular genetics of MHC class II alleles in Chinese patients with IgA Nephropathy and its relation with prognosis. *Kidney International*, **46**, 185–90.

16. Feehally, J., Beattie, J.T., Brenchley, P., Coopes, B.M., Mallick, N.P., and Postlewaite, R.J. (1986). Sequential study of the IgA system in relapsing IgA nephropathy. *Kidney International*, **30**, 924–31.

17. Lee, H.S., Choi, Y., Yu, S., Hoh, H., Kim, M., and Ko, K.W.A. (1988). Renal biopsy study of HBV-associated nephropathy in korea. *Kidney International*, **34**, 537–43.

18. Lai, K.N., Li, P.K.T., Lui, S., Au, T.C., Tam, J.S., Tong, K.L. *et al.* (1991). Membranous nephropathy related to hepatitis in adults. *New England Journal of Medicine*, **324**, 1457–63.

19. Lai, K.N., Ho, R.T.H., Tam, J.S., and Lai, F.M. (1996). Detection of hepatitis B DNA and RNA in kidneys of HBV-related glomerulonephritis. *Kidney International*, **50**, 1965–77.

20. Kitagawa, T., Fujita, H., Hibi, I., Aageneas, O., Laron, Z., Laporte, R.E. *et al.* (1984). A comparative study on the epidemiology of NIDDM between Japan, Norway, Israel and the United States. *Acta Pediatrica Japonica*, **26**, 275–81.

21. Kitagawa, T., Owada, M., Urakami, T., anpd Tajima, N. (1994). Epidemiology of type I and type II diabetes mellitus in Japanese children. *Diabetes Research and Clinical Practice*, **24**, S7–13.
22. Kuzuya, T., Akanuma, Y., Akazawa, Y., and Uehata, T. (1994). Prevalence of chronic complications in Japanese diabetic patients. *Diabetes Research and Clinical Practice*, **24**, S159–64.
23. Chugh, K.S., Jain, S., Sakhuja, V., Malik, N., Gupta, A., Sehgal, S. *et al.* (1992). Renovascular hypertension due to Takayasu's arteritis among Indian patients. *Quarterly Journal of Medicine*, **85**, 833–43.
24. Lai, K.N., Chan, K.W., and Ho, C.P. (1987). Glomerulonephritis associated with Takayasu's arteritis. Report of 3 cases and a review of the literature. *American Journal of Kidney Diseases*, **7**, 197–204.
25. Cheng, I.K. (1996). Peritoneal dialysis in Asia. *Peritoneal Dialysis International*, **16**, S381–5.
26. Li, L.S. (1996). End-stage renal disease in China. *Kidney International*, **49**, 287–301.
27. Lo, W.K., Jiang, Y., Cheng, S.W., and Cheng, I.K. (1996). Survival of CAPD patients in a center using three two-liter exchanges as standard regimen. *Peritoneal Dialysis International*, **16**, S163–6.
28. Szeto, C.C., Lai, K.N., Yu, A.W.Y., Leung, C.B., Ho, K.K.L., Mak, T. *et al.* (1997). Dialysis adequacy of asian patients receiving small volume continuous ambulatory peritoneal dialysis. *International Journal of Artificial Organs*, **20**, 428–35.
29. Teraoka, S., Toma, H., Nihei, H., Ota, K., Babazono, T., Ishikawa, I. *et al.* (1995). Current status of renal replacement therapy in Japan. *American Journal of Kidney Diseases*, **25**, 151–64.
30. Kim, M.J. (1996). Nephrology and renal replacement therapy in South Korea, a brief report on the Korea Society of Nephrology and Korean Society of transplantation. *Nephrology, Dialysis, Transplantation*, **11**, 979–81.
31. Liu, K.D. (1985). Demography of renal transplantation therapy in China. *China Journal of Organ Transplantation*, **6**, (Abstract), 12.
33. Guanyu, W., Nan, C., Jiaqi, Q., Shanyan, L., Quinjun, X., and Dechang, D. (2000). Nephrology Dialysis and Transplantation in Shanghai, 1999, *Nephrology, Dialysis, Transplantation*, **15**, 961–3.

INDEX